Eating Traditional Food

Due to its centrality in human activities, food is a meaningful object that necessarily participates in any cultural, social and ideological construction and its qualification as 'traditional' is a politically laden value. This book demonstrates that traditionality as attributed to foods goes beyond the notions of heritage and authenticity under which it is commonly formulated.

Through a series of case studies from a global range of cultural and geographical areas, the book explores a variety of contexts to reveal the complexity behind the attribution of the term 'traditional' to food. In particular, the volume demonstrates that the definitions put forward by programmes such as TRUEFOOD and EuroFIR (and subsequently adopted by organisations including FAO), which have analysed the perception of traditional foods by individuals, do not adequately reflect this complexity. The concept of tradition being deeply ingrained culturally, socially, politically and ideologically, traditional foods resist any single definition.

Chapters analyse the processes of valorisation, instrumentalisation and reinvention at stake in the construction and representation of a food as traditional. Overall the book offers fresh perspectives on topics including definition and regulation, nationalism and identity, and health and nutrition, and will be of interest to students and researchers of many disciplines including anthropology, sociology, politics and cultural studies.

Brigitte Sébastia is Researcher in Anthropology at the French Institute of Pondicherry, India.

Routledge Studies in Food, Society and Environment

A full list of titles in this series is available at: http://www.routledge.com/books/series/RSFSE/

Recently published titles:

Food Literacy
Key concepts for health and education
Edited by Helen Vidgen

Sustainable Urban Agriculture and Food Planning
Edited by Rob Rogemma

Transforming Gender and Food Security in the Global South
Edited by Jemimah Njuki, John R. Parkins and Amy Kaler

Urban Food Planning
Seeds of Transition in the Global North
Rositsa T. Ilieva

Food Consumption in the City
Practices and Patterns in Urban Asia and the Pacific
Edited by Marlyne Sahakian, Czarina Saloma and Suren Erkman

Eating Traditional Food
Politics, Identity and Practices
Edited by Brigitte Sébastia

Feeding Cities
Improving local food access, security and sovereignty
Edited by Christopher Bosso

The Right to Food Guidelines, Democracy and Citizen Participation
Country case studies
Katharine S.E. Cresswell Riol

Eating Traditional Food

Politics, identity and practices

Edited by Brigitte Sébastia

Routledge
Taylor & Francis Group
LONDON AND NEW YORK

earthscan
from Routledge

First published 2017 by Routledge

2 Park Square, Milton Park, Abingdon, Oxfordshire OX14 4RN
711 Third Avenue, New York, NY 10017

Routledge is an imprint of the Taylor & Francis Group, an informa business

First issued in paperback 2018

British Library Cataloguing-in-Publication Data
A catalogue record for this book is available from the British Library

Library of Congress Cataloging in Publication Data
Names: Sébastia, Brigitte, editor.
Title: Eating traditional food : politics, identity and practices / edited by Brigitte Sébastia.
Description: London ; New York : Routledge is an imprint of the Taylor & Francis Group, an Informa Business, [2017] | Includes bibliographical references and index.
Identifiers: LCCN 2016021306| ISBN 9781138187009 (hbk) | ISBN 9781315643410 (ebk)
Subjects: LCSH: Food habits--Cross-cultural studies. | Food consumption--Cross-cultural studies. | Nutrition--Cross-cultural studies. | Food--Cross-cultural studies. | Social psychology--Cross-cultural studies.
Classification: LCC GT2850 .E37 2017 | DDC 394.1/2--dc23
LC record available at https://lccn.loc.gov/2016021306

ISBN: 978-1-138-18700-9 (hbk)
ISBN: 978-0-367-02983-8 (pbk)

Typeset in Bembo
by HWA Text and Data Management, London

Contents

Figures and tables

Figures

Tables

Contributors

Elise Billiard holds a PhD in Anthropology from the University of Provence, France. After studying at several French universities, she settled in Malta where she teaches anthropology, sociology and food culture at the University of Malta. Her main interest is material culture and food culture which are at the centre of her present research. She is also involved in research regarding nationalism, urbanism and the construction of heritage. She has published *Tkecnir, Kitchen Work* (2011) and co-published books on urban art, among which are *Transit* (2012) *and Day & Night* (2014). She is the author of some ten articles and chapters in French and international journals and of books on urban culture and food heritage and identity in Malta.

Detlef Briesen is a professor at the department of contemporary history at Justus-Liebig University, Gießen, Germany. His research and publications focus on political and cultural history, such as city systems, urban identities, consumerism, youth culture, and health and nutrition in Europe and North America. He has also shown growing interest in including Asian countries into these studies, as he is currently visiting professor at the National University of Vietnam, University of Science and Humanities, Hanoi, and a DAAD (Deutscher Akademischer Austauschdienst) counsellor for Vietnam, Laos and Cambodia. He has published and co-edited seven books, among which are Warenhaus, *Massenkonsum und Sozialmoral. Zur Geschichte der Konsumkritik im 20. Jahrhundert, Department Store, Mass Consumption, and Moral. On the History of Consumerism in the 20th century* (2001) and *Das gesunde Leben Ernährung und Gesundheit seit dem 18. Jahrhundert, The Healthy Life. Nutrition and Health since the 18th Century* (2010), as well as three books dealing with politics and religion in India (with Sigrid Baringhorst), spatial planning (with Wendelin Strubelt), and the state of law in South-East Asia (with Ulrich von Alemann), and many articles and chapters in German and International journals and books.

Nicolas Commune completed his doctorate in sociology at the University of Rouen, France, in 2015. His dissertation is a socio-anthropological approach to ayurvedic therapists in France, in association with which he is investigating the process of appropriation of ayurvedic knowledge and the discourses on health of these practitioners. His previous research concerned the practice of ayurveda in England. He is a postdoctorate fellow in the Philippines where he conducted research on the internationalisation of local therapeutic knowledge and its encounter within international tourism and the wellness industry. The publication of several papers from his communications in international conferences is pending.

Tristan Fournier is a sociologist researcher in at the Interdisciplinary Research Institute on Social Issues (IRIS) within the French National Centre for Scientific Research (CNRS) in Paris, France. His previous work focused on eating choices and food changes, and questioned the status of scientific knowledge as well as the role of the socio-cultural dimensions of food regarding chronic disorders, aging, and the sanitary crisis. Presently, he leads two research programs: the first one on the social, political and scientific issues of nutritional (epi)genomics, and the second, on the obstacles to heritagization of food in the Pyrénées mountains (France). He has published and co-published around 20 papers in French and international books and journals, and co-edited a special issue of *Journal des Anthropologues* on food and gender.

Liora Gvion is Professor of Sociology at The Kibbutzim College of Education in Tel Aviv, Israel, whose major fields of interests are the sociology of food and the sociology of the body. Her previous researches concerned cultural and political aspects of the Palestinian cuisine in Israel, the lesbian community and the professional body. Her present research is twofold: social relationships embedded in operatic production and narrative analyses of food television programmes. She is the author of *Begova Habeten* (2006), *Beyond Hummus and Falafel: Social and Political aspects of Palestinian food in Israel* (2012). She has over 40 articles and chapters on different topics in English and Hebrew in Israeli and international journals and books.

Esther Katz is a French anthropologist and senior scientist at the IRD (Institut de Recherche pour le Développement). She is a member of the IRD/MNHN joint research unit "Local Heritage and Governance", based at the National Museum of Natural History (MNHN) in Paris. Her main research topics deal with anthropology of food, ethnobiology/ethnoclimatology and cultural identity. She has been doing fieldwork in Mexico since 1983 and in Brazil since 2007, and she has worked as well in the Congo, Indonesia and Laos. She is presently leading a project on food heritage and culinary practices and is involved in several projects on food heritage, agrobiodiversity and climate change. She was the co-editor of *Food Models and Social Recompositions in Latin America* (2008), *Aires y lluvias* (2008), *Entre ciel et terre. Climat et Sociétés* (2002), and *Antropología del clima en el mundo hispanoamericano* (1997). She has published about 90 articles and book chapters (30 dealing with food in Latin America) and presented 70 papers at international conferences. She is a member of the editorial board of the online journal *Anthropology of Food*.

Elena Lazos is professor and full time researcher at the Institute of Social Sciences at the UNAM: Universidad Nacional Autonoma de México, Mexico, since 1992. She has a PhD in anthropology and socio-economic of development from the École des Hautes Études en Sciences Sociales, Paris. She has conducted research in different regions of Mexico, Ecuador, Bolivia, Brazil, Bolivia, Nicaragua, Switzerland and France, in collaboration with international and national researchers. In recent years, her main research explores traditional knowledge of maize management, food sovereignty, climate change and agrodiversity, and environmental governance. She has taught around 60 courses in universities in Mexico, Switzerland, Greece, Bolivia, and Canada. She is the author and co-author of around 30 papers in national and international journals and books.

Delphine Marie-Vivien is a researcher in law, in the UMR Innovation, at CIRAD, Montpellier, France. She graduated in chemistry and intellectual property law from the University of Strasbourg. After five years working on intellectual property and genetic resources issues, she became a visiting researcher at NLSIU, Bangalore, India. Her PhD thesis was entitled "The law of geographical indications in India compared to French, European and International laws". Since 2012, she has been based in Vietnam, working on research projects on the protection of geographical indications (GIs) in South-East Asia and worldwide. She is the author of *Geographical Indications in India, a new perspective on the French and European experiences* and has published around 20 articles in French and international journals and books on the governance of GIs, the protection of GIs for handicraft goods, the link between GIs and biodiversity, and GIs and world heritage.

Sandrine Ruhlmann is an anthropologist. Her PhD thesis was on the food culture of the Mongolian Halh that she studied in relation to various concepts such as death and birth, and the sharing of food in domestic and festive spaces. She was a post-doctoral researcher at the Laboratoire d'Anthropologie Sociale (Collège de France, Paris), and is presently at the Centre d'anthropologie sociale (LISTT, Toulouse) where she is conducting research on the perception of animal diseases by Mongolian herders, on health surveillance and control of animals and humans. At the same time, she is continuing to study Mongolian food culture, especially by exploring the changes which are affecting food patterns in the Mongolia capital, Ulan Bator. Her thesis, under the title *L'appel du bonheur. Le partage alimentaire mongol*, was published in 2015, in the collection *Nord-Asie*. She has published around 20 articles on Mongolian culture and food in French and international journals and collective books.

Brigitte Sébastia is a medical anthropologist at the French Institute of Pondicherry and an associate member of Ecole des Hautes Etudes en Sciences Sociales, Paris (CEIAS and Centre d'anthropologie sociale,

Toulouse). Her previous researches concerned therapeutic pluralism in India in the treatment of mental health, and the practice and knowledge of siddha medicine. Her present research is an exploration of the evolution of food habits and patterns in South India according to changes in agricultural policy and practices, and its impact on health. She is currently developing a programme, entitled Food and Nutrition in Indian contexts, aimed at reviving traditional food for the improvement of health and agrodiversity. She is the author of *Māriyamman-Mariyamman. Catholic Practices and Image of Virgin in Velankanni (Tamil Nadu)* (2002), *Les rondes de saint Antoine* (2007), and is the editor of *Restoring Mental Health in India. Pluralistic Therapies and Concepts* (2009). She has published around 25 articles and chapters related to her researches in India (medical, food, culture) published in French, Indian and international journals and books. She is a member of the editorial board of the online journal *Anthropology of Food*.

Charles-Édouard de Suremain is an anthropologist conducting research at the IRD/MNHN joint research unit "Local Heritage and Governance" (UMR PALOC), based at the National Museum of Natural History (MNHN) in Paris and is presently seconded to the CIESAS in Mexico City. His previous research concerned the construction of socio-ethnic prejudice and of the identity of workers in the coffee plantations of Guatemala, followed by the process of ethnogenesis by groups of Quechua-speaking settlers in Ecuador. His current research examines the representations, discourses and practices, including body care and daily food, related to the development of young children in the context of the restructuring of health systems in Latin America. He has also conducted research in Congo, Bolivia and in Peru on the social and cultural dynamics for fighting infant malnutrition. He is co-editor of the online journal *AnthropoChildren*, specialising in the anthropology of children, and a member of the editorial board of the online journal *Anthropology of Food*. He has published and co-edited several books including *Modèles de l'enfance* (2012) and *Enfance et enfants dans les sociétés andines contemporaines* (2014). He has published around 20 articles and chapters in French and Spanish in international journals and books.

Foreword

'Eating Traditional Food: politics, identities and practices' wrestles down the concept and practices of producing and consuming 'traditional foods', without falling either into the ethnocentric, nationalist rendering of tradition, or the blanket denunciation of the very concept of tradition by critical scholars, who thereby abandon any notion of common practices over time, which can be used to contain invented traditions and criticise market and state manipulation of heritage. We are reminded that tradition is the production of the past in the present. The authors do a great service in trying to draw the boundaries of the modern and traditional, the past and present, community and consumer practices. They, thus, enable us to protect what comes from a long duration and is widely shared by the commons without the protection of intellectual property rights, against the encroachment of private, commodified, consumer culture, undertaken primarily for profit and for social prestige. Nevertheless, the authors complicate the effort by drawing lines of filiation between the apparent polar opposites such as the modern and the traditional. We are made aware that tradition, like authenticity, is both practically and politically necessary, while conceptually fraught, in terms of whose tradition is being valorised and whose customs slighted. There is no easy way to identify tradition without engaging with insidious epistemologies of power, and the power to erase practices, or make some practices more visible than others at a particular conjuncture.

For instance, in the exemplary case of meat eating in India, which of the many traditions among Vedic texts, Brahmin teachings, Muslim custom and Dalit practices can and must be valorised, practices that were often deployed against each other? How long does a practice have to be practised to become traditional? The chapter on Malta underlines the exquisite paradox where olive oil and wine production, that were abandoned a millennium ago, are re-introduced as traditional practices, while the seven-decade-old production of a soft, fizzy, drink that is widely consumed, such as Kinnie, is ignored in the consecration of the traditional among a newer cosmopolitan class, in alliance with organisations such as the European Commission and UNESCO, with an acute awareness of their new-found and newly valued Mediterraneanness. There is some sense that a practice has to be good by some definition to be protected. Who gets to decide what is good and what is the process of doing that?

Other questions remain: do 500 years of the continuous presence of Islam make halal an Indian tradition? Can a mere century of tea drinking, in spite of its ubiquity, be adequate to mark it as a quintessentially Indian tradition? Does a millennium of intoxication of various fermented and distilled drinks, count towards an Indian tradition, even if there is minimal textual evidence for it? When do invaders become settlers, and settlers, natives? Much hinges on drawing a temporal line of belongingness across social fields. Many of these questions are interrogated in this book, along with epistemological issues of visibility and invisibility, textual residue, the power of paperwork, and the evanescence of oral practices, both in the realm of taste and of talk.

One thing we learn repeatedly is that contingency is crucial: the threat of transgenic maize was the trigger for the mobilisation of the idea and state policy of Mexican gastronomic tradition as submitted and accepted by UNESCO; the recent wave of Hindu nationalist mobilisation and polarisation has been vital to revivifying the question of beef-eating's Indianness; and the crisis of confidence in modern science and the distribution of risk is key to the emplacement of Ayurveda in France; while the reinvigorated disenfranchisement of Palestinians is fundamental to the contestation around traditional Palestinian foods, such as hummus. So, the authors struggle to find a tradition, if they are to speak at all of dispossession and appropriation by others, no matter how fraught that definition. Which leads immediately to further questions of methods of preservation of legitimate traditional practices – is it best to do so by everyday practice, market power or state policy?

Dietary prescription, apparently ubiquitous today, is in fact an old social habit. Nutritional advice is a venerable tradition of the dissemination and imposition of expert knowledge, to inform and contain lay practices. The history of the production and consumption of amaranth, *chapulines*, and *pulque*, in Mexico's Central Highlands, for instance, are entangled with questions of class and race, tourism, national politics and indigeneity. As illustrated in the compelling chapter by Katz and Lazos, *pulque*, the fermented beverage from the agave plant, which typically grows above altitudes of 1500 metres, was an important traditional indigenous drink and food (children often consumed it for breakfast); it was appropriated by Spanish elites (as an intoxicant along with wine) in the seventeenth century, but came to be thought of as a "primitive" drink of the "savage" Indians by the end of the nineteenth century. In particular, the antipathy towards *pulque* deepened when the *hacendados* from the South were the target of the revolutionaries of 1910. By 1923, the new regime enacted alcohol taxes that disadvantaged *pulque* over the newly emergent urban and cosmopolitan beer. The alliance between the post-revolutionary government, religious authorities and German immigrants reconfigured beer as a more modern, healthy and hygienic drink, because it was bottled and refrigerated, and it became the most popular alcoholic beverage, even in indigenous villages.

Substantively, the various chapters show us how dietary traditions are embroiled in contingent struggles between classes, races and political factions. Epistemologically, they demonstrate how much richer the story can be when researchers have access to Spanish, French, Portuguese and German sources, and can master modes of data visualisation for beautifully illustrative maps and graphs, for instance of amaranth, *pulque* and insect consumption.

Finally, this book is the product of an illuminating failure. The idea emerged from an international conference on traditional foods in the Department of Food Sciences at the University of Puducherry, India, convened in December 2010. But it turned out that most of the submitted papers ignored the social and cultural aspect of the question and drove headlong into the more fashionable question of nutritional values of traditional foods, after a desultory discourse on indigenous food practices, a discourse confined to two dominant traditions of nutritionism (nutrient-oriented exclusion of social questions) and the political economy of hunger and malnutrition. It is only very slowly, in spite of its importance in revealing the logic of actually lived life, that everyday food practices of various classes and ethnicities are beginning to emerge as a site of scholarly engagement, and this book is a testimony to the power of such an analytic.

Krishnendu Ray
Associate Professor, New York University, USA
Chair, Department of Nutrition, Food Studies & Public Health
President of the Association for the Study of Food & Society

1 Eating traditional food

Politics, identity and practices[1]

Brigitte Sébastia

Traditional food: a term which resists definition

The idea of editing a book on 'traditional foods' emerged from a three-day international conference entitled 'Traditional foods' organised by the Department of Food Sciences of the University of Puducherry, India, 1–3 December 2010. I was invited, as an anthropologist, to chair the introductory session entitled 'Diversity of traditional foods'. This panel aimed at approaching the subject in the context of the social sciences. However, except for one chapter, the contributions have not been included in this book because of their lack of involvement with food culture. Indeed, after a brief presentation of the communities (mostly tribal) which consume the targeted traditional foods, and some historical outlines, the presentations immediately shifted to the field of nutritional sciences, focusing on the nutritional values of these foods. The failure of most of the speakers to develop their presentation on the cultural aspect of traditional foods has to be understood as due to the absence of awareness of food studies in disciplines other than those of biotechnology and nutritional sciences. The historical background of famine, hunger and undernourishment in India which continues to pervade the imagination, as pointed out by Sunil S. Amrith (2008),[2] may justify the focus on nutritional sciences in the field of food studies, as well as that on economic sciences in the domain of the social sciences. Apart from the pioneer studies by R.S. Khare (1976a, 1976b, 1992)[3] and R.S. Khare and M.S.A. Rao (1986), few Indian researchers have examined the practices of preparing and consuming food in contemporary India from the perspective of tradition, either on a daily basis or during biographical and religious festivities and rituals. The works of Anil Kishore Sinha on traditional sweetmeats (2000), of Chitrita Banerji (2001, 2006, 2007) and Manpreet K. Janeja (2010) on memories of dishes prepared by grandmothers and mothers, the studies on evolution of consumption of foodstuffs and dishes by Om Prakash (1961), K.T. Achaya (1998a, 1998b) and Tuk-Tuk Kumar (1988), and on the adaptation of Indian foods in colonial cuisine (Brown 1998; Sangar 1999), are exceptions.[4]

The infeasibility of compiling a book of chapters by the panel constrained me to search for experts exploring traditional foods in diverse cultural areas and contexts. The chapters which compose this book, by the plurality of their approaches, political, identity, religious, symbolic and medical, allow not only for deepening the recurrent values attributed to traditional foods evoked by the panellists (identity, religious and nutritional), but also for debating the relevance of definitions of the subject developed by two extensive European programmes, EuroFIR and TRUEFOOD; of these, that of EuroFIR has been retained by the FAO.

The first question that arises with regard to the term 'traditional foods' is what people have in mind when they employ it. According to what criteria do they qualify a foodstuff or a dish as traditional? In which situations and contexts, whether social, religious, ideological or political, may a food be given traditional value, positive or negative? In the sixth synthesis report of EuroFIR on Traditional Foods in Europe, Elisabeth Weichselbaum and her colleagues argue that "Although the term 'traditional foods' is widely used, and everybody has a rough idea of what is meant by it, there are hardly any definitions that clearly define traditional foods." (2009: 4). In common belief, traditional foods often evoke cultural heritage, the know-how shared and transmitted, quite often by word of mouth, amongst a more or less wide group of people (family, clan, territory, country or a geographical region covering several countries, such as rice in Asia or olive oil in Mediterranean areas). They suggest an extensive past which defines them as being tasty, healthy and in harmony with nature; many of these attributes are rooted in memory and imaginary. Lin T. Humphrey states that "In memory culture, where we find traditional recipes and food stories, 'traditional foods' may refer to either the kind of heritage or history that we actually had or the one we only wish we had. When we label food traditional, it is usually a mark of approval." (1989: 163). Nevertheless, as the author emphasises, "'tradition' is a value-laden word" and "food depends on total context in our memories and with our associations to develop such meanings and identification and such positive and tasty connotations" (Samuelson quoted by Humphrey *ibid.*): this leads to a certain blurring, elasticity and heterogeneity of what may be perceived as a traditional food. The recipes that Humphrey has collected from her students,[5] who had investigated what they understood by traditional foods, are particularly illuminating on the conceptual variability of the term. The students qualify their selected recipes as traditional either because they are used by their mother or grandmother, they are hand-made, they include some unusual ingredients, they are served on special occasions (religious or biographical celebrations) or they are 'good to share' with their peers. Humphrey comments that the choice of recipes by students is not oriented according to long-term use and cultural relationship, but to the role they play in their social life, to "create and enforce a sense of identity with both past and present family and friends." (*ibid*: 168).

Compared to Humphrey's students, the representation of traditional foods by the contributors of the panel 'Diversity of Traditional Food' was conventional: they inscribed this category, explicitly as well as implicitly, within long-term use. They explicitly supported the long-term consumption of traditional foods by mentioning historical evidence drawn from ancient texts such as the Ṛg Veda[6] or from normative literature such as Manusmṛti or Gṛha Dharma which codify food consumption and patterns according to the eater's identity[7] or biographical rituals, respectively. On the other hand, they implicitly called upon the long use of traditional foods as they associated them with indigenous communities, predominantly tribes, who produce, collect and consume them. Another criterion which emerged from most of the papers was the healthy, even medical, value that their authors attributed to these foods. This relationship is not surprising as, on the one hand, food in Indian traditional medicine is fundamentally allied to medication for preventing and treating diseases,[8] and on the other, studies on food in India, as mentioned above, focus predominantly on the field of dietetics and biotechnology.

To return to the fundamental question 'what is a traditional food', it is surprising that few countries have proposed a definition although it might be an added-value for marketing. The only attempts come from European countries which have carried out two extensive cross-national/cultural surveys, both funded by the Sixth Framework Programme of the European Commission. The first study, TRUEFOOD, involving six regions selected in seven European countries (Belgium, France, Greece, Italy, Norway, Poland and Spain), aimed to develop innovations in the food industry in order to help producers of traditional foods "to maintain and expand their market share in a highly competitive and increasingly global food market" (Guerrero *et al.* 2009: 345). The objective was to make agricultural products financially attractive in order to alleviate rural depopulation. An understanding of the way in which consumers from rural as well as urban areas defined and perceived traditional food products was the first step of this programme (Almli *et al.* 2011; Guerrero *et al.* 2009; Pieniak *et al.* 2009). A definition was produced based on interviews (Guerrero *et al.* 2009):

> [a traditional food] is a product frequently consumed or associated to specific celebrations and/or seasons, normally transmitted from one generation to another, made with care in a specific way according to the gastronomic heritage, with little or no processing/manipulation, that is distinguished and known because of its sensory properties and associated to a certain local area, region or country.

The analysis of cross-national/cultural data resulting from the TRUEFOOD programme revealed important differences in the perception of traditional foods between the seven countries involved in the programme. Although the general apprehension of traditional foods was very positive (from 5.51 to 6.03 on scale 1–7), the reasons for which each European country valorised them varied significantly in terms of organoleptic properties and environmental and economic advantages, as well as in their inscription in the patrimonial field and in religious and biographical celebrations. This significant variability adds to the paramount difficulty of finding a consensual definition for a term as abstract and culturally-connoted as that of traditional foods.

The second study is the programme EuroFIR (European Food Information Resource) involving 13 European countries. With the objective of investigating the health value attributed to traditional foods through interviews on selected ingredients, cooking methods and dishes, the programme endeavoured to develop a definition of 'traditional foods' (Trichopoulou *et al.* 2006; Weichselbaum and Costa 2009). The definition by which 'tradition' means "conforming to established practice or specifications prior to the Second World War",[9] is presented by Weichselbaum *et al.* (2009: 4–6):

> [...] a food with a specific feature or features, which distinguish it clearly from other similar products of the same category in terms of the use of 'traditional ingredients' (raw materials or primary products) or 'traditional composition' or 'traditional type of production and/or processing method'.

This definition was developed by clarifying three terms. 'Raw material or primary product' is understood as "either alone or as an ingredient, which has been used in identifiable geographical areas and remains in use today (taking into account cases where use was abandoned for a time and then reinstated) and its characteristics are in accordance with current specifications of national and EU legislation". 'Traditional composition' is defined as "the uniquely identifiable composition (in terms of ingredients) that was first established prior to the Second World War and passed down through generations by oral or other means (taking into account cases where composition was abandoned for a time and then reinstated) and when necessary is differentiated from the composition defined by the generally recognised characteristics of the wider group to which the product belongs". Lastly, the 'traditional type of production and/or processing' is specified as "the production and/or processing of a food that 1- has been transmitted from generation to generation through oral tradition or other means and 2- has been applied prior to the Second World War and remains in use (taking into account cases where composition was abandoned for a time and then reinstated) despite its adjustment to binding rules from national or EU food hygiene regulations or the incorporation of technical progress, under the condition that production and /or processing remains in line with methods used originally and that the food's intrinsic features such as its physical, chemical, microbiological or organoleptic features are maintained." This definition was adopted by the Food and Agriculture Organization (FAO) during the 26th FAO Regional conference on Europe in Innsbruck, Austria, on 26th–27th June 2008 (ftp://ftp.fao.org/docrep/fao/meeting/013/K2473E.pdf).

The definition given by EuroFIR is, admittedly, more elaborate than that of TRUEFOOD, but it calls for comment. First, the definition delimits the time prior to which a food consumed today can be classified as traditional. This time limit, as emphasised by Elise Billiard in this book, tends, however, to be ethnocentric and does not fit in with the representation of traditional foods by people. As demonstrated by Sandrine Ruhlmann in her chapter, the Mongolians consider dumplings as belonging to their food culture, even though these products, which originated in China, have entered their diet recently. Secondly, the inclusion of "restated food" into the EuroFIR definition, i.e. dishes and ingredients having benefited from a revival after a period of abandonment, is all the more uncertain when other elements of the definition are considered. Certainly, the goal of "maintaining the physical, chemical, microbiological features" is difficult to respect due to the changes that have affected production of foodstuffs (agricultural methods, environmental issues) and of dishes (processing and cooking methods) and, when "restated foods" are concerned, it is simply unrealisable as data from the past are missing. Thirdly, "maintaining organoleptic features", i.e. characteristics such as taste, flavour, odour, consistency, etc. which are subjective, is all the more impossible where "restated foods" are concerned as their perception is distorted by memory and imaginary. Lastly, the definition fails to take into consideration the fact that traditional knowledge and know-how are far from being homogenous and fixed. In cuisine, as in siddha medicine on which I have been conducting research, recipes, like formulas, may have evolved according to the creativity of the cook or the practitioner, often with a competitive aim. Cooks, like traditional practitioners, are not always eager to reveal their recipes, omitting, sometimes deliberately, to mention ingredients which make their dish or remedy different in taste or in efficacy. In a certain way, secrecy may be a component of cuisine, as it is a feature of alchemy.[10] Compared to the EuroFIR definition, that of TRUEFOOD, despite its weakness, corresponds better to the common representation of traditional foods, as it specifies: the continuity between generations, transmission of knowledge and know-how, seasonality of food (with reference to nature) in daily consumption and during festival time, sensory properties of food and relationships between traditional foods and cultural heritage whether local or national. In other terms, the definition of EuroFIR is clearly directed by a legal intention, perhaps with a commercial objective even though the aim of the programme was to examine the healthy aspects of traditional foods. That of TRUEFOOD, although its objective was precisely commercial, has a much more anthropological dimension; its failure to mention the time period during which a food or ingredient may be called traditional may reflect discrepant perceptions of traditional foods by consumers. Nevertheless, the research papers of the teams involved in these two programmes provide some information on the representations of traditional foods by consumers that complement the definitions. For example, while terms such as local, territory, community, culture, are omitted in the definition of EuroFIR, Trichopoulou and her colleagues (2007: 426) specify that "traditional foods include foods that have been consumed locally or regionally for an extensive time period." While the definition of TRUEFOOD is silent on the consumption period necessary to classify a product as traditional food, Luis Guerrero and his colleagues (2009: 345–346) specify: "Traditional [related to food] means proven usage in the community market[11] for a time period showing transmission between generations; this time period should be the one generally ascribed to one human generation, at least 25 years". This period, significantly shorter than that proposed by EuroFIR, is obviously debatable as it is oblivious of the boom in the food industry, transport, catering, tourism, migration and communication tools which accelerate circulation of products, people and recipes. The relevance of these two programmes is justified by their teams as a means for protecting traditional foods against the risk of their disappearance. However, one may deplore the lack of investigation into the reasons why some traditional foodstuffs or dishes are being abandoned while others have been granted national or international recognition, such as ratatouille, a vegetable dish originally from Provence which is now prepared all over France and neighbouring countries, curries originally from India declared a national dish in England, or pizza from Italy consumed, admittedly with variations according to local taste, all over the world (Bell and Valentine 1997). Moreover, these programmes have not sought to grasp the broadness of the concept of traditional food that people use, according to context, for supporting or, inversely, for counteracting economical, political, medical and identity claims. The following excerpt from Uma Narayan's work related to food, quoted by David Bell and Gill Valentine (*ibid*.: 2), expresses the plurality and ambiguity of representations attributed to traditional foods:

> Thinking about food has much to reveal about how we understand our personal and collective identities. Seemingly simple acts of eating are flavoured with complicated and sometimes contradictory cultural meanings. Thinking about food can help reveal the rich and messy textures of our attempts at self-understanding; as well as our understanding and problematic understandings of our relationship with social Others.

Food in general, and traditional foods in particular, are providers of personal or collective identities, and markers of social and cultural representations as varied as aesthetics, pleasure, ethics, memory, politics, lifestyle and well-being. The multilayered representations of traditional foods, and the diversity of contexts in which they are appropriated by a group, a community or a nation, are the focus of this book.

The construction of the concept of traditional food through ten cases studies

The book presents ten case studies, rooted in different cultural areas, which analyse the processes of valorisation, instrumentalisation, adjustment, adoption and reinvention, at stake in the construction of a food – ingredient as well as dish – as traditional. In order to reproduce the diversity of attributes of traditional foods developed in each of these studies, the arrangement of the book has been to avoid any classificatory topics which might reduce the chapters to their major focus. The book, rather, unwinds like a thread on which an important attribute of traditional foods tackled in one chapter is then deepened by the following chapter(s). The thread uncoils through three aspects of traditional foods: construction, dispossession and appropriation or invention, engaged with more or less deeply in each chapter, definition and regulation, nationalism and identity, and relation to health.

The three categories of products – amaranth, insects and *pulque* – explored in Chapter 2 are unquestionably traditional: their consumption by prehispanic communities is reported by Spaniards who established themselves in Mexico, and has continued thank to the intermixing of Spaniards with indigenous people. However, as discussed by Esther Katz and Elena Lazos, their consumption has never been linear: according to period, it faced some restriction for religious, moral and/or social reasons. If these products have survived till today, it is partly because they have benefited from a revival movement fostered by their nutritional quality which promotes them to the rank of what the authors name "super-foods". The revitalisation of traditional ingredients, recognised for their nutritional values, agricultural advantages or their sustainability with regard to the food security, is a worldwide movement made necessary by the repeated crises which, each time, throw light on inequities regarding food affordability in terms of access and cost, detrimental effects of intensive cultivation and irreparable loss of biodiversity, etc. As crucial as the revival of traditional food ingredients is, their benefit to the populations who have the most need of them is diminished: while the promotion of amaranth has profited indigenous people of Mexico who, not having stopped consuming it, have now revived its cultivation and sold amaranth-based products to the well-off, promotion of insects has not had the same result. Indeed, how is it possible to convince marginalised communities to consume foods which have contributed to their ostracism? The reluctance to consume insects echoes what I have observed in South India concerning the revival of millets for improving the nutritional quality of the diet of poor. As millets were deprecated as 'food of poor', 'food of villagers' or 'coarse cereals', the poor and villagers avoid consuming them as much as possible while higher classes, sensitised by nutritional discourses, turn to them to improve their health, especially to prevent or treat diabetes. Following a process similar to that described by Katz and Lazos, the enthusiasm of higher classes for millets has led to a significant increase in their price which make them barely affordable for the poor. While the insects' price inflation stems from the combination of a degraded environment that has reduced drastically the availability of insects and from the valorisation of insects as gastronomic components, that of millets results from the fact that their production, not supported by government programmes, does not face the new requirement from the food industry, restaurants and food markets that attract the health conscious higher classes.

In contrast to the three Mexican foods which, even though they have experienced periods of fluctuation, have been cultivated, produced and consumed since time immemorial in Mexico, the Chapter 3, by Elise Billiard, based on the case of Maltese cuisine, shows that the meaning accorded to the term 'traditional' is hardly fixed. Her chapter contributes with relevance to the debate on the definition of a traditional food. It deals with the impossibility of establishing a clear definition of the term 'tradition' and, concomitantly, of its association with food. Rather than defining these elusive terms, which might be counterproductive, it proposes to examine the way knowledge and practices are transmitted within a community. Relying on Timothy Ingold's work (1997), the author argues that the transmission and preservation of culinary know-how including gestures and experiences, is more relevant than the recipes in books.[12] The author's opinion does not support the EuroFIR and TRUEFOOD projects which, promoting the standardisation of recipes for marketing purposes, risk reducing the diversity of knowledge and skills. Her statement resonates with the situation I have observed in the field of siddha medicine, where industrialisation of remedies, modelled on bio-pharmaceutical practices, leads to a transformation and a significant decrease in the repertoires of traditional formulas (Sébastia 2010). While the formulation of remedies in ayurvedic or siddha medicine relies upon a combination of multiples ingredients, ayurvedic and siddha pharmacies have developed new formulas by using only two or three ingredients selected for their active properties. If such ingredients are used in these medical systems, may these remedies still be called traditional? Such a transformation raises questions about the impact of the industrialisation process on traditional foods in terms of authenticity and recognition compared to those made at home or in restaurants. The industrialisation process is selective and reductive: it ends up imposing uniformity on traditional dishes which are essentially as variable in composition and taste as they are dependent on the virtuosity and improvisation of the cook, and on the regional identity from which they originate. Observations in the field of traditional foods do not allow merely investigation of how skills are transmitted and how a dish may differ from the original, but also shed light on discrepancies in discourses and in political debates articulated from a nationalist perspective. The production of olive oil, the iconic product of Mediterranean countries, has recently been introduced into Malta with the help of the European Union. Although in the distant past, olive trees were cultivated there, the use of olive oil in cooking has not been attested. The reintroduction of olive trees has allowed the Maltese to produce an oil that they called 'traditional'. By inscribing their culture in the list of Mediterranean countries recognised for their healthy diet,[13] they rewrite the history of their country, erasing traces of the people (Arabs, British) who colonised them and transformed their agriculture by developing cotton crops (Arabs) and sheep breeding (British), even though these influences are still present in their dietary pattern. In an identity construction, the question of the time prior to which a food may be labelled 'traditional' is not an issue. On the contrary, historical facts may be denied and reconstructed in order to support the claims as is cogently demonstrated by Ruhlmann in her chapter on the valorisation of dumplings by Mongolia. However, the historical background is one of the proprietary criteria for a traditional food to be recognised, and thus the historical evidence is meticulously examined in documents for obtaining a certification of traditional food at the national and international levels, as Chapter 4 by Delphine Marie-Vivien, on geographical indications (GIs) shows in the Indian context.

The classification of foodstuffs and dishes under the "traditional" label undoubtedly offers advantages for both producers and consumers. Antonia Trichopolous and her colleagues (2007) argue that the designation of marketed traditional foods protects products, producers and consumers. The products and producers may benefit from a newly booming market due to the fact that 'traditional' is an added-value for consumers in search of authenticity, and certification protects the consumers from false claims. Obviously, as mentioned above, a certification does not always guarantee the authenticity of a product as the choice of the ingredient or the recipe has been defined by the person or company who has submitted his/its application. The examples of products proposed for obtaining the GI designation in India are particularly relevant to the analysis of the issues raised by certification. European countries have been first in creating designations, among which some are used worldwide. These designations, defined in 1992 and redefined in 2006 by the European Council Regulation, aim to prioritise either the link between a food and its place of origin and production (Protected Designation of Origin, PDO; Protected Geographical Indication, PGI) or the method (culinary patrimony) used to produce it (Traditional Speciality Guarantee, TSG). Although certain food products would fit the TSG designation, the GI is the one India has chosen and for which it enacted the GI Act in 1999. The GI designation has been accorded to several agricultural products cultivated in a delimited territory such as Darjeeling tea, Coorg oranges, Virupakshi Hill Banana, Malabar pepper, etc.; sometimes the designation name corresponds to the variety of a plant such as Navara rice (Kerala). It has also benefited some food products, known and made all over India but particularised by a recipe developed by a manufacturer, such as the two sweetmeats, Dharwad *peḍha* and Tirupati *laddu*. As discussed by the author, this designation may be misused due to the fact that the commercialisation of *peḍha* and *laddu* under the label Dharwad *peḍha* and Tirupati *laddu* is the monopoly[14] of only one family and the temple committee of Tirupati-Tirumalai who applied for the designation, while the recipe and the processing mode of preparing these sweetmeats is shared by other manufacturers of the region. On the other hand, when a product is not clearly designated by a geographical name obtaining the label is complicated. The case of Basmati rice presented in the chapter is particularly illustrative as repeated applications for GI designation have been rejected.[15] Compared to Navara rice for which the applicants succeeded in demonstrating a link with the region and culture of Kerala, the cultivation of Basmati rice covers too wide a territory to benefit from the GI designation. Indeed, while Basmati refers to a variety of rice which was cultivated in Pakistan, North India and Bangladesh, several cultivars have been developed from the aromatic Basmati 370 variety developed from a local rice in 1933 at a rice research station now located in Pakistan (Singh 2000). The first attempts to certify Basmati rice resulted from the necessity of protecting it from biopiracy when the US Patent and Trademark Office granted a patent on Basmati rice developed by Rice-Tech Inc., Texas (Mukherjee 2008). While India had to enact laws to protect its collection of rice germoplasts from biopiracy by international seed agencies such as Syngenta (Lutringer 2012), it had no law for protecting its foodstuffs within the World Trade Organization. The enactment of the GI Act in 1999 was initiated at this critical period. Interestingly, the author mentions that the political party which enacted the law was the Bharatiya Janata Party. This party, made up of ultra-right members, is well known for its nationalist positions and reinterpretations of history aiming at denouncing outsiders who pervert Indian culture (see Sébastia Chapter 6 in this volume) and sack the richness of the country. If the interest of the GI designation is born from a will to protect the knowledge, know-how and natural resources of the country, the objectives of the applicants in registering a product are today driven by the same intentions for which these designations were established, that of commercial benefits for producers. This especially concerns those aiming at the international market, and consumers too, as the Indian middle and upper classes are increasingly attracted by the concept of tradition, be it applied to foods or to any goods such as sari, shawl, textile or soap.

The valorisation of traditional foods with a political and nationalist intention highlighted in the two previous cultural contexts, and also evoked in Chapter 2, as Mexico had inscribed prehispanic food to its patrimony to gain recognition from UNESCO, is one of the major topics developed in this book. Dumplings in Mongolid, as discussed by Ruhlmann, are regarded as "authentic" and "true" Mongolian foods, although introduced only in the 1970s and are certainly of Chinese origin. Having progressively entered the food system of Mongolians, dumplings have acquired the same attributes and values, physical, symbolic and soteriological, as those with which traditionally consumed foods were endowed, especially mutton and dairy products. Due to these attributes, they hold a prevalent role in the festive meals whose symbolic function is to maintain the order of the universe. In addition, whereas Buddhism with its hierarchical system was combatted by the socialist regime, the democratic regime which emerged after the collapse of the USSR has been promoting Mongolian identity, with Genghis Khan as the emblematic figure of nomadism, as well as Buddhism. In this political and religious reconfiguration, dumplings have acquired a preeminent place as Mongolians use them to express certain Buddhist karmic conceptions, especially those of distributing accumulated happiness and, in return, gaining merit towards auspicious rebirth. Such a process of construction is a contemporary example of invented traditional foods in line with the ideas of invented tradition presented by Eric Hobsbawm and Terence Ranger (1983). In his introduction, Hobsbawm argues that invented traditions "give to any desired change (or resistance to innovation) the sanction of precedent, social continuity and natural law as expressed in history" (*ibid*: 2). The denial of the origin of dumplings which stems from a long period of conflict with, and domination by, the Chinese, allows the Mongolians not only to legitimise their contemporary practices, but also to support their representation of the world and their beliefs and ethics.

The process of appropriation of a food, with claim to a traditional origin, is at the heart of the actions led by Dalit students (lower castes in Hindu stratification) of the Osmania University at Hyderabad documented by Brigitte Sébastia. In contrast, however, with the dumplings of Mongolia or the olive trees of Malta, the food the students claim is beef, a product which is neither borrowed from another food culture, nor whose consumption was interrupted for a long time. Qualifying beef as a traditional food may seem as strange as inadequate, as this ordinary ingredient is consumed all over the world. But in

India its consumption gives rise to a very peculiar situation. Due to progressive restriction on cow slaughter influenced by Buddhism and Jainism, and its vehement condemnation since the early nineteenth century by Hindu nationalist movements, consumption of beef was given up by castes of middle and upper status, and became a marker of Muslim and Dalit identity. While Muslims and Dalits have been encouraged to change what the nationalists interpreted as an 'evil' habit, the present day situation is reversed as, thanks to an improvement in their socio-economic status, lower Dalits are able to raise their voices to claim their rights to eat what they called their traditional food. However, the beef *biriyāni*, they select to support their claim is far from being a traditional Dalit dish. It is an invented tradition or, to quote Claude Levy-Strauss, a '*bricolage*' (see also Ruhlmann) which serves, not to legitimise contemporary practices or to support a representation of the world, as in the case of dumplings, but rather to de-stigmatise a foodstuff and make it appreciated, nutritional values participating significantly in this construction.

The strategy adopted by Dalits students to endorse a positive image of a traditional food which has contributed to their marginalisation is rare. More common, as demonstrated above through the consumption of insects or millets, is to renounce to the foods which are ostracised or are ostracising. The situation examined by Liora Gvion shows that this is not always possible, as a traditional food may be an effective instrument to subdue a community. Analysing the reality TV programme Israeli 'MasterChef', the author shows how the Israeli Chefs construct and reproduce the stereotypical image of the Palestinian community of Israel, as being seldom disposed to change their conservative attitude. Unlike the Dalits, the Palestinian contestants resist throwing back the image expected by the Israeli society. But to stay in the competition, they have no alternative but to admit their inability to adapt to the modern values of the society in which they are living and to demonstrate their attachment to their food heritage. The Palestinian food patrimony is presented by the chefs as poor; this ignores the fact that certain of its dishes have participated in the creation of the Israeli cuisine which is a combination of recipes and know-how borrowed from diverse cultures within which Jews lived before establishing themselves in Israel (Ranta 2016). This story of the dispossession of a traditional food is not different from that of the dumplings originating in China: in these two situations of conflict, to deny any quality to the adversary, such as being the creator of a traditional food, permits those who act in this way to position themselves as superior.

In other contexts, the appropriation of food patrimony from others is not accompanied by their dispossession. It is because high values are attributed to them that some traditional foods are appropriated or borrowed. These values may be reflect cultural preference and closeness as in the case of olive oil in Malta, or their nutritional qualities,[16] or the quest for authenticity as demonstrated by the Indian food recommended by French ayurvedic practitioners (see Commune in this volume). The former two, cultural preference and nutritional properties, are the values that the Bolivians, studied by Edouard de Suremain, emphasise in expressing their nostalgia for a time of abundance when they lived in Argentina as migrants, and in describing their miserable life since their return to Bolivia. Nostalgia, and more precisely the nostalgia for food, has been widely designated as a contribution to the nationalist and identity construction of migrants (Holtzman 2006). Foods from the motherland, quite often qualified as traditional, are highly valued compared to the foods of host countries. For example, in the context of migration studies of Indians, the works on food culture have especially benefited from the contributions of Indian migrants. The nostalgic memories of the food consumed at home, either analysed (Mannur 2010; Ray 2004) or expressed (Banerji 2001, 2006, 2007; Brown 1998) hold an important place in this context. Such feelings are in line with a construction, even an idealisation, of the nation[17] in which Indian culinary culture is one of the components, whether in a situation of migration (Mannur 2010; Srinivas 2006) or at home (Appadurai 1988; Srinivas 2006). Anita Mannur, underlining the valorisation of Indian food in diasporic milieus, calls it "culinary citizenship", i.e. "a form of affective citizenship which grants subjects the ability to claim and inhabit certain subject positions via their relationship to food" (Mitra 2011: 434–5). This identity construction through the mirror of memory is a feature shared by migrants. As John D. Holtzman asserts, "ethnic identity forms a central arena in which food is tied to notions of memory, although not necessarily framed in those terms." (Holtzman 2006: 366). However, the repertory of traditional foods of the motherland, sometimes imagined, invented or reconstructed, is not always as valorised as it is for the Bolivian returnees. In their poor country, migration is a means to escape poverty and food insecurity, and the return home is an experience all the more bitter in that they do not find any work as would allow them access to good food, i.e, food available only to rich people. Such a situation is obviously far from that of Indian migrant writers. Belonging to elite groups, these writers know about Indian food culture only from the varied and rich food they ate in childhood, and eat during their holidays at home. The books of Chitrata Banerji, for example, full of tastes and smells, relate her food discovery of India. In contrast, de Suremain points out that the return home for the Bolivians entails difficulties in coping with a monotonous and scanty diet and the deprivation of what they call Argentinean traditional foods, especially beef and bread, two valued items accessible in Bolivia only by prosperous people. The discourses of Bolivian returnees between the food of "there" and the food of "here", to use the dichotomy of the author, point to the decline in their socio-economic status due to their impoverishment; they have become *indiecitos* (small Indians) again, and have also lost legitimacy as they are no longer able to nourish their children adequately. While, "there", the place of plenty, the children's bodies, fed with nutritious and fatty foods, were strong and well developed, "here", the place of scarcity, their body is deteriorating and becoming weak. The main food featured in their memories of "there" is meat, especially beef. Mirroring the Dalit students' claims, they attribute a high nutritional value to it. Even though their consumption of beef in Argentina was limited to Sunday and festive days, their deprivation in Bolivia is regarded as very detrimental to the health of their children.

The question of healthy foods is at the heart of the final three chapters which approach these foods from the point of view of the diet recommended by a governmental policy, by dieticians or by ayurvedic practitioners. A model of a sustainable and healthy diet is all the harder to define as each country has its own conception of food, oriented according to ideological and socio-cultural criteria, as clearly epitomised in this book. This complexity leads to a cacophony of dietary recommendations, fuelled by diverse ideologies and often contradictory or unsuitable for the food pattern of the targeted people, with the result that they are poorly observed. Dietary concepts, so popular today, are in fact an old story. They form a significant part of traditional medical thought (Farquhar 2002; Sébastia 2015; see also de Suremain and Commune in this volum); to this extent that they have entered the discourses of lay people. They have also influenced theories on the prevention of disease, as Detlef Briesen demonstrates in his chapter on Germany. He is not concerned with traditional foods because Germany does not, properly speaking, have a food culture; the German tradition lies in its strong and lengthy involvement in creating a healthy diet. It played a pioneer role in the nutritional sciences which were applied in agro-industry for developing processed food affordable by all socio-economic groups. While meat consumption, especially pork, was promoted to enhance the nutritional quality of the diet of the poor, vegetarianism found a fecund field in this country preoccupied by the health of its population. Drawing on theories and influences as diverse and heteroclite such as: the humoural balance of the Hippocratic physiological system, the vitalism movement, derived from the *'principe vital'* of Jean Jacques Rousseau, the ideology of National Socialism aimed at elevating moral German behaviour by eradicating smoking, drinking and meat-eating and, more recently, the Negative Nutrition, concept used by Warren J. Belasco to describe a movement that emerged in the 1960s in US inciting consumers to eat less and to question their own food habits, the valorisation of the vegetarian diet, or at least, of a diet based more on plant food, has been progressively spreading. The inclination of Germany towards a healthy diet has favoured the development of organic agriculture that started in the 1920s, as a result of which the country is the second biggest market for organic products in the world after Denmark. The historical, sociological and medical conditions which lead to a valorisation either of meat consumption or of vegetarianism differ. But these theses, all aiming at promoting good health through a diet supposedly nutritional, confuse the representation of an ideal diet or, playing with the terminology of Warren J. Belasco (1989), what a positive diet is. This confusion partly explains why people tend not to be compliant with the food recommendations prescribed for preventing or treating food-related disorders.

A marked resistance to following dietary recommendations is epitomized by French people with hypercholesterolemia. The difficulty nutritionists face in convincing their patients to comply with their food prescriptions leads them to turn to sociologists in order to understand the causes. The chapter by Tristan Fournier reveals that attachments to traditional foods and to eating habits and environment are the main factors hindering compliance. This gives rise to two observations. First, traditional foods to which "patients" are attached are not always healthy, cheese and processed meat being the two products inherent to French food culture that are most mentioned. This observation stands as a counterpoint to common sense about the healthy value attributed to traditional foods as was focused on by the EuroFIR programme and mentioned by Indian panellists at the conference "Traditional food". The fact that traditional foods may have some consequences for health, or are too calorific compared to the energy requirement of modern life, may lead to their being abandoned. The agro-industry has been penetrating this field to develop more healthy traditional foods, but the organoleptic properties of these foods meet with lukewarm appreciation from consumers. Secondly, the social and familial environment in which food habits are rooted is a significant obstacle to following food recommendations. While people are prone to comply with prescriptions when they are alone in front of their plate, compliance becomes a real challenge when the sharing of food takes place in the circle of family, social or professional relationships. The sharing of food being an important part of the commensal relationships which link an individual to a group, the observance of food recommendations is all the more difficult in that the food culture in which these relationships are inserted accords great importance to the sharing of meals. This is the case in France, well known for its sophisticated *manières de table* centred on culinary hedonism as a value favouring dialogue and conviviality (Poulain 2002). This is also the case in India where, although its *manières de table* are entirely opposed to the French model, the meal being swallowed rapidly quite often with scant conversation, the repeated invitations which are intrinsic to the commensal obligations of people expose those with diabetes to breaking their regimen frequently and to consuming the rich food they are served.[18] Not only is temptation high when people on a particular regimen are exposed to their favourite dishes while the rest of the family is not constrained by the same regimen, but also the refusal of a dish or the impossibility of sharing the same menu during a friendly meal or a business lunch creates awkwardness.[19] Medication is, in these cases, the best recourse to treat food-related diseases and to avoid health complications. But medication, notably in the long-term, as in the treatment of chronic diseases, is not always accepted because of its iatrogenic effects, either real or anticipated. Failure to take medication is common, at least till secondary problems occur, and resort to another medical system, called in western countries alternative or complementary, may become a second option. This is the topic explored in the last chapter of this volume.

The practice of ayurvedic medicine in France, as Nicolas Commune observes in his contribution, is hardly visible. Compared to Germany, for example, where pharmacies sell Chinese medicine and spas, run by graduate ayurvedic practitioners, offer Indian medicines and massages, ayurvedic centres and clinics are limited in their practice. Although unconventional medical systems increasingly enter hospitals, and unconventional remedies pharmacies, French legislation is reluctant to support medical systems other than biomedicine and homeopathy and imposes restrictions, one in particular being the obligation not to treat diseases. This restriction obliges ayurvedic practitioners to invest in the field of prevention and thus to develop their knowledge of foods, and especially traditional foods, which form an important part of the therapeutic universe of this medicine. But, using the food repertoire of India when practising in France is not without difficulty. Today exotic foods are increasingly available in France, facilitated by the import market developed by ethnic or specialist wholesalers to respond to the demands of foreign communities, and of French consumers, enthusiasts for new products. But the diversity of these imported products is not sufficient for the needs of ayurvedic practitioners, so that they are obliged to create a new repertoire of 'traditional foods' able to replace those recommended in the ayurvedic texts. The process of replacement described by Nicolas Commune that uses complex and subtle tools, exposes the inventiveness and the dynamic work of innovation, adaptation and re-appropriation of certain practitioners in juggling with diverse sources of knowledge in order faithfully to practise ayurveda according to the tradition, and/or to distinguish themselves from their peers. The process of replacement also reveals the plasticity of 'Indian traditional foods' which may be substituted for by French foods in order to fit in with ayurvedic tenets. However, not all ayurvedic practitioners support this form of adaption which, according to them, does not respect the pure ayurveda.

The large variety of contexts supported by rich ethnographic material explored in the articles presented in this book shows that the reality behind the valorisation of a food or dish as traditional is more multiple and complex than the criteria used by the two European programmes for evaluating the perception of traditional foods by individuals would suggest. The concept of tradition is so deeply ingrained emotionally, culturally, ideologically and politically, that the definition of traditional food resists any simplification or standardisation.

Notes

1 The language editing of this book has been partly funded by the French Institute of Pondicherry. My heartfelt thanks to the Institute and to my colleague and friend, Mary Boseman, who did her best to improve the quality of the texts written by authors, in many cases not Anglophone.

2 Here, I refer to the remark by Sunil S. Amrith (2008: 1012): "The government of food in modern India developed alongside an imagination of hunger; the language of science, and in particular nutritional science, was central to both."

3 These books by R.S. Khare doubtless concern food-related tradition in a wide sense. Nevertheless, the significant limitation of these books, intrinsic to the Brahmin identity of their author, is that they focus only on the consumption of, and attitudes to, foods of the vegetarian upper castes of North India. As Jack Goody argues regarding Khare's food study carried out in Lucknow, a town famous for its rich and elaborate Mughal cuisine: "Wherever he can, Khare takes a 'cultural' view; and culture for him has its 'orthodox' expression in Hindu cosmology" (Goody 1982: 123).

4 Compared to the scarcity of research on food in social sciences, as Arjun Appadurai had already pointed out in 1988, the production of cookbooks is rapidly expanding. While the author argued that this literature, stemming from the middle classes (corresponding to today's upper classes), tended to distinguish itself from the moral and medical concepts related to Indian food culture; this is less true today as many

cookbooks, relying on the rapid development of metabolic diseases, aim to promote a healthy diet quite often valorised through vegetarianism.

5 The study was conducted at Citrus College, California.

6 The Ṛg Veda is one of the four Hindu canonical texts made up of hymns written in Vedic Sanskrit which, according to philologists and indologists, were composed between 1500 and 900 AD.

7 The Manusmṛti or Mānava dharmaśāstra (Codes of Manu) is a legislative text dated 200 BC on the etiquette of social classes, mostly of the three first *varṇa* or brahmanical categories (Brahmaṇa, Kṣatriya and Vaiśya). Subjects related to food such as what, how and when to eat, with whom to eat and how to prepare food hold an important place as food is ambivalent: it nourishes as well as pollutes (symbolically) the body and mind.

8 Food and diet, from one point of view, is a vehicle for maximising the efficacy of a remedy (for example, ingredients such as honey, milk, warm water, etc. or eating an unsalted or cooling diet, etc.), and from another, foods interfere in the body balance maintained by the three *doṣa*, *vāta-pitta-kapha* (flux of energy and substances, generally translated as humours).

9 According to Trichopoulous *et al.* (2006: 503), the historical event of the Second World War has been chosen because it is considered as "a time barrier before the food industry revolution, where populations still applied simple and time-honoured approaches." Compared to the definition of 'traditional' which was formulated first by the Commission of the European Communities, 2005, "Traditional means proven usage on the Community market for a period at least equal to that generally ascribed to a human generation" (*ibid.*), that of EuroFIR is more precise from the point of view of time.

10 The association between food/cuisine and medicine/alchemy is all the more pertinent in the Indian context. As well as close relations with matter, spirituality and the psyche, many ingredients of medicinal preparations and dishes (spices such as pepper, ginger, turmeric, etc., lemon, milk, honey, dates, *ghī*, green leaves etc.) and apparatus (pots, grinders, mortars), are common (Sébastia 2012).

11 The usage of "community market" in this sentence and elsewhere in TRUEFOOD articles is not clear.

12 Arjun Appadurai (1988: 3) has pointed out that cookbooks presuppose "often an effort on the part of some variety of specialist to standardize the regime of the kitchen, to transmit culinary lore, and to publicize particular traditions guiding the journey of food from marketplace to kitchen to table."

13 The Mediterranean diet, considered as healthy for the balance of its components, was inscribed in 2010 on the Representative List of the Intangible Cultural Heritage of Humanity. On the website of UNESCO, the Mediterranean diet is defined as: "characterized by a nutritional model that has remained constant over time and space, consisting mainly of olive oil, cereals, fresh or dried fruit and vegetables, a moderate amount of fish, dairy and meat, and many condiments and spices, all accompanied by wine or infusions, always respecting beliefs of each community." http://www.unesco.org/archives/multimedia/index.php?s=flvplayer&pg=33&vl=Eng&vo=2&id=1680 (download January 17.02.2014)
See also the website of a Maltese company, producer of olive oil, which makes copious use of health and medical arguments in promoting its oil: http://wardija.tripod.com

14 The term 'monopoly' is borrowed from an article by Meghna Banerjee and Susanah Nausahd (2010) which argues that GI registration "may encourage formation of undesirable monopolistic practices" (*ibid.*: 109). The authors criticise the use of the GI designation of Tirupati *laddu* as an abusive form of the commercialisation of faith that profits the temple organisation. This designation is obviously a case of misuse, but it is not surprising: the commodification of rituals and religious goods has significantly developed in India, *prasad* being just one example of the transformation of a sacred gift from the deity into a commercial item supposedly sanctified by the deity.

15 The GI has been, however, granted to seven North Indian states in February 2016.

16 Although not evoked by Elise Billiard, olive oil has acquired its very high reputation from research on the benefits of the Mediterranean diet which has pointed to the chemical properties of the oil for preventing cardiovascular diseases. However, this oil has always been highly valorised in Mediterranean cultures, as food as well as medicine. In Ancient Greece, it was used to massage the bodies of athletes as a means of preventing and healing injuries (Domikos *et al.* 2010); olive oil and olive leaves were recommended as food and as remedies by the Prophet Muhammad for preventing and treating many health conditions (Saad and Said 2011).

17 Nation is used in the sense of a collective sharing of a set of idioms, representations and practices which gives it its uniqueness compared to other nations (Anderson 1991; DeSoucey 2010).

18 As I have noticed during my open discussions with patients with diabetes about their perception of the diet recommended by siddha practitioners or by dieticians, and with dieticians working in various clinics, the frequency of social invitations is one of the factors most often mentioned to justify non-compliance with the regimen.

19 Regarding my experience as a French woman who dislikes the taste of cheese, each time cheese is served I am systematically questioned about why I do not eat it. My response has quite often been followed by a discussion on such an aberration.

References

Achaya, K.T. (1998a). *A Historical Dictionary of Indian Food*, New Delhi: Oxford University Press.

Achaya, K.T. (1998b). *Indian Food: The Historical Companion*, New Delhi: Oxford University Press.

Almli, V.L., Verbeke, W., Vanhonacker, F., Næs, T. and Hersleth, M. (2011). "General image and attribute perceptions of traditional food in six European'countries", *Food Quality and Preference*, Vol. 22: 12–138.

Amrith, S.S. (2004). "Food and welfare in India, c. 1900–1950", *Comparative Studies in Society and History*, Vol. 50(4): 1010–1035.

Anderson, B. (1991). *Imagined Communities: Reflections on the Origin and Spread of Nationalism*, London and New York: Verso.

Appadurai, A. (1988)."How to make a national cuisine: cookbooks in contemporary India", *Comparative Studies in Society and History*, Vol. 30(10): 3–24.

Banerjee, M. and Nausahd, S. (2010). "Grant of geographic indication designation to Tirupati Laddu: commercialization of faith", *National University of Juridical Sciences Law Review*, Vol. 3: 10–121.

Banerji, C. (2007). *Eating India. Exploring a Nation's Cuisine*, New Delhi: Penguin Books.

Banerji, C. (2006). *Feeding the Gods. Memories of Food and Culture in Bengal*, Calcutta: Seagull Books.

Banerji, C. (2001). *Memories of Women, Food and Ritual in Bengal*, Calcutta: Seagull Books.

Belasco, W.J. (1989). *Appetite for Change. How the Counterculture Took on the Industry*, New York: Pantheon Book.

Bell, D. and Valentine, G. (1997). *Consuming Geographies. We Are Where We Eat*, London and New York: Routledge.

Brown, P. (1998). *Anglo-Indian Food and Customs*, New Delhi: Penguin Books.

DeSoucey, M. (2010)."Gastronationalism: food traditions and authenticity politics in the European Union", *American Sociological Review*, Vol. 75(3): 432–455.

Domikos, N.N., Nomikos, G.N. and Kores, D.S. (2010)."The use of deep friction massage with olive oil as a means of prevention and treatment of sports injuries in ancient time", *Archive of Medical Science*, Vol. 5: 642–645.

Farquhar, J. (2002). *Appetites. Food and Sex in Post-socialist China*, Durham, NC and London: Duke University Press.

Goody, J. (1982). *Cooking, Cuisine and Class. A Study in Comparative Sociology*, Cambridge: Cambridge University Press.

Guerrero, L., Guàrdia, M.D. *et al.* (2009)."Consumer-driven definition of traditional food products and innovation in traditional foods. A qualitative cross-cultural study", *Appetite*, Vol. 52(2): 345–354.

Hobsbawm, E. and Ranger, T. (1983). *The Invention of Tradition*, Cambridge: Cambridge University Press.

Holtzman, J.D. (2006)."Food and memory", *Annual Review of Anthropology*, Vol. 35: 261–278.

Humphrey, L.T. (1989)."Traditional foods? Traditional values", *Western Folklore*, Vol. 48 (2): 162–169.

International Institute for Population Sciences (IIPS) and Macro International (2007). *National Family Health Survey (NFHS-3), 2005–06: India: Volume I*, Mumbai: IIPS.

Ingold, T. (1997). *From the Transmission of Representations to the Education of Attention*. http://lchc.ucsd.edu/mca/Paper/ingold/ingold1.htm (retrieved on 12.09.2011).

Janeja, M.K. (2010). *Transactions in Taste. The Collective Lives of Everyday Bengali Food*, New Delhi: Routledge.

Khare, R.S. (ed.) (1992). *The Eternal Food. Gastronomic Ideas and Experiences of Hindus and Buddhists*, Albany, NY: State University of New York Press.

Khare, R.S. (1976a). *The Hindu Hearth and Home*, New Delhi: Vikas Publishing House.

Khare, R.S. (1976b). *Culture and Reality. Essays on the Hindu System of Managing Foods*, Simla: Indian Institute of Advanced Study.

Khare, R.S. and Rao, M.S.A. (eds.) (1986). *Food, Society and Culture. Aspects in South Asian Foods Systems*, Durham, NC: Carolina Academic Press.

Kumar, T.-T. (1988). *History of Rice in India. Mythology, Culture and Agriculture*, Delhi: Gyan Publishing House.

Lutringer, C. (2012). *Gouvernance de l'agriculture et mouvements paysans en Inde*, Paris: Karthala and Genève: Institut de hautes études internationales et du développement.

Mannur, A. (2010). *Culinary Fictions: Food in South Asian Diasporic Culture*, Philadelphia, PA: Temple University Press.

Mitra, R. (2011). "Crossing the border and tasting the nation: the Indian experience in Chitrita Banerji's *Eating India: Exploring a Nation's Cuisine*", *Rupkatha Journal on Interdisciplinary Studies in Humanities*, Vol. 3(3): 434–439.

Mukherjee, U. (2008). "A study of the basmati case (India-US basmati rice dispute): the geographical indication perspective", *Social Sciences Research Network*. www.papers.ssrn.com/sol3/Delivery.cfm/SSRN_ID1143209_code936691.pdf (retrieved on 12.12.2014).

Pieniak, Z., Verbeke, W., Vanhonacker, F., Guerrero, L. and Hersleth, M. (2009)."Association between traditional food consumption and motives for food choice in six European countries", *Appetite*, Vol. 53: 101–108.

Poulain, J.-P. (2002). *Sociologies de l'alimentation*, Paris: Presses Universitaires de France.

Prakash, O. (1961). *Food and Drinks in Ancient India: From Earliest Times to 1200 A.D.*, Delhi: Munshiram Manoharlal Publishers.

Ranta, R. (2016). "Re-Arabizing Israeli food culture", *Food, Culture and Society*, Vol. 18(4): 611–627.

Ray, K. (2004). *The Migrant's Table. Meals and Memories in Bengali-American Households*, Philadelphia, PA: Temple University Press.

Saad, B. and Said, O. (2011). *Greco-Arab and Islamic Herbal Medicine: Traditional System, Ethics, Safety, Efficacy, and Regulatory Issues*, Upper Saddle River, NJ: John Wiley & Sons.

Sangar, S.P. (1999). *Food and Drinks in Mughal India*, New Delhi: Reliance Publishing House.

Sébastia, B. (2015)."Coping with diseases of modernity: the use of Siddha medical knowledge and practices for diabetics' care", in K.A. Jacobsen, *Routledge Handbook of Contemporary India*, pp. 474–489. Abingdon: Routledge.

Sébastia, B. (2012)."Competing for medical space. Traditional practitioners in the transmission and promotion of Siddha medicine", in V. Sujatha and L. Abraham (eds), *Medicine, State and Society: Indigenous Medicine and Medical Pluralism in Contemporary India*, pp. 165–185. Delhi: Orient Black Swan.

Sébastia, B. (2010). "Governmental institution versus associations. Multifaceted expression of siddha in Tamil Nadu". http://rcsi.hypotheses.org

Singh, V.P. (2000). "The basmati rice of India", in R.K. Singh, U.S. Singh and G.S. Khush (eds.), *Aromatic Rices*, pp. 135–153. New Delhi: Oxford and IBH Publishing.

Sinha, A.K. (2000). *Anthropology of Sweetmeats*, New Delhi: Gyan Publishing House.

Srinivas, T. (2006)."'As mother made it'. The cosmopolitan Indian family, 'authentic' food and the construction of cultural utopia", *International Journal of Sociology of the Family*, Vol. 32(2): 191–221.

Trichopoulou, A., Vasilopoulou, E., Georga, K., Soukara, S. and Dilis, V. (2006)."Traditional foods: why and how to sustain them", *Trends in Food Science and Technology*, Vol. 17: 498–504.

Trichopoulou, A., Soukara, S. and Vasilopoulou, E. (2007)."Traditional foods: a science and society perspective", *Trends in Food Science and Technology*, Vol. 18: 420–427.

Weichselbaum, E., Benelam, B. and Costa, H.S. (2009)."Traditional foods in Europe", Synthesis report No. 6, *European Food Information Resource EuroFIR*, under the 6th Framework Food Quality and Safety thematic priority. Contact FOOD-CT-2005-513944. www. Eurofir.net (retrieved on 10.01.2013).

2 The rediscovery of native 'super-foods' in Mexico

Esther Katz and Elena Lazos

Introduction

In Latin America, Mexico is the country where the food has retained more Amerindian traditions than elsewhere. At the beginning of the sixteenth century, just after the conquest, the Spaniards discovered, in Mexico, edible plants and animals unknown to them. They immediately adopted some local foodstuffs, while disregarding others.

In this chapter, we will examine the fate of three traditional foodstuffs and beverages specific to the indigenous cultures of Mexico which were rejected, despised or prohibited by the colonisers or, later, by the upper classes, but are presently eliciting enthusiasm as health or gourmet foods: a pseudo-cereal, amaranth (*Amaranthus* spp., *Chenopodium* spp.), edible insects and a fermented drink, *pulque*, drawn from the sap of the century plant (*Agave* spp.). Due to the quality of their nutrients, these three products may be considered as 'super-foods', and definitely be classified as 'traditional foods', since they have been consumed by the autochthonous people of Mexico for centuries. We will analyse reasons why these foods were rejected at some point, while the consumption of other traditional foods, such as maize and beans, was never questioned. We will show that such dynamics varied according to periods and places: at the beginning of the sixteenth century, the Spanish clergy prohibited 'pagan' offerings, often made of amaranth, and probably disdained its consumption; most Spaniards rejected insects, while they adopted *pulque*, a drink that the elites started to despise only at the end of the nineteenth century. Why and how a change in the appreciation of these foods and drinks has occurred over time and why they are valued today, also constitute questions we aim at developing in this account.

We will base our analysis on bibliographical data, as well as on fieldwork conducted over the last 30 years with Amerindian and *mestizo* populations residing in rural areas: by Esther Katz, in the state of Oaxaca (mainly the Mixtec highlands) and by Elena Lazos, in the states of Yucatán, Veracruz, Jalisco, Tlaxcala and Oaxaca.[1] We will add to this material, diffuse observations made in different parts of the country. In order to understand the context of the traditional indigenous foods, we will present first the historical context of the constitution of Mexican cuisine, starting with the meeting of the indigenous and Spanish cultures, as the fusion of Amerindian and Spanish culinary traditions is a salient feature of Mexican cuisine.

The historical context of Mexican food

After the discovery of the West Indies by Christopher Columbus in 1492, the Spaniards landed, in 1519, on the Atlantic coast of Mexico, and explored the vast territory of the Aztec empire, densely populated and composed of different ethnic groups who had many cultural features in common. In particular, they were sedentary cultivators, while their neighbours in northern Mexico were mainly hunter-gatherers.[2] In 1521, the Spaniards conquered the Aztec empire, which they renamed 'New Spain'. They eliminated the Aztec elites, but maintained the Aztec organisation of the empire, including the tribute system.[3] In spite of the epidemics that eliminated a high percentage of the population (Cook and Borah 1979), the indigenous people remained more numerous than the Spaniards who, at the beginning of the colonisation, were mainly men, either friars or soldiers. The ecclesiastics evangelised the indigenous population and struggled against pagan beliefs and practices. However, agrarian rites were so crucial that they kept being performed in the form of Catholic saints festivals (Lammel *et al.* 2008). The friars played a major role in the diffusion, in Mexico, of plants such as wheat and barley, fruit trees and herbs, and animals such as cows, sheep, goats, pigs and hens, that the conquerors judged essential to their subsistence and introduced from Spain (Berthe 1988). At the end of the sixteenth century, the Spaniards imported tropical plants from their other territorial possessions, especially Peru and the Philippines (Patiño 1969). The introduction of all these new crops and animals modified the ecosystems, but the indigenous people kept cultivating the *milpa*, a crop association of maize (*Zea mays*), beans (*Phaseolus* spp.) and squash (*Cucurbita* spp.) (Wolf 1959). Maize, beans and chilli pepper (*Capsicum annuum*) constituted their staple food and numerous cultivated and wild plants as well as mushrooms complemented the diet. Regarding animal products, game and domesticated dog and turkey played a minor role in the diet, but insects were consumed regularly (Casillas and Vargas 1984; Sugiura and González de la Vara 1996). Through the 'Columbian exchange', the indigenous people adopted foodstuffs from the Old World, but without changing their diet pattern, while the Spaniards adopted some from the New World and contributed to their diffusion all over the planet. In the eyes of the Spanish conquerors, maize was similar to wheat, *tortilla* (maize flat cakes) to bread, American beans (*Phaseolus* spp.) to fava beans (*Vicia faba*) and chilli pepper (*Capsicum annuum*) to black pepper (*Piper nigrum*). The first colonisers adopted local foods because indigenous women, keepers of the culinary traditions, cooked for them. Nevertheless, the Spaniards did not adopt all the indigenous food habits.

At the end of the sixteenth century, the hybridisation of the Mexican culinary system accelerated with the foundation of convents. Spanish nuns invented new dishes combining local and introduced ingredients and cooking techniques, mixing Arab-Andalusian and Aztec cuisines.[4] They participated in the elaboration of a refined cuisine at the New Spain vice-royal court, probably inspired by the culinary traditions of the Aztec court (Long 1996, 1997). The Spanish language integrated new terms from the language of the Aztecs, Nahuatl, for previously unknown plants, animals, dishes and cooking utensils.[5]

Despite intermarriages between Spaniards and indigenous people during the colonial period, the latter still constituted more than half of the total population at the beginning of the nineteenth century (Navarrete 2004). Their pre-eminent presence, as well as the role of indigenous women as cooks and the existence of a refined court cuisine, contributed to the preservation of many more Amerindian cooking traditions in Mexico than in other Latin American countries.

After the Independence of the country in 1821, the *mestizo* population grew tremendously due to two main reasons: increase of mixed marriage compared to the colonial period, and the official designation of the *mestizo* category to people who did not speak an indigenous language; this included people of Spanish descent as well as the numerous Indians who no longer spoke their native language (Pitt-Rivers 1992). The invention of a national cuisine was a political project for the new nation. Rejecting Spain, the elites first took France and its cuisine as a model, but progressively integrated into the national cuisine, all through the nineteenth century, the culinary traditions of central Mexico, the region of the capital city (Bak-Geller 2008). The Mexican Revolution of 1910 enhanced the glorification of the indigenous roots of the country. Many traditional dishes served today are considered as belonging to the indigenous heritage, even though the recipes include foodstuffs introduced by the colonists.

Nowadays, speakers of native languages, mainly located in the centre and the south of the country, constitute only 6.5% of the total population (INEGI 2010), but a much higher number of people, difficult to evaluate, are actually Indians who have lost their native tongue, but often keep indigenous culinary traditions. Moreover most Mexican people have, to some degree, indigenous roots, thus, many elements of the indigenous food culture have been transmitted to the whole society and integrated into the national cuisine. Nevertheless, many Mexican people give credit to the Indians of the past, but do not want to be assimilated to present-day Indians who are often poor and live in so-called 'marginal' mountain areas. In the second half of the twentieth century, many of them were attracted by the modernity model of their giant neighbour, the United States, and rejected aspects of Mexican culture perceived as backward. In 1992, at the 500th anniversary of the discovery of America, Mexican people wondered whether it was legitimate to celebrate an event that had led to genocide and cultural loss, and became more conscious of their indigenous roots. In 1994, the Zapatist rebellion in Chiapas raised more questions on the present situation of the Amerindians, their struggle for land and for their subsistence. In 2000, facing maize pollution by transgenic seeds, many indigenous and peasant organisations as well as NGOs centred their socio-political demands on food sovereignty and the right to cultivate traditional food. They demanded that the right to food be included as a human right in the Mexican Constitution. In the meantime, the Conservatory of Mexican Gastronomy submitted to UNESCO an application for inscribing Mexican cuisine as an intangible heritage, enhancing the role that indigenous people played in preserving over centuries a diversity of foods and dishes. This declaration was effective in 2010, generating tremendous enthusiasm among chefs, entrepreneurs, government institutions and communities, eager to promote both Mexican gastronomical traditions and innovations. Mexican chefs, trained in haute cuisine, are now integrating regional ingredients and recipes, and creating new dishes inspired by these traditions.

In the context of these socio-political and cultural movements, we will now examine three contrasting examples of traditional indigenous foods, previously rejected, despised or forgotten, that have recently been rediscovered by the elites and part of the mainstream population.

Amaranth: from 'lost crop of the Aztecs' to health food

In the sixteenth century, the Spanish chroniclers described under the name of *bledo* a plant with edible grains and leaves that the Aztecs called *huauhtli*. It was identified as belonging to the botanical genus *Amaranthus* only at the beginning of the twentieth century and therefore called amaranth, in Spanish *amaranto*. Scientists, such as the botanist and geographer Jonathan Sauer (1950), found out later that the term *huauhtli* actually covered two botanical genera, *Amaranthus* spp. (*Amaranthaceae*) (with either black or white seeds) and *Chenopodium* spp. (*Chenopodiaceae*) (with red seeds).[6] The Argentinian scientist Armando Hunziker (1952) defined amaranth as a 'pseudocereal', a grain similar to cereals, but not belonging to the same botanical family (the *Poaceae*, also called *Gramineae*). Recently, in the framework of a project of the National Commission of Biodiversity (CONABIO), the botanists Cristina Mapes and Eduardo Espitia (2010) achieved a complete revision of these species in terms of taxonomy, domestication, cultivation, geographical distribution and uses: *Amaranthus cruentus* and *A. hypocondriacus* are the main grain *Amaranthus* species cultivated – and domesticated – in Mexico; some non-cultivated species of amaranth are only used for their leaves, such as *A. hybridus*, known as *quintonil* (from Nahuatl *quiltonilli*) and usually gathered as a weed from the maize fields; the main grain *Chenopodium* considered as an amaranth is *Chenopodium berlandieri* var. *nuttalliae*; its young inflorescences, called *huauhzontli,* are commonly eaten in the Central Highlands (*Altiplano Central*).[7]

In central Mexico, at the beginning of the sixteenth century, *huauhtli* was a staple and a ritual food, as important as maize. It was not only cultivated in the Basin of Mexico, location of the Aztec cities, but also brought as tribute to the Aztec rulers from other parts of the Central Highlands (present-day states of Mexico, Morelos, Hidalgo) (see Figure 2.2). The tribute of amaranth reached almost the same quantity as that of maize (Sauer 1950). The Spanish friar Bernardino de Sahagún (1999 [1570–1582]), who had lived in central Mexico for several decades, and mastered the Nahua language, provides us with a detailed description of the different types of *huauhtli* consumed by the Indians as well as the dishes prepared with the grains (*huauhtli*) and with the leaves (*huauhquilitl*). The Aztecs consumed *huauhtli* in the same way as maize, in *tortillas*, in *tamales* (steamed dough wrapped in leaves) or in *atole* (gruel). Amaranth leaves were mixed with maize in *tortillas* and *tamales,* or used to prepare *moles* (thick chilli sauce). Sahagún, quoted by Sauer (*ibid.*: 567–570), described how, during their rituals, the Aztecs shaped images of their gods into a dough called *tzoalli*, made of amaranth seeds, toasted maize and agave honey, that they consumed at the culmination of the ceremony.

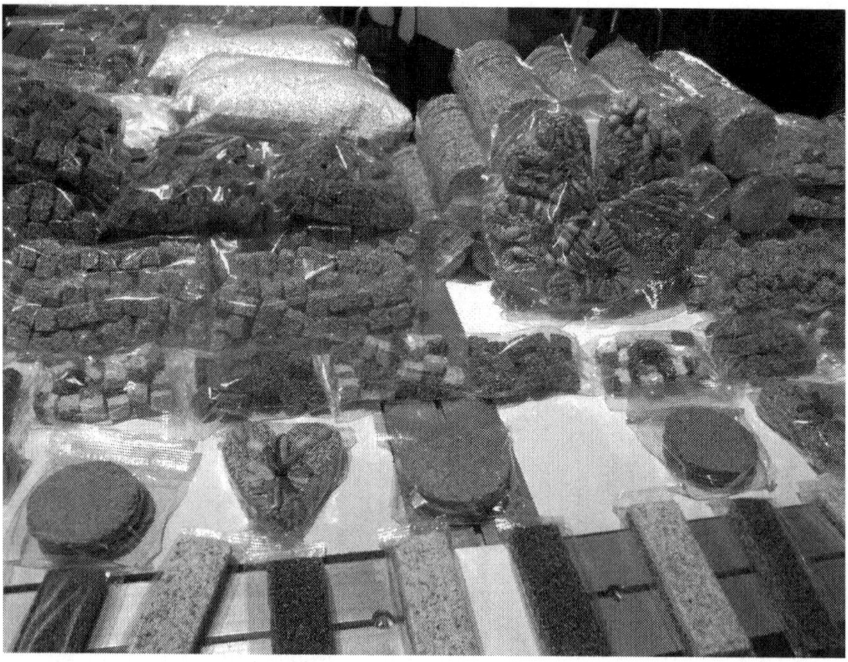

Figure 2.1 Amaranth: popped seeds (in the back) and candy

Source: © Esther Katz

The Spanish clergy, fighting against 'idolatry', prohibited such offerings. There is no evidence that the Spaniards banned the everyday consumption of *huauhtli*, but the prohibition of the offerings may have contributed to the decline of its cultivation. Moreover, the demographic decline due to epidemics resulted in abandonment of land and loss of knowledge, and the introduction of wheat and barley possibly led to a displacement of amaranth (Martínez-Alfaro *et al.* 1994). Amaranth could have been adopted as a grain crop, the same way as maize, but this did not happen. Although maize was often mixed with amaranth to make *tzoalli*, it kept on being cultivated and consumed as a staple food. Was it more difficult for the Spaniards to deal with a very small seed that needed to be popped in order to be consumed? The historical accounts have not yet given even a tentative answer to this question.

Several decades after the conquest, according to the *Relaciones Geográficas*, a survey conducted by the government of New Spain in 1577–1580, amaranth was still a staple in central Mexico and other regions of the country. It was cultivated mainly in the Central Highlands and in smaller quantities from Veracruz in the east, to Jalisco in the west (see Figure 2.2). At the beginning of the seventeenth century, a priest reported that the Indians in his parish in the present state of Guerrero still made offerings of *huauhtli,* but from then on, amaranth cultivation declined, without, however, totally disappearing (Sauer 1950: 571–575).

Amaranth is very rarely mentioned in documents of the late colonial period, but Sauer (*ibid.*) notes that the word *alegría*, defining a sweet made of popped amaranth seeds, was in use in 1698. This candy was the main form in which amaranth was

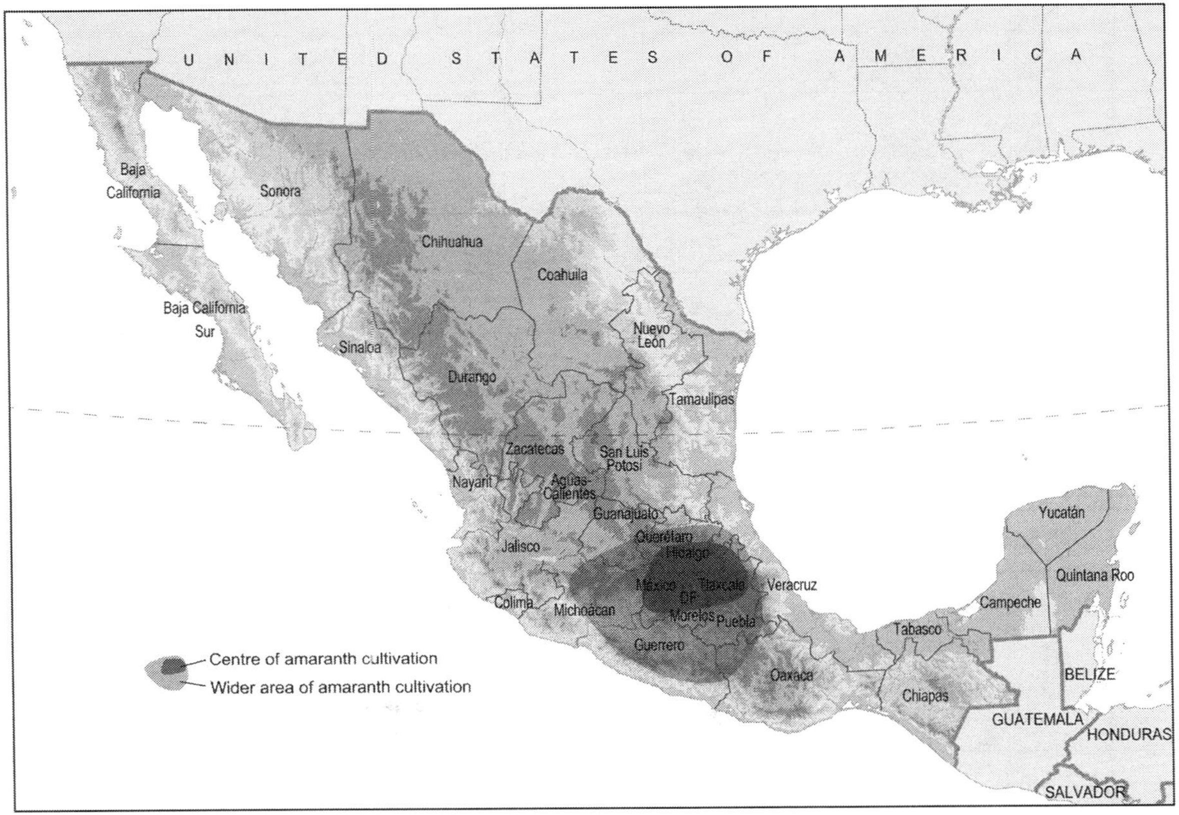

Figure 2.2 Main areas of amaranth production in Mexico

consumed. Then the plant itself began to be called *alegría* too. In an agronomy journal, an article published in the 1880s indicated 'the cultivation of *alegría*' in the state of Mexico, and its sale as manufactured candies in the nearby market of Texcoco, located just north of Mexico City (*ibid.*). Nevertheless, amaranth had disappeared from the official statistics: not a single village indicated its cultivation in the agricultural survey conducted in the 1890s by the Mexican government (República Mexicana, Secretaría de Fomento, 1893–1895, quoted by Sauer *ibid.*).

At the beginning of the twentieth century, scientific curiosity was raised again about *huauhtli*, the lost crop of the Aztecs, what allowed its botanical identification, as mentioned above. In the 1940s, Sauer dedicated extensive research to this plant and found out that it had not disappeared. He pointed out that "although reduced to an inconspicuous relic of the once great staple, the crop has been conserved by a surprisingly large number of Mexican communities", and "sizeable fields of amaranths are planted by only a few *pueblos* today; generally a few plants are sown near the houses or scattered through the maize fields; often only a small minority of the families still grow them." (*ibid.*: 578). He showed that amaranth was still cultivated, and also, was commercialised as *alegría* candy, in the Central Highlands (the Federal District and the states of Mexico and Morelos –the Aztec cradle –, as well as the states of Puebla and Tlaxcala) and the Valley of Oaxaca, but only a few communities of the Central Highlands consumed the grains in a traditional way, i.e. in the form of *atole* and *tamales*. Communities in the state of Michoacán still consumed it in that way, but there cultivation showed a decline. In the remote area of the Montaña de Guerrero (Guerrero Mountain), the anthropologist Hendrichs (1945, quoted by Sauer 1950: 579) observed that the custom of sowing a little amaranth in the maize fields had persisted throughout these mountains, where it was consumed as *atole.*[8] Sauer found very scarce evidence of amaranth cultivation in Guatemala, but his colleagues observed it in Jalisco (in the west), Sonora, Chihuahua and Sinaloa (in the north).

In the 1950s, Hunziker (1952:78), studying the Andean amaranth, emphasized that amaranth grain was superior to cereals in protein and fat content. However, the nutritional content of amaranth began really to attract research attention in the 1970s. In 1972, an Australian scientist showed that amaranth seeds contain a high level of lysine, an amino acid usually low in cereals. Soon afterwards, in 1976, the Rodale Research Center in Pennsylvania started a major research project on amaranth: its scientists collected samples from different parts of the world and developed breeding and agronomic research in order to adapt amaranth cultivation to modern agricultural techniques (NRC 1984). In the meantime, scientists of the National Research Council of the United States, worried by the risks of starvation as the world food resources rely mainly on about 20 crops, conducted research to diversify the food base and to attract attention to plants considered as 'non-conventional' (NRC 1975). Considering its high potentialities, they dedicated a monograph to amaranth and suggested its incorporation into breakfast cereals or confectionary (NRC 1984).

In the 1970s, the production of amaranth in Mexico was still very low. However, its potential for health favoured its revival. An annual fair devoted to *alegría* (and olives) was created in 1971 in Tulyehualco, Federal District, a semi-rural area adjacent to Mexico City, located in the cradle of amaranth cultivation and, supposedly, of *alegría* candy.[9] In 1983, the cultivation of amaranth for commercial use was estimated to cover 300 hectares. In 1985, this had already increased to 1,500 hectares, mostly in the state of Morelos (Mapes and Espitia 2010: 52–55). Since then, it has been increasing (Figure 2.3) and amaranth now reaches a very good price on the market. The commercial production of amaranth is now concentrated in four states in the Central Highlands: Morelos, Tlaxcala, Puebla and the Federal District. There is also some commercial production in the states of Mexico, Guerrero, Oaxaca and Durango; recently, it started also in Chihuahua (Figure 2.2) (Mapes and Espitia 2010: 55, 141–146).

Since the 1990s, further investigations have been carried out on finer aspects of the nutritional content of the different species of amaranth: the quality of protein, lipids and starch, anti-oxidant properties, dietary fibre, vitamins, minerals and other micro-components (squalene, tocopherol, phenolic compounds, etc.) (Venskutonis and Kraujalis 2013).[10] The balanced amino acid composition of amaranth is estimated to be close to the optimum protein reference pattern in the human diet, the combination of amaranth and maize flour (50:50) almost reaches the perfect score of 100 on the nutritionist's scale, and the combination of amaranth and wheat flour increases the nutritional value of baked products. It is now used for protein enrichment of food products. Moreover, amaranth grains have higher lipid content than most cereal grains and contain large amounts of squalene (a lipid used in cosmetics). It is also gluten-free and is therefore suitable for the diets of coeliac disease patients (Grobelnik-Mlakar *et al.* 2009).

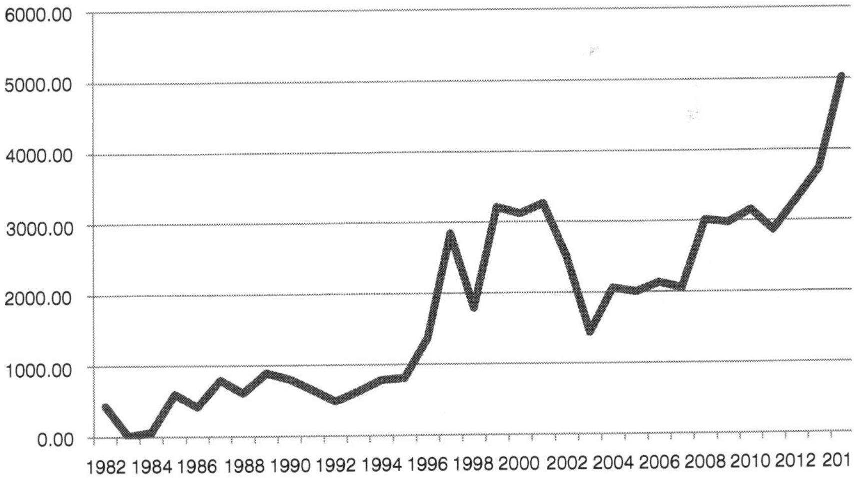

Figure 2.3 Cultivated area of amaranth (1982–2014)

Source: SIAP-SAGARPA, 2015, Estadísticas Agropecuarias Nacionales http://www.siap.sagarpa.gob.mx (retrieved on 09 November 2015).

Since the beginning of the twenty-first century, Mexican people from all social classes have become aware of the need for healthier food habits. The statistics showing a relationship between bad nutrition and diabetes, which has tremendously increased in the country, as well as the incidence of overweight and obesity (Gutiérrez *et al.* 2012), have been widely commented on. Amaranth has attracted part of the population by its nutritional qualities.

In Mexico, amaranth is still commonly consumed as *alegría* candy. For the last decade, it has also been included in mixed breakfast cereals, sold as plain popped seeds in local markets, health food shops and some supermarkets, and new types of amaranth candies have been created. It is consumed mainly by health-conscious people of the urban intellectual middle class. For instance, the supermarket in the National Autonomous University of Mexico (UNAM), where students and professors shop, displays a much wider variety of packs of popped amaranth seeds than other supermarkets. In small tourist towns of the state of Morelos, where people from the intellectual middle class of Mexico City spend weekends, women from villages of Western Morelos sell packs of popped seeds of amaranth from their family production. The 45th *Alegría* and Olive Fair in Tulyehualco was held in February 2016. As observed by anthropologist Charles-Edouard de Suremain (personal communication), the fair is mainly attended by local people, but some people from Mexico City go there too. Many stands display the prehispanic origin of the product. All kinds of amaranth products are exhibited, including new types of candies such as chocolate amaranth bars. Such products were also exhibited at the third World Forum of Mexican Gastronomy in November 2015 (See Figure 2.1). It looks like a growing sector, where creativity is enhanced. Amaranth is now sold in health food shops, not only in Mexico, but also in the United States, where it was first promoted, and in many other countries. As a health food, amaranth is finally conquering the world.

Insects: food for 'savage people' or a delicacy?

In the sixteenth century, at the beginning of the colonial period, the consumption of insects by indigenous population was described by Spanish friars and naturalists. The friar Bernardino de Sahagún (1999), in particular, delivered a precise account of some insect species eaten by Indians: grasshoppers/crickets, ants and their larvae, caterpillars from agave and maize, and aquatic bugs and their eggs. Unlike the friar who lived close to the Indians and found these insects "good to eat", most of the Spanish colonists probably rejected this food. However, the friar's example shows that some people are ready to taste and appreciate foods not considered as edible in their own culture.

Today, the Mexican population is divided between consumers and non-consumers of insects; many non-consumers consider the insect eaters as uncivilised people: Indians eat them and descendants of Spaniards do not. However, in a country where European and indigenous populations were mixed, the division between eaters and non-eaters is blurred. As mentioned above, people classified as *mestizos*, because they no longer speak an indigenous language, often keep many indigenous cultural features and food habits, including the consumption of insects; and Mexico has the most Amerindian cuisine in Latin American. For the same reasons – a high proportion of population of Amerindian descent and a national cuisine integrating indigenous ingredients and dishes – it is also the Latin American country where insects are eaten the most (Katz 2016).

The Mexican entomologist Julieta Ramos-Elorduy, who has been conducting major research on edible insects since the late 1970s, has shown that a wide range of insects species, much larger than the list provided in the sixteenth century, is consumed in Mexico nowadays: in 2012, she had recorded 547 species of edible insects from all over the country, but had collected more species in the central and southern part of Mexico (Figure 2.5), where there is a higher indigenous population (Ramos-Elorduy 1982, 1997; Ramos-Elorduy *et al.* 2012).[11] Since the beginning of her studies, she has been promoting a wider consumption of insects and even published an insect recipe book for a general audience. She has also shown that insects constitute a good source of proteins, minerals and vitamin B and have high digestibility (Ramos-Elorduy 1982, 1997). The high nutritive potential of the insects recently attracted the attention of the FAO, which promotes insect consumption in order to fight against hunger and ill-nutrition, as insects are not only rich in protein, minerals and vitamins, but are also low in fat. Insects are now being raised for animal feed and human consumption (Huis *et al.* 2013).

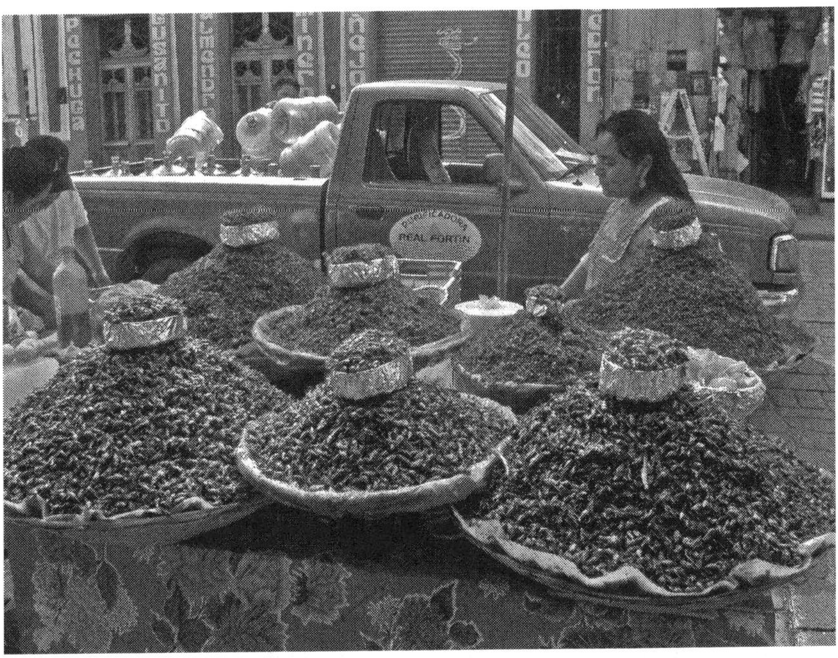

Figure 2.4 Insects: Grasshoppers sold in a market in Oaxaca.

Source: © Esther Katz.

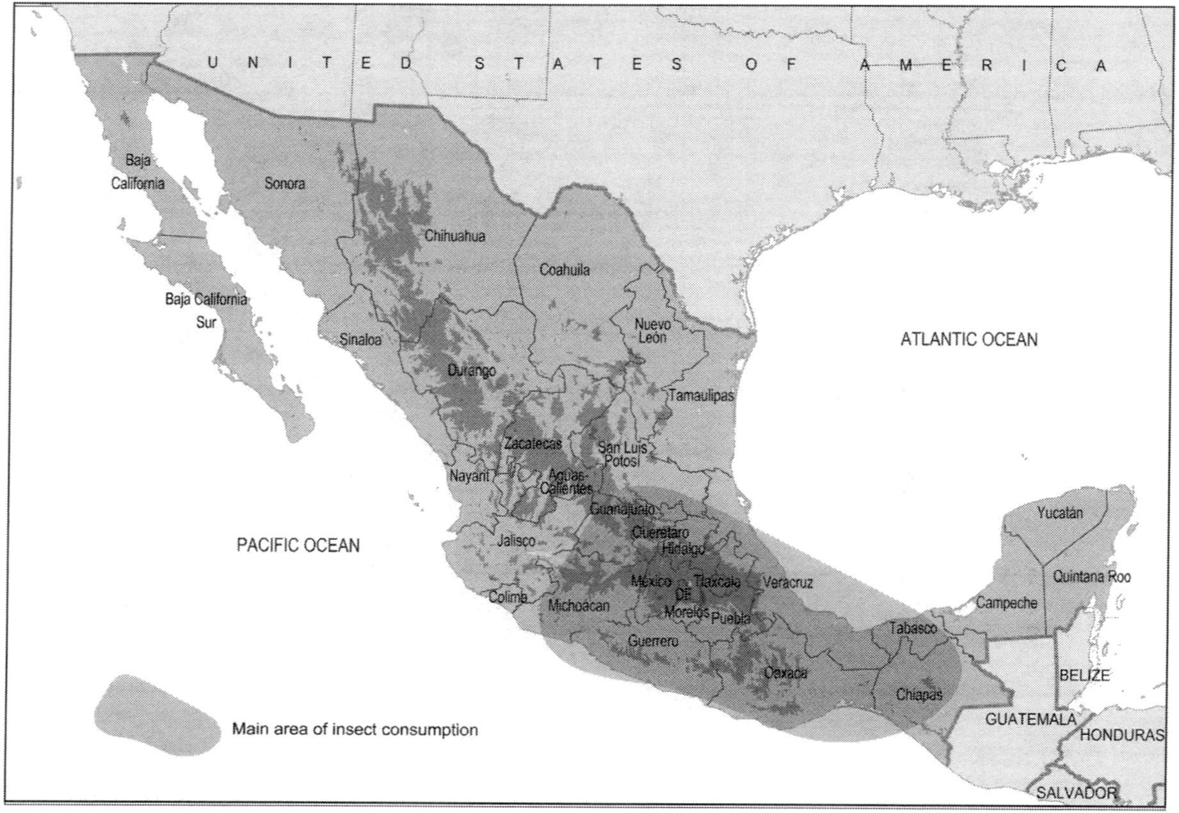

Figure 2.5 Main areas of insect consumption in Mexico

People who do not eat insects tend to think that the consumption of insects is consequent to poverty. Actually, insects are too small to fill hungry bellies. However, in Mexico, they compensate the poor intake of animal products in indigenous people's diet. In most Indian villages, animal breeding is a minor backyard activity and hunting is very occasional. Usually the farmers kill a chicken once a week or every two weeks, and bigger animals for festivals. Only over the last 20 years, has meat consumption in rural areas experienced an increase, due to the remittances from migrants residing in the United States. For indigenous people, insects are not perceived as an emergency food or a poor people's food (as for instance, wild greens): they are a tasty food (Katz 1996).

The problem with insects is that they are available in small quantities or in specific periods. As we observed in the field, people might find, during the maize harvest, one maize caterpillar (*Heliothis zea*) in a maize cob, a few grasshoppers or crickets in the grass, while at another time, they will harvest ten *Coleoptera* larvae from a tree trunk, three caterpillars from an agave leaf or will catch a wasp's nest to grill the larvae. Collecting an insect does not occur every day, but is relatively frequent all through the year.

Only some species (social insects) are found in large quantities (Ramos-Elorduy 1997). In the Mixtec highlands, in the dry season, when it is windy, forest bugs (*Hemiptera*) of different species (*Edessa* spp.), called *chinches*, or in other regions *jumiles,* can be collected in epiphytic *Bromeliaceae*. Children climb the trees, grab the epiphyte, bring it down to the ground and shake it until all the bugs fall from it. They eat them alive; and appreciate them for their spicy taste, reminiscent of chilli pepper. If they bring the bugs home, their mother grills and then grinds them in a mortar to make a hot sauce. At the very beginning of the rainy season, below 1500 metres of altitude, the nuptial flight of big ants, called *arrieras* (*Atta mexicana*, *A. cephalotes* and *Pogonomyrmex* sp.), takes place for a few days. Braving ant bites, people are eager to catch the *alate* adults, called *chicatanas*, while they are mating (Katz 1996). At that period, as people can collect one to two kilograms, grilled *chicatanas* can be found in local markets. *Jumiles* (bugs) and *chicatanas* are particularly appreciated in the states of Guerrero and Oaxaca (Ramos-Elorduy 1982). *Jumiles* are also sold in the markets of the states of Mexico and Morelos and *chicatanas* in the state of Veracruz.

In the Valley of Oaxaca, the Zapotec farmers have techniques for collecting large quantities of grasshoppers (*Tettigoniidae*) and crickets *(Acrididae)*, both called *chapulines*, that are sold in city and villages markets, and grilled with salt, chilli pepper and lemon. They are also consumed, and occasionally sold in small quantities in markets of the central highlands (Ramos-Elorduy *et al.* 2012). Another local treat is the red agave worm (*gusano rojo de maguey*), a caterpillar *(Comadia redtenbacheri)* well known for flavouring *mezcal* (a local agave distilled alcohol) (Ramos-Elorduy 1982). *Chapulines* and red agave worms have been known for decades as regional specialties in Oaxaca (Moedano 1988). Another caterpillar, the white agave worm (*gusano blanco de maguey*; *Aegiale hesperiaris*), is traded in Oaxaca, as well as in Mexico City. It is exploited in all the highlands, from the state of Jalisco in the west, to the state of Oaxaca in the east, to San Luis Potosí in the north (Ramos-Elorduy 1982).

Some insect species are typical of, and unique to, the Central Highlands. Two types of insects, in particular, have been highly appreciated and traded for centuries, *escamoles* and *ahuautli*, but are threatened by environmental degradation and overexploitation. *Escamoles* (in Nahuatl *azcamolli*) are ant larvae (*Liometopum* spp.). They are mainly traded from the state of Hidalgo, and are now the insects most often served in Mexico City gourmet restaurants. *Ahuautli* are the eggs of different species of aquatic bugs (*Hemiptera*), called *axayacatl* (*Krizousacorixa* spp., *Corisella* spp., *Notonecta* spp.) (Ramos-Elorduy 1982). *Ahuautli* means 'water amaranth', as these tiny white eggs resemble amaranth seeds. According to the ethnoarcheologist Jeffrey R. Parsons (2006), in the sixteenth century, *ahuautli* was produced in abundance on the lakes of the Central Highlands and traded to the capital city. It was considered as a delicacy by the Aztec emperor and used as offerings in some Aztec rituals. Interestingly, after the conquest, it was even eaten, notably on Fridays (days without meat), by some Spaniards who, according to chroniclers, found it very tasty. At that time, different types of aquatic bugs were exploited, but only *ahuautli* was highly valued, while other species were consumed by poor people. As most of the lakes of the Basin of Mexico have been progressively dried out since the colonial period, *ahuautli* production has drastically diminished. Part of Mexico City has been built over the drained lakes, only small portions of lakes still exist in the Federal District, and *ahuautli* now comes mainly from lakes in the state of Hidalgo, at a very high price (*ibid.*).

In regions where some insect species have been considered as gourmet food or regional specialties, not only Indians, but also a wider range of the population value them. Tourists to Oaxaca, for instance, are recommended to give the *chapulines* a try. Insects have therefore an ambiguous status: they symbolise the food of 'savage people', but they are regarded as valued foodstuffs. Indian people in the countryside continue to eat insects, but are sometimes limited by the degradation of the environment. People from rural areas who migrated to Mexico City, or whose villages were absorbed by the city, were used to eating insects, but some of them have given up that consumption at a point in their lives, because of rejection of their culture, because they associated this food habit to village life and poverty, or because the resource became rare or expensive.

A few decades ago, the Market of San Juan, in the historical centre of Mexico City, provided the working classes with insects and game. In the same quarter, Don Chon restaurant, also patronized by working-class people, served dishes of Central Highlands insects: *ahuautli, escamoles* and white agave worms. But in the 1980s, Mexican cuisine and its regional components began to be promoted. Attractive recipe books as well as scientifically based books and booklets on Mexican food aimed at a large audience began to be published (Castelló Iturbide 1986, González de la Vara 1996-97), reinforcing the interest in typically Mexican foods, especially of prehispanic origin. Associated with this movement, Don Chon restaurant gained the reputation of serving 'prehispanic food'. As mentioned above, Mexican people became more conscious of their indigenous roots in the 1990s; Mexican cuisine was declared an intangible heritage by UNESCO in 2010, and Mexican chefs, trained in haute cuisine, began to integrate local ingredients and create new dishes inspired by these traditions. Insect species, considered for centuries as a delicacy, naturally found their way to elegant Mexican restaurants, such as El Cardenal run by one of the leading Mexican chefs. As we observed in Mexico City, Central Highlands insects, *escamoles* and sometimes *ahuautli,* are proposed, and occasionally, *chapulines* (grasshoppers) and *chicatanas* (*Atta* ants), more commonly offered in Oaxaca. Small restaurants or bars in elegant quarters of the city (Coyoacán and La Condesa) now serve insects, such as grilled *chapulines* with *guacamole* (avocado paste) as aperitif dishes. In tourist places, such as the pyramids of Teotihuacan (just outside the city), small restaurants offer aperitif dishes with *escamoles* and white agave worms, possibly collected from that area, as well as *chicatana* ants, probably imported from warmer regions. Recently, luxury chocolate makers, trained in Europe or the United States, have opened shops in Mexico, especially in Mexico City. Some of them have created 'typical Mexican' chocolates, flavoured with *chapulines* or *chicatanas*. The customers of the Market of San Juan are no longer from the working class, but rather from the upper middle class or are students of gastronomy. The market is now renowned for 'exotic foods' such as game, mushrooms and insects, mainly *escamoles*, *chicatanas*, *jumiles* and red agave worms, that the shopkeepers buy frozen and sell all year long, independently of the natural cycle of the insects. Some small companies have started over recent years to develop food products made out of insects. In the World Forum of Mexican Gastronomy, that we attended in Mexico City in November 2015, their stands presented grasshopper salt and grasshopper powder from Michoacan, and chilli sauces, in glass jars, from Hidalgo, flavoured with white agave worms or *xamues* (in this context, *Pachilis gigas, Hemiptera*), supposedly created by Otomi women. Mexican Indian people who have migrated to the United States are nostalgic for their foods and crave insects. In California, Françoise Lestage (2008) observed that *chapulines* and *chicatanas* were brought through individual networks to Oaxacan migrants; some of them even opened shops offering Oaxacan food specialties, including insects. Presently, because of strict border controls, people usually send food to their relatives in the states through private shipping companies. As a consequence, some of the valued insect species, like *chicatanas*, see their prices climbing on the regional markets and local people are now unable to buy them.

So, on the one hand, fewer Mexicans of the working classes consume insects than before, and many Mexicans still reject this consumption, while on the other hand, the demand for specific insect species, considered as gourmet food, has increased. In the meantime, environmental degradation has often led to a decrease of insects. Ramos-Elorduy (2006) is sounding the alert about the risk of overexploitation of these sought-for species, especially in fragile environments. High protein insects have been a rich and tasty component of poor people's diet. Through the integration of the tastiest species into present-day gastronomy, these are likely to escape from the people who, for centuries, have maintained knowledge of them. Nevertheless, there are at least 500 less tasty species which have not attracted the attention of chefs.

Cultural and political turning-points of pulque and beer consumption

The traditional use of pulque from past to present

Pulque is a fermented beverage extracted from different species of the century plant or agave, in particular *Agave americana, A. salmiana* and *A. atrovirens*.[12] Agave (in Spanish *maguey*, in Nahuatl *octli*) is traditionally produced above 1500 metres altitude, in the highlands of the states of Hidalgo, Querétaro, Tlaxcala, Puebla, San Luis Potosí, Mexico, Michoacán, Jalisco, Guerrero and Oaxaca (Figure 2.7). It is often planted at the limit of two plots, on the edge of agricultural terraces, preventing the soil from being washed out by the rains.

To produce *pulque*, people scrape the 'heart' of the century plant, after having cut out the central floral sprout, to form a receptacle where the sap accumulates. The agave is scraped every day for several months, until the plant dies. The fresh sweet-tasting sap is called 'honey water' in Spanish (*aguamiel*) and 'honey' in several indigenous languages (for instance, *necutli* in Nahuatl).

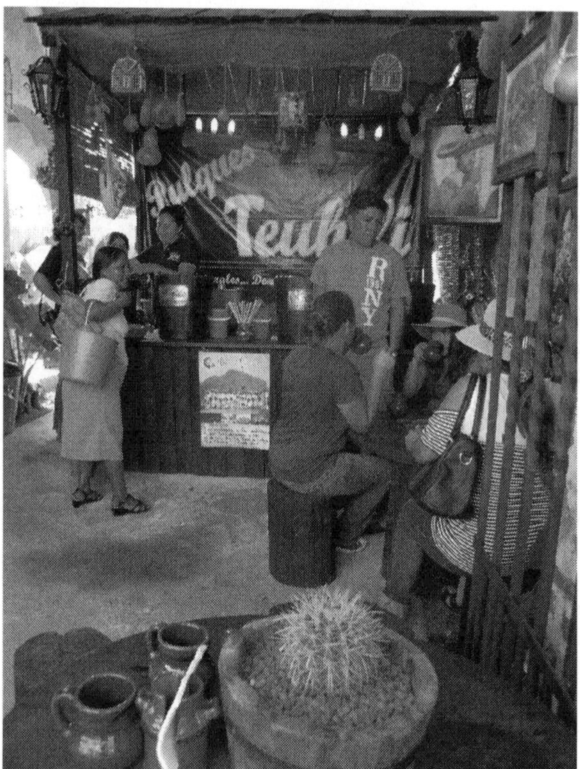

Figure 2.6 *Pulque*: a stand in a tourist town in Morelos

Source: © Esther Katz.

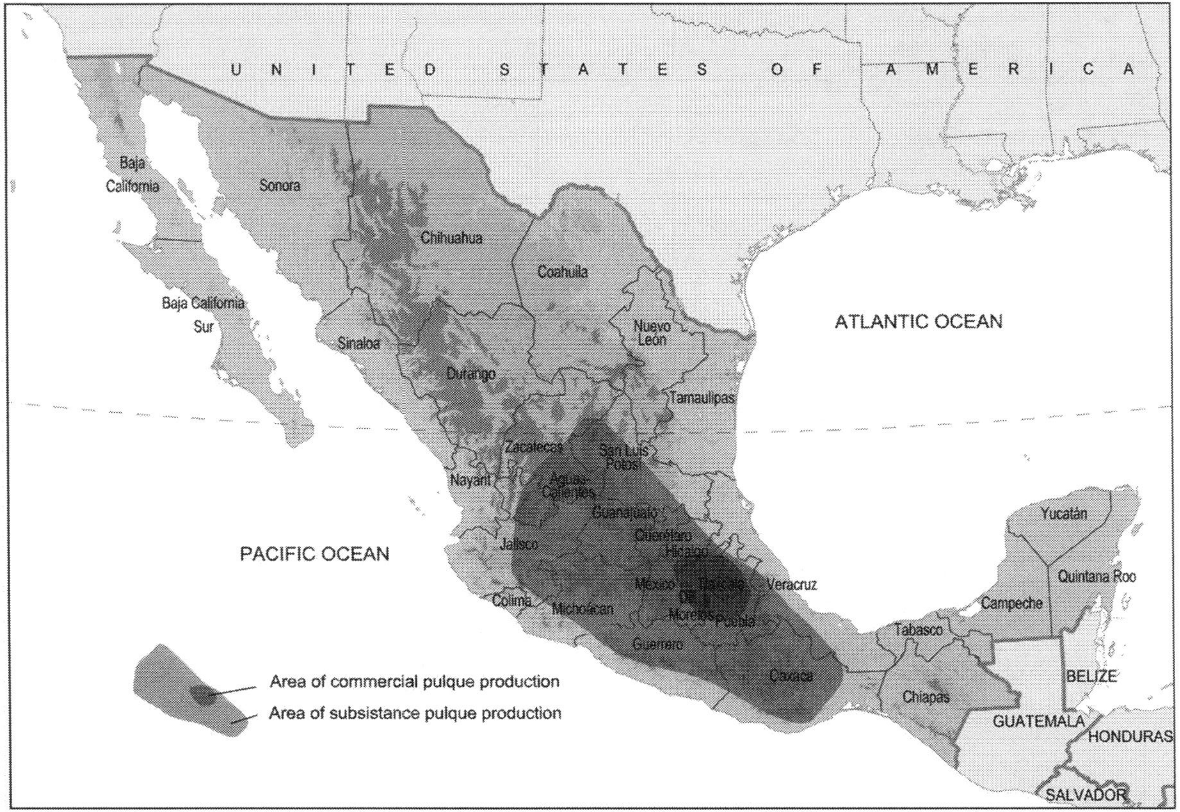

Figure 2.7 Main areas of pulque production in Mexico

is recommended for breast-feeding women. The farmers say a prayer and bless the sap on its first extraction and when the first *pulque* has fermented. They always pour it on the earth as an offering before drinking it. In some highlands villages, farmers pour it on the earth when they start planting maize. They also make an offering of *pulque* when praying for the rain, as well as in therapeutic rituals (Katz 2002). *Pulque* is not only an alcoholic beverage, it is a nutritive substance, considered as food. In the Central Highlands, children took *aguamiel* or *pulque* for breakfast, at least until recent decades (Fournier 1983), lactating women drink it too, and men drink it while working in the fields 'because it gives them strength' and keeps them hydrated (Valadez-Montes 2014), as Tlaxcala farmers explained to us.

Pulque and politics from the colonial period to the twentieth century

After the conquest, the Spaniards adopted *pulque* as an alcoholic beverage, but without taking into account its ceremonial use. During the colonial period, *pulque* and wine stood together on the table of the Spanish and Creole elites. Wine was restricted to the upper classes, but *pulque* was a very popular drink for the whole population (Becerra 1988; Fournier 1983; Ramírez 2012). At the beginning of the seventeenth century, as *pulque* had become an important economic source, the Spaniards enacted the first laws in order to regulate its production and commercialisation. The vice-king and the ecclesiastical authorities controlled the *maguey* cultivation and the *pulque* production. The Spaniards transformed lands in the centre of Mexico, with dry and poor soils, into the first *pulque haciendas*, a lucrative business. At the end of the eighteenth century, the first *pulquerías* produced and sold *pulque* on a larger scale, so as from 1785 to 1789, *pulque* was among the four products that generated the highest tax revenues (Loyola 1956).

After Independence (1821), *pulque* continued to represent a very important economic source, but its golden era occurred during the presidency of Porfirio Díaz (1876–1910). The introduction of the railway, in the 1870s, accelerated the business, as it allowed thousands of barrels to be sent to Mexico City from the *haciendas* located on the railway route between the capital city and Puebla, an area called the Apan Valley (*Llanos de Apan*).[13] Some *hacendados* of that region started occupying political cargoes, at the regional and national level. They also acquired a high number of *pulque* taverns all over Mexico City. The federal government could not ignore the power of the *pulqueros* and their investments in big companies. The *Compañía Expendedora de Pulques*, owned by *hacendados*, Mexican deputies and government officials, monopolised the production. In 1895, there was a *pulque* production of almost 3 million hectolitres that represented 80.3% of all the alcohol consumption, and in 1903, it reached a peak of 7 million hectolitres representing 86.7% of all the alcohol consumption (Ramírez *ibid.*: 90–91).[14] At the beginning of the twentieth century, the *pulque hacendados* were rich and powerful people. Around 275 *haciendas,* from small to enormous, covered 250,000 hectares, growing 150 to 200 million agave

An agave plant produces from 2 to 7 litres of sap per day, and from 200 to 500 litres over a period of 3 to 4 months. The sap is left to ferment naturally for two or three days, attaining an alcoholic content of 5 to 7 degrees proof. In the Central Highlands (*Altiplano Central*), small farmers, called *tlachiqueros,* take care of the agave plants, scrape them and collect the sap. In that region, in the 1970s, *haciendas* produced *pulque* in much larger quantities; there the sap was left to ferment in large barrels called *tinacales* (Fournier 1983). As we have observed in the Mixtec highlands, either men or women collect the sap, prepare the *pulque* and sell it in the market. In the state of Tlaxcala, we have noticed that some farmers leave the sap to ferment inside the century plants around the maize fields, so when they work in the fields they can drink the *pulque* straight from the plant.

When we started our fieldwork at the beginning of the 1980s, *pulque* was frequently consumed in villages and small towns of regions with a high percentage of indigenous populations, such as the Central Highlands or the Mixtec highlands. However, in Mexico City, *pulque* had very adverse connotations. It was associated with rural habits; it was considered as unhygienic and *pulquerías* (*pulque* taverns) were regarded as dirty working-class bars. In villages of the Central Highlands, Dominique Fournier (1983) observed in the late 1970s that this negative feeling was affecting the local farmers who were becoming ashamed of drinking a 'beverage of Indians' and that *pulque* production in *haciendas* was significantly decreasing. Why was *pulque* so despised while it was on the table of the Spanish elites in the colonial period?

In the Central Highlands, archaeological evidence of *maguey* scraping dates back to the fourth century BC (Parsons and Parsons 1990). Since prehispanic times, the century plant has been playing an important part in the economy and subsistence of the native people. It is a multi-use plant embedded in multi-dimensional aspects (social, economic, cultural, ecological, political). Now, as in the past, people eat the leaves and the flowers when cooked, draw starch, sugar, liquid, alcohol out of the plant, wrap food to be cooked in the leaf cuticle (*mixiote*), use the leaves to hold or cover food or other substances, even to protect roofs, use them as medicine, and use the fibre to weave or sow and the thorns as needles (Parsons and Parsons *ibid.*; Ramírez 2012). After the Spanish conquest, the chroniclers, in particular de Sahagún (1999), described the use of *pulque* in its cultural context. On a daily basis, among the Aztecs, old men strictly regulated its consumption to avoid excessive drunkenness among young people, but both men and women drank it during festivals. Offerings of *pulque* were performed in many ceremonies and agricultural rituals (Sahagún, 1999). According to myths or legends collected among the Aztecs at that period, the *pulque* gods, the *Centzon-Totochtin* (the 400 rabbits) took care of the agave, the harvests and the abundance of food resources (Fournier 1983; Fournier and Mondragón 2014). The Aztecs conceived of *pulque* as blood. The agave plant has its 'heart' opened to extract blood symbolically, and after giving all its blood, it dies (*ibid.*). Similar symbolism persists among contemporary indigenous people. For the Mixtecs, *pulque* (called 'white liquid', *nute kwixi*) is compared to sperm, milk, blood and rain. It is supposed to be 'pure blood' and plants *(ibid.*: 52–53). But in 1907, *pulque* production decreased to 4.6 million hectolitres (*ibid.*: 90).

Federal deputies who feared the *hacendados'* escalating power, as well as various ecclesiastic authorities criticising the high alcoholism rate, started to make a case against the consumption of *pulque*. The Catholic and laic press published articles describing the Mexican population as physically and mentally degraded because of *pulque*. But at that time, *pulque*, like maize, beans and chilli pepper, was considered as part of the basic diet of peasants and workers, as well as of the middle class. If a worker earned a salary of 30 pesos per month, he spent an average of 5 pesos on *pulque*, 5 pesos to buy maize, beans and chilli pepper, 5 pesos for the house rent and 3.5 pesos to buy meat.[15] The use of this sort of information, the anti-alcohol campaigns, and the defamation of *pulque* triggered the downward spiral of its production (*ibid.*: 61). Moreover, part of the political elite of the North tried to destroy the *pulque* empire by publishing articles about violence in Mexico City due, according to them, to the high consumption of *pulque*. Scientists reinforced the idea of a relationship between high criminality rates and alcohol consumption, in particular *pulque* (*ibid.*: 68; Nemser 2011).[16] As it was difficult to control the cleanliness of the barrels, the quality of the fermentation and the illegal commercialisation, the *pulque* industry received many attacks because of its non-hygienic processing (Valadez-Montes *ibid.*). With all this negative publicity, from the 1,300 *pulquerías* that existed in Mexico City at the beginning of the twentieth century, only 700 were left in 1910 (Mercadotecnia 2010).

Moreover, the Mexican Revolution, starting in 1910, provoked the dismantling of the *haciendas* associated with the former Porfirio Díaz regime. The new regime represented by Venustiano Carranza, clearly favoured the beer industry, as the wheat and barley were produced in the north of Mexico where Carranza supporters predominated. The new political elite tried to destroy the 'ancien régime' represented by the *pulque hacendados*: they redistributed *haciendas* lands, led anti-alcohol campaigns, regulated the *pulquerías*, increased the taxes on *pulque,* and marginalised *pulque* as a 'poor' or Indian beverage. Afraid of being jailed, many *hacendados* fled to Europe. From the late 1920s onwards, the area of land dedicated to growing agave plants, as well as the *pulque* production, significantly decreased, while the beer industry started to develop (Escalante and Gosset 2008; Medellín 1980). In 1923, a change was exacted on alcohol taxes, to the disadvantage of *pulque* and the advantage of beer, and taxes on *pulque* further increased in the 1930s and 1940s (Valadez-Montes *ibid.*).

Beer production had been for a long time a very minor industry. In the sixteenth century, under the rule of Emperor Charles V, the New Spain government gained authorisation to produce beer, but as barley and wheat were scarce, this production remained on a minor scale. During the colonial period, the Spaniards imported beer from Europe, but people hardly consumed it as it was scarce and expensive. Beer production started to develop only by 1875, thanks to German immigrants who brought their specific know-how and technology. By 1903, the Germans – and a few other people – had already created 19 beer factories in different parts of the country. The biggest brewery, Cuauhtémoc, in Monterrey, already produced

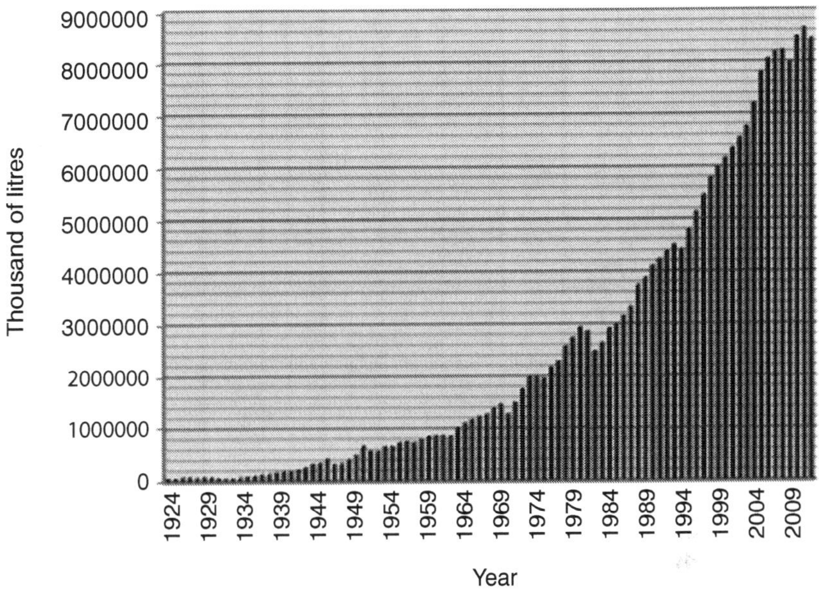

Figure 2.8 Production of beer in Mexico (1924–2014)

Source: SIAP-SAGARPA, 2015, Estadísticas Agropecuarias Nacionales http://www.siap.sagarpa.gob.mx (retrieved on 09 November 2015).

1 million litres in 1893 and kept on growing (Reyna and Krammer 2012). Unlike *pulque*, beer could be bottled and easily transported and stocked. The alliances between the post-revolutionary government, the religious officials and the beer industry reinforced the image of beer as a better, healthier and more hygienic product than *pulque*. The promoters of beer recommended consuming it during meals, so it started to be introduced in restaurants (while *pulque* was only served in taverns). After the 1920s, beer production started to increase until it became the most popular alcoholic beverage everywhere in the country, even in indigenous villages, as shown in Figure 2.8.

In the 1920s, *pulque* definitely lost the battle against beer. Nevertheless, the *pulque* production, although decreasing, was still resistant, as it benefited from new consumers, the peasants migrating to Mexico City. In 1933, the first patent to bottle *pulque* triggered the creation of several small industries, but from then on, *pulque* was considered a 'dirty' alcoholic beverage, drunk only by poor farmers, workers and indigenous people. With the land reform carried out under the government of Lázaro Cárdenas (1934–1940), the distribution of the lands of the *pulque haciendas* provoked a more serious crisis in production. The agave cultivation area diminished to more than half between 1930 and 1970 (Figure 2.9), although in the 1960s, the government of President López Mateos tried to boost agave cultivation. In 1953, in Hidalgo and Tlaxcala, the taxes of the *pulque* production still represented respectively 30 and 50% of the total government revenues, but in the 1970s, they

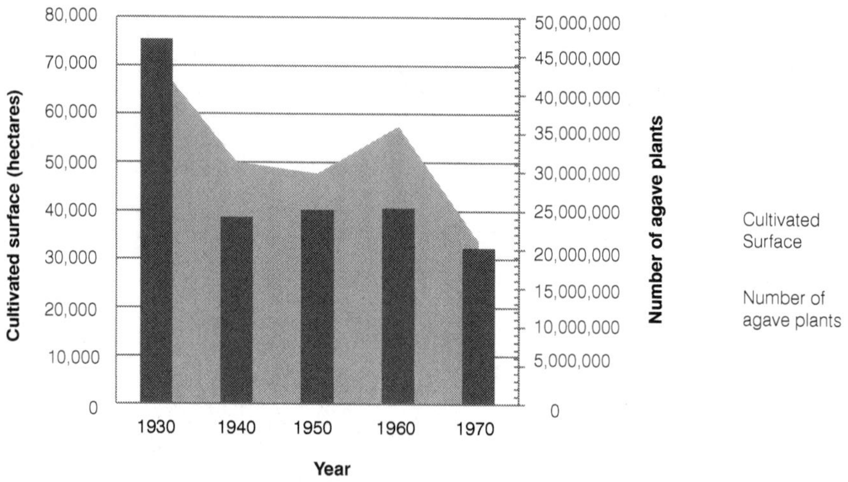

Figure 2.9 Cultivation of agave (maguey) between 1930 and 1970

Source: Censos Agrícola, Ganadero y Ejidal; Anuario Estadístico de los Estados Unidos Mexicanos; Oficina de Estadísticas de la Contaduría de la Federación y Patronato del Maguey (Comercio Exterior 1978: 1314).

did not even reach 1% (Loyola, 1956; Comercio Exterior 1978). Here, we go back to the situation of the 1980s described above: *pulque* was despised, beer was inundating the market, but *pulque* was still consumed although in much smaller quantities than beer, in so-called marginal areas such as the Mixtec highlands, and even in rural areas near Mexico City, such as Milpa Alta.

Pulque revival

However, nutritional studies brought to light the fact that *pulque* contained proteins, vitamins B, D and E, and a high proportion of vitamin C, minerals and sugars (Correa-Ascencio *et al.* 2014). At the beginning of the 1990s, as the indigenous roots of the country again started to be appreciated, *pulque* was valued as a traditional beverage. The *maguey* started to be cultivated once more in Hidalgo, Tlaxcala, Puebla, Querétaro and, to a lesser extent, in Veracruz, Michoacán, Guerrero and Oaxaca (Figure 2.10).

In regions of traditional *pulque* production, many annual *pulque* fairs have been created after 2005: in the Federal District ('Gastronomic Maize and *Pulque* Fair', Milpa Alta, since 2011; 'I love *pulque*', Mexico City, since 2016) and the states of Mexico ('The Rabbit and *Pulque* Fair', Huixquilucan, since 2006), Hidalgo (Ocampo, Apan Valley, since 2006), Puebla (Ozolco, since 2012), Michoacán ('Beverage of the Gods' Fair, Tupataro, since 2013) and Oaxaca (Tlaxiaco, since 2007). In 2016, the organisers of Tlaxiaco *pulque* fair pointed out that agave production was decreasing in their region and that they were hoping the fair would help to boost it.[17] Around the same period, chic *pulquerías,*

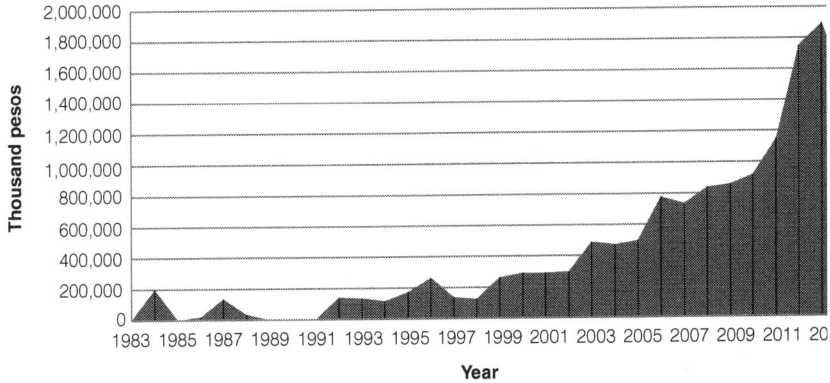

Figure 2.10 Production value of maguey

Source: SIAP-SAGARPA, 2015, Estadísticas Agropecuarias Nacionales, http://www.siap.sagarpa.gob.mx (retrieved on 09 November 2015).

attended by young people, appeared in Mexico City, Tlaxcala and Puebla. They are very different from the old style *pulquerías* that were mainly attended by men of the working classes. *Pulque* is sold in these bars as an organic and nutritious alcoholic beverage, frequently mixed with fruit juices. In the villages where *pulque* has always been consumed, people occasionally mix *pulque* with fruit juice (called *pulque curado)*, but it is more commonly drunk pure. The fruit juice probably attenuates the fermented taste of *pulque* and makes it more acceptable to a sector of the population who was not raised drinking it. This new gourmet market has provoked an important increase in the value of the production over the last 10 years (Figure 2.10), although it does not reach the production rates of the previous decades. In Guadalajara, a small catering company run by militant young people is promoting *pulque* tasting with different flavours and offers *pulque*-based cocktails, with tortillas chips and a *pulque* and cheese chilli sauce, which was traditionally made in some villages of that region.

Since Mexican cuisine was labelled a 'World intangible heritage' by UNESCO, *pulque,* as a traditional drink and heritage, is more valued. *Pulque* stands, from Puebla and Hidalgo, were present at the last World Forum of Mexican Gastronomy in Mexico City in November 2015. The vendor from Puebla emphasised the nutritional values of *pulque*, arguing that his company had been a pioneer in seeking scientific research collaboration.

Producers in Hidalgo, state of Mexico, Federal District (Milpa Alta) and above all Puebla and Tlaxcala are producing *pulque* for commercial purpose, especially to sell it in Mexico City. Producers from Milpa Alta also sell *pulque* on week-ends in tourist towns of the state of Morelos visited by people from Mexico City. Puebla producers do not actually completely fulfil the demand. Puebla traders buy *pulque* in village markets in the Mixtec highlands from small farmers, estimating it to be of very high quality (Diana Lope Alzina, personal communication) (see Figure 2.6).

In Tlaxcala, *pulque* producers who persevered and kept cultivating agave in spite of adversities, argued that *pulque* was a local heritage, a collective asset of the people, with nutritive and medicinal properties (Valadez-Montes, 2014). In 2012, when we visited the Industrial Magueyera Mexicana, a small *pulque* industry in Altzayanca, Tlaxcala, the owner, Víctor Manuel Cervantes, explained: "there are many alcohols, but we are producing *pulque*, the only alcoholic beverage representative of Tlaxcala. [In prehispanic times] this product was the beverage of kings; other people who dared to consume it were sacrificed". He is referring to the glorious prehispanic past, presenting *pulque* as an elite drink, and enhancing regional identity. This company produces 3,000 litres per month of *pulque*; 60% of the production is kept in oak barrels for three years, 20% is flavoured with aniseed, and the rest with other flavours. This company sells its products in tourist places such as the archaeological site of Cacaxtla (Tlaxcala). Manuel Sánchez Armas, the owner of another company, Industrial Magueyera, struggles for the cultural re-appropriation of *pulque* by Mexicans. Twenty years ago, he canned *pulque* that he distributed in supermarkets and sent to the border city of Tijuana for North American and Mexican consumers (Ceballos 2001). Now, he is producing fine *pulque* and agave honey targeted at the gourmet market of Tlaxcala and Mexico City. During an interview, he confided: "We are looking for a new broker to export it, but we do not have much capital and we do not receive any financial support from the government." Nevertheless, he continues to look for commercial alternatives (Ceballos *ibid.*). All these small, family enterprises are trying to recover *pulque* as the 'nectar of the gods' and to reintroduce it as an ethnic and organic product in the Mexican food culture.

Pulque is therefore re-conquering the consumers, but it will probably never regain the importance it had at the end of the nineteenth century. Above all, it has tremendously decreased in the consumption of the poorest people who have replaced it by less nutritious or stronger alcohols and less nutritious industrial foods.

Conclusion

According to Parsons (2010), in the Mexican Central Highlands, in the prehispanic period, the combination of maize/beans/amaranth with agave cultivation and, moreover, exploitation of lake resources (including aquatic insects, spirulina, fish, ducks, frogs, etc.) was very efficient in providing an adequate diet. After the Spanish conquest, amaranth was suppressed as a staple, and the lakes around Mexico City were progressively drained, depriving the surrounding population of highly nutritious foods. Scientific analyses of nutrient components of these prehispanic foods have, in the last decades, shown that amaranth, insects and *pulque* were definitely super-foods. As such, their consumption is now promoted, but we doubt that it will regain to the importance it used to have during the prehispanic period, or even at the beginning of the twentieth century. It does not seem either that the lower classes who consumed them will fully reintegrate them into their diet. The fluctuating fate of these super-foods over the last five centuries reveals relationships of power, first between the colonisers and the colonised, then between social classes, ethnic groups and political parties, based on economic interests. Nowadays, diets are being homogenised, industrial food is more and more consumed, most crops are grown with pesticides, and poor nutrition is causing major health problems. Going back to the super-foods of the past and the deep roots of Mexican identity is a good solution, as long as everybody, rich or poor, benefits from it. As usual, these foods are likely to escape the poorest people who need them more.

Notes

1 Acknowledgements for the most recent fieldwork: The fieldwork conducted in 2011 in the Mixtec highlands (Oaxaca) (both authors) was funded by the European Union project 'Engov-Bek(onal)', *Environment and Governance in Latin America-Building and Exchanging Knowledges on Natural Resources* (2011–2015) (FP7-2010) (SSH-CT-2010-266.710) ; fieldwork in Tlaxcala (Elena Lazos) by CONACyT/CIBIOGEM project *Impactos sociales, económicos y culturales de la posible introducción de maíz genéticamente modificado en* México (2012–2015) ; fieldwork in Mexico City, Morelos and Oaxaca in 2015 (Esther Katz) by Sorbonne-Universités project 'PALIM' *Patrimoines alimentaires et Pratiques culinaires* (2014–2016); This part of Katz's research is also included in ANR project 'FoodHerit' *Food Heritage and Gastropolitics* (2013-2017) and Sorbonne-Universités project 'PALSAN' *Patrimoine Alimentaire et Santé* (2014-2015).

2 The area of central and southern Mexico and the north of Central America, which corresponded roughly with the Aztec empire, were defined as the 'Mesoamerican cultural area' by Paul Kirchhoff (1992). The arid areas of northern Mexico were mainly, but not exclusively, populated by hunter-gatherers, called 'Chichimec' by the Aztecs.

3 For instance, foodstuffs from the lowlands, such as chilli pepper and cocoa beans, were brought as tribute to the Aztecs.

4 Most early colonisers came from southern Spain (Andalusia and Extremadura) where the Arab-Andalusian culture developed until the expulsion of the Arabs in 1492. Colonial Mexican cuisine, like colonial architecture, has inherited elements from the Arab-Andalusian influence.

5 Nahuatl was used as a *lingua franca* in the Aztec empire, and then in New Spain. It is still spoken today by about a million and half indigenous people (INEGI 2010). For example, the Spanish words for 'chilli pepper' (*chile*), 'tomato' (*tomate*) and 'avocado' (*aguacate*) originate from the Nahua names *chilli, tomatl* and *ahuacatl*; on the other hand, plant names like *maíz* (maize) or *maguey* (agave, century plant) come from Taino, an Arawak language spoken in Hispaniola (Santo Domingo/Haiti) where Colombus landed in 1492 (Torres 1985).

6 According to Jonathan D. Sauer (1950), *Amaranthus* and *Chenopodium* species can be recognized and differentiated on the illustrations of the sixteenth century: the plants with entire leaves are amaranths and those with dentate leaves chenopods.

7 Related species with small grains were domesticated in the Andes: *kiwicha (Amaranthus caudatus), quinoa (Chenopodium quinoa)* and *qañiwa* (*Chenopodium pallidicaule)* (Hernández-Bermejo and León 1994).

8 Recently, the anthropologist Françoise Neff (2005, and personal communication 2015) confirmed these observations and, moreover, has observed that amaranth is still used by the Nahua Indians of that region in offerings, called *tzoalli*: as the Aztecs did, they shape maize and amaranth dough into mountains or snakes, to pray for rain.

9 http://www.mexicodesconocido.com.mx/santiago-tulyehualco-y-la-feria-de-la-alegria-y-el-olivo-distrito-federal.html; http://www.fiestasdemexico.com/2015/12/feria-de-la-alegria-y-el-olivo-2016.html (retrieved on 22 February 2016).

10 It is now known that a seed of grain amaranth is on average composed of 13.1–21.0% crude protein; 5.6–10.9% crude fat; 48–69% starch; 3.1–5.0% (14.2%) of dietary fibre and 2.5–4.4 % ash. Proteins have high digestibility (approx. 90%) and are rich in lysine (4.9–6.1 g per 100 g of protein) (Grobelnik-Mlakar *et al.* 2009).

11 Curiously, as observed by E. Lazos, the Yucatec Maya Indians eat very few insects, compared to Indians of other regions.

12 There are more than 200 species of agaves in Mexico, some have specialised use in the production of sap for alcoholic beverages (*tequila, mezcal, pulque*), others in the production of fibres and sisal.

13 In 1896, around 400,000 litres were brought daily to Mexico City, which had a population of 400,000 people. In those days, the *pulque* industry involved around 128,000 workers (Loyola 1956).

14 *Anuario Estadístico de la República Mexicana* 1895, Dirección General de Estadística, Dr. Antonio Peñafiel, Oficina Tipográfica de la Secretaría de Fomento, 1896, México, pp. 798–799 and 809.

15 Information from *Memoria que presentó el Secretario de Hacienda al Congreso de la Unión*. 1909–10, México, Tipografía de la Impresora de Estampillas, 1911 (González 1970: 391).

16 It echoed a previous action led by the colonial government who, during the revolt of 1692, blamed the violence on *pulque*, and attempted to regulate it. However, at that time, as everybody drank *pulque*, the government distinguished the pure 'white *pulque*', drunk mainly by the elite, from the 'mixed *pulque*', consumed by the plebeian masses. The elites used the 'mixed *pulque*' as a metaphor of race mixing (*mestizaje*) and condemned it as a threat to political stability. These feelings and ideologies permeated the centuries (Nemser 2011).

17 http://alianzanahuaca.org/2014/09/27/feria-gastronomica-del-maiz-y-el-pulque
http://ciudadanosenred.com.mx/feria-del-pulque-i-love-pulque
http://www.24-horas.mx/inauguran-feria-del-pulque-en-hidalgo
http://alianzanahuaca.org/2013/02/27/2da-feria-del-pulque-en-ozolco
http://www.flotrawww.ignaciomartinez.com.mx/noticias/1a_feria_de_la_bebida_de_los_dioses_en_tupataro_29384
https://oaxaca.quadratin.com.mx/Anuncian-Feria-del-Pulque-en-Ojo-de-Agua-Tlaxiaco (retrieved on 22 February 2016).

References

Bak-Geller, S. (2008). "Les livres de recettes 'francisés' au Mexique au XIXe siècle. La construction de la nation et d'un modèle culinaire national", *Anthropology of Food,* no. S4. http://aof.revues.org/index2992.html (retrieved on 19 December 2015).

Becerra, L. (1988). "El pulque, ancestral bebida obtenida del árbol de las maravillas", *Nueva Antropología*, Vol. 10(34): 195–198.

Berthe, J.-P. (1988). "L'évangile et l'outil : le changement technique dans un village indien du Mexique au XVIe siècle", *Techniques et Culture*, Vol. 11: 65–82.

Casillas, L. and Vargas, L.A. (1984). "La alimentación entre los Mexicas", in A. López-Austin and C. Viesca (eds), *Historia general de la medicina en México*, Vol. 1: *México antiguo,* 133–156. México: UNAM.

Castelló Yturbide, T. (1986). *Presencia de la comida prehispánica*, México: Fomento Cultural Banamex.

Ceballos, Y. (2001). "Industria del pulque: Futuro bajo presión", *Agencia Reforma*, May 30: 1–8.

Comercio Exterior. (1978). "El maguey y el pulque. Había una vez…", *Sección Nacional, Sector Agropecuario*: 1312–1317.

Cook, S. and Borah, W. (1979). *Essays in Population History, Mexico and California,* Berkeley: University of California.

Correa-Ascencio, M., I. Robertson, O. Cabrera, R. Cabrera and Evershed, R. (2014). "Pulque production from fermented agave sap as a dietary supplement in Prehispanic Mesoamerica", *Proceedings of the National Academy of Sciences of the United States of America*, Vol. 111(39): 14223–14228.

Escalante, A. and Gosset, G. (2008). "El pulque, una bebida con un gran pasado y ¿un futuro incierto?", *Unión de Morelos (Academia de Ciencias de Morelos)*: 22–23.

Fournier, D. (1983). "Façons de boire, façons de voir…", *Social Science Information*, Vol. 22(3): 411–434.

Fournier, P. and Mondragón, L. (2014) "El pulque", *Arqueología Mexicana*, No. 57: 66–75 (special issue).

González, N.M. (1970). *Historia moderna de México. El porfiriato. La vida social*, México: Hermes.

González de la Vara, F. (ed.) (1996-97). *La cocina mexicana a través de los siglos.* Vol. 10, México: Clío / Fundación Herdez.

INEGI (2010) *Censo de Población y Vivienda 2010*, México: INEGI. www.cuentame.inegi.org.mx (retrieved on 05 November 2015).

Grobelnik-Mlakar, S., Turinek, M., Jakop, M., Bavec, M. and Bavec, F. (2009). "Nutrition value and use of grain amaranth: potential future application in bread making", *Agricultura*, Vol. 6: 43–53.

Gutiérrez, J.P., Rivera-Dommarco, J., Shamah-Levy, T. S. *et al.* (2012). *Encuesta Nacional de Salud y Nutrición 2012. Resultados nacionales*, Cuernavaca: Instituto Nacional de Salud Pública.

Hernández-Bermejo, J.E. and León, J. (eds) (1994). *Neglected crops. 1492 from a different perspective*, Rome: Food and Agriculture Organization.

van Huis, A., van Itterbeeck, J., Klunder, H., Mertens, E., Halloran, A. *et al.* (2013). *Edible Insects. Future Prospects for Food and Feed Security*, Rome: Food and Agriculture Organization.

Hunziker, A.T. (1952). *Los pseudocereales de la agricultura indígena de América*, Buenos Aires: Acme Agency.

Katz, E. (1996). "Insectes comestibles du haut pays mixtèque (Mexique)", *Anthropozoologica*, Vol. 23: 77–84.

Katz, E. (2002). "Rites, représentations et météorologie dans la Terre de la Pluie (Mixteca, Mexique)", in E. Katz, M. Goloubinoff and A. Lammel (eds.), *Entre ciel et terre : Climat et sociétés*, pp. 63–88. Paris: Ibis Press/IRD Editions.

Katz, E. (2016). "Insectes comestibles en Amérique Latine: de nourriture d'Indiens à patrimoine alimentaire", in E. Motte-Florac and P. Le Gall (eds.), *Savoureux insectes. De l'aliment traditionnel à l'innovation gastronomique*, pp. 87–115. Rennes/Tours: Presses Universitaires de Rennes/ Presses Universitaires François Rabelais.

Kirchhoff, P. (1992). "Mesoamérica. Sus límites geográficos, composición étnica y caracteres culturales", in J. Vivó (ed), *Una definición de Mésoamérica*, pp. 28–45. México, IIA-UNAM.

Lammel, A., M. Goloubinoff. and Katz, E. (eds.) (2008). *Aires y lluvias. Antropología del clima en México* México: CIESAS/CEMCA/IRD.

Lestage, F. (2008). "De la circulation des nourritures", *Anthropology of Food*, No. S4. http://aof.revues.org/2942 (retrieved on 19 December 2015).

Long, J. (ed.) (1996). *Conquista y comida: consecuencias del encuentro de dos mundos,* México: UNAM.

Long, J. (1997). *La cocina mexicana a través de los siglos. IV. La Nueva España*, México: Editorial Clío.

Loyola, E. (1956). *La industria del pulque*, México: Banco de México, Departamento de Investigaciones Industriales.

Mapes-Sánchez, E. C. and Espitia-Rangel, E. (2010). *Recopilación y análisis de la información existente de las especies del genero* Amaranthus *cultivadas y de sus posibles parientes silvestres en México* (final report). Project: Centro de origen y diversidad genética, México: DGSPRNR-SEMARNAT/CONABIO.

Martínez-Alfaro, M.A., Ortega-Paczka, R. and Cruz-León, A. (1994). "Introduction of flora from the Old World and causes of crop marginalization", in J.E. Hernández-Bermejo and J. León (eds), *Neglected Crops. 1492 from a Different Perspective*, pp. 23–33. Rome: Food and Agriculture Organization.

Medellín, R. (1980). "Los campesinos cebaderos y la industria cervecera en México", *Comercio Exterior*, Vol. 30(9): 927–936.

Mercadotecnia (2010). "¿Pulque? – No, gracias, mejor una cerveza", *Expansión*, September 2010: 109–110, 1st publication 1910.

Moedano, G. (1988) (ed.). *Atlas cultural de México. Gastronomía*, México: SEP/INAH/Planeta.

National Research Council (NRC) (1975). *Underexploited Tropical Plants with Promising Economic Value.* Washington, D.C.: National Academy Press.

National Research Council (NRC) (1984). *Amaranth. Modern Prospects for an Ancient Crop*, Washington, D.C.: National Academy Press.

Navarrete, L.F. (2004). *Las relaciones interétnicas en México*, México: Universidad Nacional Autónoma de México.

Neff, F. (2005). *Mouvement et intensité dans la pensée indienne : mythes et rituels de l'Etat de Guerrero, Mexique*, PhD Thesis in Anthropology, Nanterre: University of Paris 10, unpublished.

Nemser, D. (2011). "'To avoid this mixture': rethinking pulque in colonial Mexico City",*Food and Foodways*, Vol. 19: 98–121.

Parsons, J.R. (2006). *The Last Pescadores of Chimalhuacán, Mexico. An Archeological Ethnography*, Ann Arbor, MI: University of Michigan, Museum of Anthropology.

Parsons, J.R. (2010). "The pastoral niche in Pre-Hispanic Mesomerica", in J.E. Staller and M.D. Carrasco (eds.), *Pre-Columbian Foodways*, pp. 109–136. New York/London: Springer.

Parsons, J.R. and Parsons, M.H. (1990). *Maguey Utilization in Highland Central Mexico. An Archaeological Ethnography*, University of Michigan: Museum of Anthropology.

Patiño, V.M. (1963–1974). *Plantas cultivadas y animales domésticos de la América equinoccial*, Vol. 1–4, Cali: Imprenta Departemental.

Pitt-Rivers, J. (1992). "La culture métisse : dynamique du statut ethnique", *L'Homme*, Vol. 32(122–124): 133–148.

Ramírez, R. M. (2012). *El Rey del Pulque. Ignacio Torres Adalid y la Industria Pulquera*, México: Ed. Quinta Chilla IIS-UNAM.

Ramos-Elorduy, J. (1982). *Los insectos como fuente de proteína en el futuro*, México: Limusa.

Ramos-Elorduy, J. (1997). "The importance of edible insects in the nutrition and economy of people of the rural areas of Mexico", *Ecology of Food and Nutrition*, Vol. 36(5): 347–366.

Ramos-Elorduy, J. (2006). "Threatened edible insects in Hidalgo, Mexico and some measures to preserve them", *Journal of Ethnobiology and Ethnomedicine.* http://www.ethnobiomed.com/content/2/1/51 (retrieved on 19 December 2015).

Ramos-Elorduy, J., Pino, M., Jose, M. and Martínez, C. (2012). "Could grasshoppers be a nutritive meal?", *Food and Nutrition Sciences*, Vol. 3: 164-175.

Reyna, M. C. and Krammer, J. P. (2012). *Apuntes para la historia de la cerveza en México,* México: INAH.

Sahagún, B. de (1999). *Historia general de las cosas de Nueva España*, México: Porrúa, 1st public 1570–1582.

Sauer, J.D. (1950). "The grain amaranth: a survey of their history and classification", *Annals of the Missouri Botanical Garden*, Vol. 37: 561–616.

SIAP-SAGARPA (2015). *Estadísticas Agropecuarias Nacionales.* http://www.siap.sagarpa.gob.mx (retrieved on 09 November 2015).

Sugiura, Y. and González De La Vara, F. (1996). *La cocina mexicana a través de los siglos. I. México antiguo,* México: Editorial Clío.

Torres, B. (1985). "Las plantas útiles en el México antiguo según las fuentes del siglo XVI", in T. Rojas Rabiela and W. Sanders (eds), *Historia de la agricultura. Epoca prehispánica-Siglo XVI. Vol. 1*, pp. 53–128. México: INAH.

Valadez-Montes, M. (2014). "'Pulque limpio'/ 'pulque sucio' : disputas en torno a la legitimidad y la producción social del valor", *Revista Colombiana de Antropología*, Vol. 50(2): 41–63.

Venskutonis, P.R. and Kraujalis, P. (2013). "Nutritional components of amaranth seeds and vegetables: a review on composition, properties, and uses", *Comprehensive Reviews in Food Science and Food Safety*, Vol. 12: 381–412.

Wolf, E. (1959). *Sons of the Shaking Earth*, Chicago: University of Chicago Press.

3 Lost in tradition

An attempt to go beyond labels, taking Maltese food practices as a primary example

Elise Billiard

Introduction: an overview on defining tradition

Tradition is the bread-and-butter of anthropologists. Their expertise assures the traditional origin of crafts, customs and objects, such as cooking techniques, recipes, and food which is the subject of the present chapter. In recent years, this expertise has been increasingly employed by diverse organisations and national bodies. In many countries, the tourism industry is a major beneficiary of the labellisation of traditions since it depends on exhibitions of local heritage, stamped as traditional, to offer the uninitiated visitor an appealing, and often heavily romanticised, image of the host country. Folklore museums, indebted to anthropology, sometimes adopt the title of 'ethnographic museum'. Small enterprises and large corporations alike use or abuse the word tradition (or its adjective 'traditional') to attract costumers in search of the ever-elusive hallmarks of authenticity, quality and nostalgia. Politicians also speak about tradition, but they do so using the term with versatility and logistical tact. Their intent is to reassure voters of their loyal intentions to preserve the best of their culture and to defend such values against foreign invasion, or sometimes, on the contrary, they declare their will to establish a democratic and progressive state in opposition to a dictatorial and backward traditional society. Either way, as we shall see, tradition is an effective political tool. Nowadays, the term 'tradition' has become a label that is highly sought after by small food producers who are often considered the last guarantors of an endangered heritage. Unable to compete with multi-national giants, they need to certify the traditional quality of their products so as to obtain the financial and administrative protection that is vital to their commercial sustainability.[1]

Tradition has been the object of study for anthropologists from the earliest days of ethnography. Early anthropologists were keen on discovering the singularities between 'traditional societies' and comparing them with their 'civilisation' (Mauss 1990). Tradition also had another meaning in the nineteenth century: it referred to the official ethnic discourse on origins.[2] Nowadays, traditions are everywhere, in all societies, and are no longer the domain of anthropologists alone. Observation of rituals, beliefs and norms of behaviour passed on through generations continues nonetheless to be precisely what anthropologists are looking for and what enables them to describe the singularity of a society or 'culture'.

As an anthropologist, I should therefore be at ease in defining one of the key concepts of my discipline, yet such a definition defies any simplistic approach, and obstinately, challenges the inquisitive mind. I would like to suggest here that the massive trend towards using the word 'tradition' with such pervasive and reckless abandon has revealed the many pitfalls the search for an academic definition holds. In support of my wish to identify 'tradition' as an objective tool, I will carefully outline the various assumptions that expose the unstable fundamentals upon which tradition is constructed and defined. My main observation is that traditions, as a category of thought, can only be the offspring of a particular temporality. To free the notion of tradition from a misconstrued entanglement of theories of globalisation consequences, or with renewed fervour for national identity, a brief epistemological critique is necessary. I shall sum up only the key points – giving references to authors for further development and discussion.

It might be impossible accurately to define 'tradition' but one can focus on its essential meaning: the transmission of skills and practices between individuals or groups. How do individuals or groups transmit the knowledge acquired in a lifetime? Can we 'preserve' recipes in books? Can we learn to cook relying solely on the Internet? To what extent are gestures and habitus an essential part of the transmission of tradition? (Bourdieu 1984). Anyone who uses tradition as a methodological tool in his everyday research should investigate these crucial elements. Drawing my hypothesis from the work of Timothy Ingold (1997, 2001, 2010), I shall introduce some remarks that will help to enable a sounder study of the way that skills are passed on. I consider that the critique of tradition is a necessary milestone on the path towards a better understanding of the dynamic of cultures since the transmission of practices carries with it the reproduction and transformation of culture. I will argue this critique on the basis of examples taken from my PhD fieldwork, undertaken in Malta, on the topic of food discourses and practices.[3] Food traditions are a particularly rich topic since the need to eat is universal, and as such, is a relevant subject for comparisons. Food practices are particularly interesting as they convey two areas of life: they are present both in mundane domestic practices and in political nationalist discourse. However, my perspective on traditions is not limited to food but should be taken as a general critique of the concept of traditions.

My main interest in Maltese food culture is that it gathers together tradition and modernity and plays inconsistently with this dualism. The diversity of cultural influences is astonishing and one cannot but wonder how the Maltese have managed to remain a people after having integrated so many different civilisations, so many times. A small archipelago, located in the middle of the Mediterranean Sea, Malta has integrated this colourful mix into its food practices, whilst keeping distinctive tastes and recipes by dint of digesting novelties in its own particular Maltese way. Close to Italy for geographical, historical and religious reasons, the Maltese have nonetheless absorbed with gusto ham and cheese sandwiches or lager beers from their acquaintance with the British Marines. Formerly, and for more than three centuries, the islands were converted into a fortress for the Knights of Saint John of Jerusalem, the last outpost of Christianity, fighting the powerful Ottoman Empire and sealing for good the fate of the Maltese as Europeans and Christians, qualities they are still very proud of today. However, their clearly Semitic language tells a different story and some recipes also distil the strong Arabic and Muslim influences on the Maltese way of life. The delicious *pastizzi*, a refined puff pastry stuffed with ricotta or pea-mash, is still the most popular snack, a snack also consumed in Lebanon. In food culture, ingredients and recipes are not the sole elements, their combination is crucial. In the way *pastizzi* are served one can observe the Maltese mix-and-match food habits: the *pastizzi* (which are handmade) always come with a glass of dark tea, the bitterness of which is sometimes softened by tinned milk. This cohabitation of Arabic and English *savoir vivre* also stretches itself occasionally to welcome an Italian representative in the form of a large cappuccino.

The heterogeneity that characterises most culinary habits in the world is well displayed in the Maltese cuisine. In Malta, as in many other emerging economies, the incremental increase in diet-related health risks is becoming a serious issue for the local government which, in an attempt to curb this trend, has launched several information campaigns and taken direct initiatives in public institutions, such as forbidding soft drinks in schools. During my fieldwork, I noticed that many housewives are increasingly aware of the health risks of certain foods, and some have become very strict in their observance of cooking precepts that differ from those they learnt from their mothers. As a consequence many recipes are discarded and many new gestures and products have appeared in the kitchens. Animal fat is banned and replaced by margarine; sunflower and corn oil, formerly used during festive times for frying sweet or savoury pastries, is used in very small quantities and replaced most of the time with aerosols of cholesterol-free derivative oils, and in the upper middle kitchens, with imported olive oil. In cafes, sachets of sweeteners have appeared and diet soft drinks are filling up supermarket shelves. Pressure to change Maltese food is also evident in direct cultural forms, particularly in the new wave of 'Mediterraneanism'. As a young independent state,[4] Malta is not satisfied with its national image, and its tourism industry encourages putting some of the country's cultural (military history) and geographical (beaches) assets forward. In both cases, the result is a strong drive towards a reformulation of Maltese culture as a whole, and especially of Maltese cuisine.[5] In a nutshell, the Maltese official discourse stresses its belonging to Europe, to the Christian community, and more recently, to the romanticized image of the Mediterranean (Billiard 2006). Maltese food is displayed as the genuine traditionally domestic food, the ultimate proof that the Maltese are a peaceful people whose 'backwardness'[6] only adds exoticism for the northern European tourist. It is in this context that I have become aware of the destructive capacity of instrumental traditions.

Tradition as a category of though

In his seminal book, Time and the Others, Johannes Fabian (2003) delivers a radical epistemological critique of anthropological writings as being generally based on the illusion that anthropologists are 'here and now' and their objects of study 'there and then'. Surprisingly, the geographical distance was not sufficient for early anthropologists to establish a clear boundary between the observer and the subject of observation. Fabian deconstructed the illusion that the 'others' exist in a time not contemporary with our own. Behind the idea that the 'others' are living in another world, many anthropologists added that the 'others' are living in another time. This bias is evident in the original work of evolutionist anthropologists who founded the discipline, amongst them Lewis H. Morgan (1871), who – convinced of the superiority of the 'civilization' (theirs) – worked hard to produce a time-line of human diversity applying Darwin's biologic thesis on cultures. Fabian argues that the attribution of place in an abstract time has persisted until today in many analyses. These anthropologists were not only travellers in other landscapes, but also time travellers.

Although Fabian did not refer explicitly to tradition, we can use his reflective observation in attempting to define traditional food for two reasons. Firstly, because from the beginning of the discipline, and until recently (and still for many of us), tradition has been an important subject of anthropological study. If anthropological analysis is partial, wittingly or unwittingly, it might be because concepts such as 'tradition' carry a particular vision of time. Secondly, the adjective 'traditional' by itself locates (situates) the 'others' in another time. A traditional society is one where time stands still: a society that has miraculously escaped the erosion of time; a society preserved from the decadence of modernity. We shall come back to this romantic conception of the traditional 'others', but for now, I would insist on the prejudices caused by a cultural conception of time that reproduces stereotypes of the others that anthropologists aim to deconstruct.

The first postulate is that time is linear. In western societies, time is portrayed as a straight line. On this time line, the past is forever abolished by the present. Past is behind us and future in front of us. There is no repetition of past events, except in our dreams. The future is unknown and always forthcoming. This linearity of time is the source of numerous categorisations that are constantly used with abandon. Objects and practices are always situated as past or present (or even future) when in fact they all belong to this moment in time (Latour 1993). Anthropologists are not alone in their tendency to use time categories to qualify and quantify. Language is replete with expressions that take for granted the linearity of time: 'looking back'; 'heading toward the future'. Not all societies or cultures perceive time in this way. Time can be cyclical or divided between the time of the origins and the eternal present. Linear time is no more objective than other expressions of time (often perceived as primitive). What is crucial to the understanding of the workings of tradition is that any meaningful definition of the word implies a linearity of time which imposes by its nature an irretrievable past; and therefore embedded in the meaning of tradition is the fear of loss.

A fast changing world is the cliché commonly mooted as the reason for the current resurgence of traditional values. There might be some truth in this, but the phenomenon is better understood when looked at from a different angle. The urge to 'got back to our roots' implies that one is increasingly aware of the gap between the present time and the 'roots' time or, to put it rather colloquially, 'the good old days'. This awareness is a direct consequence of the ever-increasing fervour with which we are documenting the past. In other words, it is the difference between what has been documented and what we can see happening right now that gives the impression of constant movement and an unsettling feeling of loss. The technological and institutional progress made in archiving records has made us more aware of our past. Family films and photographs are so cheap and easy to take that one soon finds oneself groaning under the weight of thousands of pictures of his or her beloved children or the endless streams of holiday photographs. Obsessed with archives (facilitated in no small measure by the huge increase in digital memory), one 'looks back' to a past which is getting closer every day. And the more one is aware of the loss of past things, the greater is the obsession with desperately trying to retain something from the past. Finally, we are increasingly nostalgic because we are focusing on the distinction between now (the unwritten) and what once was (the archived).[7] Forgetting is the condition for curing the disease of history, as Frederick Nietzsche (2005) succinctly put it.

The paradox is that the past is forever abolished yet some events 'mysteriously' survive or reappear in the present. These enduring phenomena are called 'traditions'. A traditional food or a traditional ritual is a vestige of the past in the present. From this standpoint, the analysis of traditional productions (be they artefacts or rituals) serves to clarify which practices are vestiges and why some others are not. For many NGOs, national bodies and international organisations, this is the goal of current research on traditions and this is the reason why a precise definition of tradition is crucial.

Before pointing out the problems inherent in the current definitions of tradition, I would like to insist that defining some practices as traditional and others as not, is not only inaccurate but dangerous. It is counter-productive because, by documenting the material and immaterial heritage of a society, one creates archives of the recent past and, consequently, a sense of history is projected onto individuals or societies who did not necessarily have a linear vision of time. In other words, organisations such as UNESCO, with the praiseworthy intention of protecting cultural diversity, are pushing entire cultures into a western temporality and this may result in gross distortions of the true nature of these cultures and their traditions. This pervasive consequence is, however, inevitable and I prefer here to focus my argument on the weak (or erratic) postulations of tradition as they are commonly used.

Traditions are considered vestiges of the past. Does this mean that everything else is completely new? The defenders of tradition would argue that it is a matter of degree, and if traditions are opposed to novelty, it does not necessary mean that they have not changed at all as in the case of food production processes that have to be adjusted to comply with the latest European hygiene regulations. Instead of joining the endless debate on where to place the limits between major and minor change, the temptation is to leave the assembly of legislators to their cyclical (dead end) discussions, and instead, to wander with Bruno Latour (1993) through the streets of history. Latour remarks that Western history is made up of revolutionary events, isolated geniuses and radical discoveries. History is not made of everyday repetitions and small evolutions but is a fresco of heroic wars and cruel defeats. This discontinuity between the grand and the ordinary leaves untouched a plethora of minute transformations that silently worm their way into the greater reproduction of culture. Einstein and Pasteur are portrayed as if they had invented an entirely new science from a *tabula rasa*. However, it is more accurate simply to say that they added a new idea, however grand, to the pile of knowledge that was already there. Admittedly, the metaphor of accumulation or capitalisation here is not entirely fair, but one can say that men digest old books more than they write new stories (Descartes 1996); or to use a biological metaphor: 'nothing is lost, nothing is created, everything is transformed.'

There are many examples of scalable traditions which may illustrate how acquired gestures and techniques are slowly transformed as the context changes, such as a new type of food available on the market, whilst still retaining strong links with past habits. Acculturation is a slow process that eludes our tendency to categorise everything as old or new, as traditional or modern. Social phenomena that appear 'modern' are frequently easily traceable in recent history. The high consumption of soft drinks by Maltese people is seen as a recent change, and more precisely, as a negative effect of globalisation and mass production. In my historical research, I have found that the Maltese people's love of sweet and concentrated drinks is not a recent trend at all, but was already well established in the dietary habits of the Maltese at the end of the nineteenth century when the local black, sweetened house wine was the primary drink (Billiard 2010). At that time, water was suspected of carrying infectious diseases and its dull taste made it unappetizing. The consumption of soft drinks, produced since the 1930s in Maltese villages by a diversity of small producers, seems to be a direct derivative of the ancient love of sweet wine. More generally, it is not surprising to see to what extent soft drinks are popular in the Mediterranean, knowing that sugar had been produced in this region by the Arabs, centuries before it was introduced in Europe (Braudel 1996). Taste preferences can survive in diverse forms but practices are constantly evolving. We artificially extract social phenomena from their historical context or from their cultural meaning to label them 'new trends' or 'vestiges'.

I will give three examples of contemporary Maltese products which have opposite connotations: one, *Kinnie*, is seen as modern and unhealthy, and the other two, wine and olive oil, are considered traditional, typical and a part of the 'recommended' Mediterranean diet. *Kinnie* is a uniquely Maltese soft drink which was developed in 1952 by a local firm, Simonds Farsons Cisk. Its success has made it a family staple and somewhat of a matter of pride for the Maltese. However, it is unlikely that, in the eventuality that Simonds Farsons Cisk applied for protection rights or appellation, *Kinnie* would be recognised as a traditional drink or would be protected as a typical product. Because of its high level of sugar and its belonging to the category of fizzy soft drinks, *Kinnie* may not only be perceived as unhealthy, but also as a product of globalisation, even if it is unique to Malta. On the other hand, the recent introduction of quality wine and olive oil production on the Maltese islands[8] has been encouraged by both the Maltese government and the European Union. Local producers are slowly establishing a Protected Designation of Origin (PDO) for their wine and oil. All these Maltese products contain local and imported ingredients and are processed in factories for commercialisation. They may be harmful if consumed heavily, but only the soft drink gets the blame. Most importantly, the quality of wine and olive oil products dates back hardly more than a decade whereas *Kinnie* is a long-established drink. Does a tradition need to comply with the romanticized idea of the Mediterranean diet? In an article entitled 'When traditions become trendy' (2006), I argue that the selection of Maltese traditional foods is little more than a reproduction of the 'Mediterraneanist' stereotypes.

It appears obvious that the definition of tradition is highly political. Moreover, far from being neutral, the labelling of foods as traditional produces a new reality. The institutions and individuals with the power to decree what is traditional are powerful agents of change. In Malta, the codification of traditional Maltese recipes has produced a new image of Maltese culture in general and has been adopted in government health programmes. People are told that their current cooking practices are not only unhealthy, but also unfaithful to their nation. Far from preserving old food practices, the typification of 'authentic' Maltese food has led to the plantation of thousands of olive trees and vines, mostly shipped from foreign countries.

A close look at how the European Commission (EuroFIR), UNESCO, Food and Agriculture Organization (FAO) and World Health Organization (WHO) on the definition of tradition in different contexts, reveals the difficulty of distinguishing between 'true' and 'false' traditions. For instance, it is stated that the continuity in the production and consumption of any traditional food should be testified, but this obstacle may be circumvented by a further rule that authorises the reintroduction of old abandoned practices. How traditional food production is defined is presented, for example, in the definition of EuroFIR (Weichselbaum *et al.* 2009: 5–6):

> The production and/or processing of a food that:
>
> - has been transmitted from generation to generation through oral tradition or other means and
> - has been applied prior to the Second World War and remains in use (taking into account cases where composition was abandoned for a time and then reinstated) despite its adjustment to binding rules from national or EU food hygiene regulation or the incorporation of technical progress, under the condition that production and/or processing remains in line with methods used originally and that the food's intrinsic features such as its physical, chemical, microbiological features are maintained.

In the case of olive oil in Malta, production had ceased for almost a thousand years,[9] and it was only reintroduced in the late 1990s, as a direct effect of the lucrative economic returns propelled by a new-found fashion for olive oil and tourist consumption. Yet, olive oil has earned its undisputed status as a Maltese traditional ingredient. In 2007, a partly European funded project

(PRIMO) succeeded in grafting foreign trees with a local species and came up with more than 300 'indigenous' trees. The plantation of the indigenous olive trees enabled the local producers eventually to obtain a PDO. With the aid of European funding and the enthusiasm of some Maltese olive lovers, a sudden interest spread throughout Malta in olive trees that had been forgotten for centuries. Some trees, which are said to be around 2000 years old, have become monuments of national pride. After a former jeweller and a local bank started the revival, local small producers started to be lured in. A new tradition has been created. This new tradition is, however, seldom affordable for the great majority of the Maltese population who buy quite often the oil, sold in small bottles, as souvenir. It is also debatable as there are no popular Maltese recipes containing olive oil in cookery books published before the 1990s.

Traditions are not pure vestiges, something of the past that the contemporary world receives passively as is. It appears, on the contrary, that a process of arbitrary selection of a desired self image is at play (Pouillon 1975). Tradition institutes a reversed filiation where the sons reinvent the fathers' knowledge, and where the present reconstructs the past. As Gérard Lenclud ironically states (1987: 119): 'Tradition is a process of paternity recognition..'[10] Another unresolved difficulty in the definition of EuroFir of 'real' traditions is to establish a cut-off point in time after which no practice or product can be recognised as traditional. The EuroFIR and the FAO agreed that a practice, which has originated since the Second World War, could not be recognised as traditional. The Second World War is considered as 'a time barrier before which the food industrial revolution did not exist, a time when populations still applied simple and time-honoured approaches.' (Trichopoulou *et al.* 2006: 503). According to this definition, individuals did not approach life and its vicissitudes in the same 'simple and time-honoured' way after the Second World War. This condition is not only a subjective opinion based on no recorded evidence, but is also very ethnocentric. Indeed, for many colonies, independence has probably had an impact on their populations' habits stronger than that of the Second World War.

It seems that, in the mind of many legislators, there are two distinct periods: one before the Second World War, when life was slow and pots were simmering in kitchens, and another, after the Second World War, when all of a sudden life became hectic and microwaves denatured the cooking skills of housewives now unable to transmit their knowledge to their daughters orally. This opposition finds many parallels which reinforce it, among them the dualism between local and global, or between authenticity and modernity. Why these oppositions are subjective and evasive has been extensively discussed, notably by Arjun Appadurai (1996), Jean-Pierre Warnier (2002) and Daniel Miller (2012), to quote just a few. I would, however, emphasise that the definition of tradition once again escapes any effort to reduce it to something attached to a territory or to a particular time-frame. There is continuity in time and in space, and any attempt to break it into events or regions is artificial and as such political.

The definition of tradition is political because it determines which products and local cultural heritages gain the right to be protected and to survive. The decision on the traditional quality of a practice or product is also political because it is a projection and dissemination of a national ideal or is, more broadly, based on western cultural categories. Finally, the determination of tradition is political because, linking a tradition to a territory and to a local history places it at the core of the battle for local, or national identity. However widespread the opposition between tradition and modernity may be, it tends to be unique in every society. The attributes of authenticity, industrialism or modernity take on a distinct local hue depending on the cultural context. To illustrate the way individuals play with such dichotomies, I will now describe the Maltese situation.[11]

Playing with tradition versus modernity

During the fieldwork that I conducted for my PhD, I encountered a central dichotomy in everyday food discourse: Italian food as opposed to British food. It becomes clear that, in food-related issues, 'Britishness' is associated with modernity, and for this reason, is seen by some Maltese as destructive of traditional values, and by others as progressive. Although corned beef and mashed potatoes are a welcome novel importation for many Maltese, they are rejected by the conservative elite as being unauthentic and unhealthy. On the other hand, Italian cuisine, considered the epitome of Mediterranean food, is regarded as healthy and local. In a nutshell, 'Britishness' is associated with industrialisation and modernity and 'Italianness' with tradition and family orientation.

In this cultural framework, the recent vogue for traditional resurgence and the search for a national Maltese food have been inspired predominantly by Italian cuisine. Today, Maltese cookery books are proud of being influenced by Italian cuisine and they tend to despise or ignore any British influence. However, in practice, Maltese cuisine is an eclectic mix of Mediterranean and British ingredients and techniques. Maltese people love their fried potatoes with vinegar and Worcestershire sauce as much as they love pasta and pizzas. The Maltese have more than two locally produced beers and the local soft drink, *Kinnie*. Housewives are proud to show that they know to prepare mushroom soup, and trifle[12] and pudding[13] were the most common desserts mentioned during interviews conducted in 2006. Sandwiches are also an important part of the Maltese diet: ham and cheese sandwiches or toast plastered with Bovril[14] are amongst the most common dishes for light dinners. Furthermore, the British influence on Maltese food is not even a recent phenomenon. Corned beef and potatoes were integrated into the Maltese diet at the same time that pasta was introduced, around the turn of the twentieth century (Tannahill 1988).

Nonetheless, the recent defence of traditional Maltese food promotes a romanticised, or even stereotyped, fanfare of rural recipes which is cleansing the history books of any reference to corned beef or Bovril. For instance, the old recipe for vegetable soup, *minestra*, is never described in books with an added spoon of Worcestershire sauce or Bovril concentrate, yet these ingredients have been fully integrated into the modern version of *minestra*. Another example is the habit of adding corned beef to the Sunday roast potato dish called *patata l-forn*. This vernacular variation of a revered traditional dish has been common for many years, but it would be hard to find any mention of it in cookery books. This discrepancy between discourse and practice highlights, once again, the opposition between Italian and British culture and the general inaccuracy of the beliefs attached to each nationality.

The representation of the Italian and British cultures in Malta is as schematic as the rose-tinted vision the British may have of Malta. Whereas Malta is neither modern nor backward, its extremely dense population leaves little place to wander through its Mediterranean countryside; similarly, Britain is not made up solely of gentlemen playing cricket in suits. These stereotypes can be used or misused to qualify just about anything since they bring with them all sorts of connotations. To be Maltese, one has to master the dichotomy between traditional *versus* modern, associating it with Italian *versus* British characteristics. This application of globally familiar dichotomies is adapted to the Maltese context.

In another context, Daniel Miller (2005) has shown how the opposition between tradition and modernity finds its cultural relevance in the opposition between black and red in Trinidad. Similar to the case in Malta, in Trinidad soft drinks are the most popular beverage. They are broadly divided between red and black, the latter best represented by Coca-Cola and the former comprising a wide range of orange-flavoured drinks. First imported by the US soldiers that 'freed' the archipelago from British colonial power, Coca Cola has become associated with modernity and with black Trinidadians (descendants of slaves), while the red soft drinks are associated with the minority Indian population, the bearers of traditional values. According to Miller, this cultural framework is shared by the whole population. These two case studies show the versatility of the dichotomy but Miller adds another very interesting point: he insists that this framework, which is present in everyday discourse, is not to be confused with the actual food behaviours of Trinidadians. Indeed, if Indian Trinidadians are said to drink more red soft drinks, and African Trinidadians to favour black ones, in reality this is not the case. Miller points out that, in actual fact, the African Trinidadians, considered as the representatives of 'modernity', are looking nostalgically for traditions that induce them to drink more red soft drinks than their Indian compatriots who prefer to 'ingest modernity' by consuming black soft drinks. The connotations around a food item do influence its consumption but not in a literal sense. As Miller notices (*ibid*.: 64): "Africans drinking a red sweet drink consume what for them is a highly acceptable image of Indian-ness that is an essential part of their sense of being Trinidadian." To conclude, Trinidadians as much as Maltese use the dichotomy between tradition and modernity, compartmenting the reality between the two categories. In Trinidad, tradition is linked to Indian people and to red soft drinks while modernity is associated with African Trinidadians and black sweet drinks. In Malta, tradition means Italian, family values and mother's recipes, while modernity is associated with the British and seen as progressive and industrial. The play around such references is at the core of both the Maltese and the Trinidadian collective heritage because creating and understanding categories helps people reaffirm their shared identity.

The dichotomy between tradition and modernity, however artificial, is useful in many countries to instigate an identity discourse. In this respect, tradition should be studied locally, as a category of thought, but not be used by researchers as a neutral tool.

Fixing traditions

Several authors have formulated the popular sentiment of the loss of cooking skills in a world where kitchens are built with high-tech appliances and where cooking is reduced to pressing a button (Méchin 2000; Sutton 2001). As we have seen in the previous definition of traditional process given by the EuroFIR (Weichselbaum 2009), at the core of the general understanding of tradition, there is oral inter-generational transmission. But what do people mean when they speak about oral traditions? Do people succeed in transmitting their complete knowledge through words? How is it possible to 'preserve' traditions when they can no longer be transmitted from master to apprentice, but rather through impersonal means (books, computers or museum display)? The answers to these questions will lead to a new conception of the learning processes. I shall use and take as given the various assumptions of time, which have been discussed above.

When a food product and its production are recognised as traditional or typical, the producers have to follow very detailed and fixed specifications to maintain their certification (Marie-Vivien in this volume). These directives are presumably the result of the lengthy work of digging through archives and collecting evidence to prove the typicality of a product, a documentation process that may take several years. This documentation imposes on the local producers the necessity of working with scientists, historians and anthropologists. It obliges farmers to be removed from their usual environment of food production and to deal with entrepreneurs, technocrats and heritage managers. As a consequence, the production is scrutinised from the perspective of control that has a direct bearing on the process itself. A small producer has to strike a balance between retaining the eligibility for EU protection for instance, to make a better product while remaining economically viable. Maltese farmers and hunters have been faced with such scrutiny and have been quick to adopt new practices, such as transforming their bird trapping spaces into olive orchards.[15] The traditional practice is reproduced from then onwards, not following purely ancestral methods but following instead a new regime of regulations and economic realities.

Such an institutionalised approach to preserving tradition poses two major problems. First of all, we saw that the documentation demanded for submitting an application for protection implies describing the methods, the people involved in the product and the environmental conditions, with a vocabulary and from a perspective completely alien to the original context of production. In the same way, preserving 'oral' recipes in books or displaying artefacts in museums implies an extraction from the cultural and social environment, and consequently, the aims and meanings are changed. For example, nowadays Maltese do not cook the sober vegetable soup *minestra* for economic reasons, but for reasons of nostalgia and health. Slow cooking is another example of transformation and a divergence from the traditional context. In the past, when women sat next to simmering pots for hours, it was simply because there was no possibility of doing otherwise. As David Sutton (2001) points out judiciously, it was also a way for men to keep their wives at home. Slow cooking made sense at a time and in a society with a strong gender division. Nowadays, the slow food movement has become a trendy political tool that aims to counter the fast path of modern life and the globalisation of food imports. Yet, slow cooking is done by different people for different reasons in different environments. My second concern with the establishment of fixed parameters is that it does not enable food recipes or practices to evolve by the addition of a new ingredient or the use of new utensil. When, prior to any regulation, a recipe gave rise to many diverse interpretations in different farms or kitchens, and could still be referred to by its own name, now, any change has to be duly recorded and discussed to see if it is a major or acceptable variation.

Improvisation and evolution are not welcome in the certified world of traditional food. Similar to the case of language and dialects and the establishment of standard spelling and grammar, the protected food product is now asked to follow strict specifications in order to keep its label. A tradition has become a norm. In the same way, an oral language is fixed once its spelling and grammar is standardised. In France, before the late eighteenth century, there was no fixed spelling and therefore writers such as Voltaire could write words as they wished. Now that the French orthography has been established, a student is punished for his 'mistakes' (Lenclud 1987: 49). As concerning Malta, for a long time vernacular language did not seem to interest the elite who spoke Italian or French or a *lingua franca* before speaking English, until the nationalist movement decided Maltese should be a national language. It was only in 1937 that the Maltese language was fixed by grammatical rules, a unique alphabet and spelling specifications. Nowadays misspellings are common in Malta and they are the subject of numerous jokes, since there is an institutionalised 'right' way to write Maltese.

A parallel between food traditions and language can provide insight into the integration of new elements. In Malta, many English words have been integrated into the dictionary, and it has been decided that they should be spelled in a Maltese way rather than keeping their English orthography. Therefore, a roundabout in the Maltese dictionaries is written *rawndebawt*, and cake, *kejk*. The reason behind this decision is that some English words have become part of the Maltese language and have to follow the Maltese rules of spelling. Similarly, foreign recipes have been adopted by Maltese cuisine and transformed to suit the Maltese taste according to the ingredients available.

During my fieldwork and my personal travels, I am always curious to see the many mutations of recipes such as *quiche lorraine* or pizza. Cooking traditions travel and their popularity is a direct consequence of their versatility. Sylvie Sanchez (2008) has argued that pizza became famous when it was imported by Italian migrants to the USA. Pizzas are difficult to define as they may be sweet or salty, thin and crunchy, or thick and moist, every country adding its favourite ingredient such as sausages, Emmental cheese or pineapple. I have seen *quiche lorraine* prepared in Cameroon, Malta, France, Spain, England and Italy in many diverse ways: with onions and ham, with puff pastry or short crust, with or without fresh cream or even with skimmed milk and corn flour or with ricotta cheese. It is specifically against these apparent distortions that the protection of tradition has been enforced. The case of pizza is revealing of the difficulty of fixing any recipe. Everybody agrees that the American pizza with its characteristic super-imposition of many layers of ingredients and the Hawaiian pizza which contains pineapple are neither genuine nor traditional pizzas. In 2008, the European Commission has accepted that the Neapolitan pizza was protected by a Traditional Specialty Guaranteed (TSG).[16] But for the anthropologist Sanchez (2007), the original pizza is not only far from this protected 'Neapolitan pizza', it was also strongly disliked by Italians except for the poorest Neapolitans. In the streets of Naples, the pizza was made with yeast, cheese, animal fat and a few basil leaves, and was very unpopular before it reached the new world where it was reformulated (Dickie 2007). The original recipe was not what we imagine and, moreover, it quite often became wildly appreciated in other cultural contexts through its exportation and its adaptation.

Taking a radically different standpoint from the assumption that traditions are fixed, one may argue that traditions are constantly evolving. Cooking is about finding the right balance between following the rules and improvising according to the context in which the food is prepared. It is almost unfixable, and thus, enables people from all over the world to enrich their daily cooking routine. Fixing a recipe or any process is, however, not only sad for all these reasons, but it also hinders any transmission, and thus, metaphorically speaking, kills the tradition. Cooking skills are learnt through long practice and they carry with them a whole set of values that are far more complex than the simple step-by-step methods of even the best cookbooks.

Learning to cook

> Consider a cookbook. The book is packed with information about how to prepare a selection of mouth-watering dishes. But is it in this information that the knowledge of the cook consists?"
>
> (Ingold 1997)

The recipe for Mornay sauce as presented by Tim Ingold has become a classic. Criticizing one of the favourite examples of Dan Sperber (1996), Ingold gives us a clear demonstration that "the information in the recipe book is not, in itself, knowledge" (*ibid.*: 137).

Mornay sauce is supposed to be a culinary tradition transmitted from one generation to another. The recipe is made up of a series of instructions that were transmitted orally in the past, but are written down nowadays, so that, according to Sperber, any reader can follow these instructions simply by looking in the book. Nothing more is presupposed than the ability to read. This means that the ink patterns -identified as letters- can be translated into action in the reader's mind. Ingold points out that Sperber affirms that, after having read the Mornay sauce recipes, "the reader will form a mental representation of the recipe, which he can remember, forget, or transform and which he can also follow – that is, convert it into bodily behaviour" (Sperber 1996: 61). However, Ingold argues that there is no evidence that the reader will understand what he is reading nor that he will know how to put it into practice. How does the novice come to know what it means to 'bring the milk to a boil' or how to 'make a *roux*'? In fact, specific cooking vocabulary can be relatively difficult to acquire and cooking for that reason becomes, at some stage, a profession requiring long training. Ingold's argument goes beyond the vocabulary problem. Even if the reader has learnt from books or watched videos on the Internet, he still has to acquire the precise gestures and the sensory knowledge to make the sauce.

The cook is able to follow the recipe because it speaks to his/her own prior experience. He/she must have experienced butter melting at the rate that keeps it from burning and must previously have handled such substances as flour, eggs or milk and he/she must be in an environment where he/she knows where to get them (Leudar and Costall 2009). As Ingold states (2001: 137): "The verbal commands of the recipe, in other words, draw their meaning not from their attachment to mental representations in my head, but from their positioning within the familiar context of my activity in the home". So the apprentice gets to know how to put these instructions into practice by working with skilled practitioners in the kitchen or elsewhere. Thus 'all knowledge is founded in skill' (Ingold 1997). Practice is prior to mental representation. Contrary to Sperber's concept of transmission which separates the acquisition of knowledge from its practical enactment, Ingold argues that mental representations are built from practice.

Pierre Bourdieu (1977) had previously developed the idea that our mental representations are embodied and acquired through practice. The author of Outline of a Theory of Practice developed 'a dispositional theory of action' recognising that individuals actively construct social reality through 'categories of perception, appreciation and action.' But, unlike the phenomenologists, Bourdieu insists that, while being resilient and shared, these categories are not universal, but are socially constructed. To bridge the commonly opposed conceptions of the individual either as a puppet blindly following the system of values in his/her society, or on the contrary, as an agent free to interpret the social rules to his/her best interest, Bourdieu retrieved the concept of 'habitus' from philosophers such as Aristotle and Husserl. Habitus can be roughly defined as a set of socially learnt skills that are often taken for granted, and which are acquired through the experiences of everyday life. Each social group has a way to react to life and to think about the world but, as Bourdieu stresses, this is not learnt through direct communication (in school, for instance) but through daily experience. The habitus: "ensures the active presence of past experiences which, deposited in each organism in the form of schemata of thought and action, tend, more surely than all formal rules and all explicit norms, to guarantee the conformity of practices and their constancy across time" (Bourdieu 1990: 91).

Bourdieu's analysis adds a social perspective to the work of Ingold. It gives an explanation of how each social class transmits a bodily knowledge together with a perceptual structure. Habitus is a set of acquired dispositions. No one is born a cook: the training of a professional cook consists not only of daily cooking, but also of a life in the kitchen where the apprentice learns to find his/her place in the hierarchy and where he/she acquires a pride in special tasks or a drill for the rush hour. Habitus operates beneath the level of consciousness and discourse; the cook embodies tastes and skills without necessarily being able to speak about this. Habitus varies by social location and trajectory: individuals with different life experiences will have gained varied ways of thinking, feeling and acting; their primary dispositions will be more or less distant from those required for the performance of haute cuisine, and thus, they will be more or less invested in, and adept at, picking up the craft (Wacquant 2011).

Bourdieu's theory of practice thus specifies that skills cannot be dissociated from the individual's habitus. In other words, learning to cook a Mornay sauce is not about being able to follow the instructions but about integrating a complex system of representations and bodily dispositions that structures the way the apprentice will perceive and react to his/her environment which is not limited to the kitchen. Thus traditions, understood as skills, cannot be detached from their cultural and social contexts. They are not learnt in isolation, but within a specific cultural environment. Transmitting a tradition is teaching, willingly or unwillingly, a particular vision of the world.

Sadly this is not taken into consideration by institutions that extract the aspect of practice from its cultural context to be able to 'preserve' it, in a word, to stop the erosion of time; a paradox for institutions that simultaneously declare their proud intent to protect cultural diversity.

The creativity of practice

Despite the amount shared by a social group, the system of representations and dispositions that accompanies any tradition remains, nonetheless, particular to each individual. Just as each word has a different range of meanings for each person, so each recipe has a different taste for each consumer. For this reason people discuss at length the meaning of a word or the best way to make Mornay sauce or to cook stuffed calamari (squid) or the wine they have tasted with the best reputation. In a similar way, in Malta, old people divulge the secret spot on the coast where they find sea urchins, and each individual will have his own reminiscences attached to the place and to the taste of a particular sea urchin. This is exactly what a recipe, precise as it may be, can never transmit. In this sense, recipes are rather like stories: a narrative structure that gives steps to be followed: bring the milk to a boil, then pour it into the melted butter… etc. However, stories are not the vehicle for intergenerational transmission of encoded messages which, once deciphered, reveal an all-embracing system of mental representations, because stories do not come with their meaning attached, they have different meanings for different people. What they actually mean is rather something that the listener has to discover for him/herself by placing the narrative in the context of his/her own life history. Knowledge is not transmitted 'to' the apprentice but rather knowledge grows 'in' the apprentice (Ingold 2010). What the apprentice actually acquires is not a perfect replica of his/her master's knowledge. What the apprentice wishes to do is to copy the master's production (and along the way develop his/her own personal touch).

Learning is a matter of copying. A daughter wants to achieve the same stuffed calamari as her mother did. However, she knows, or will learn, that she can never succeed. She tries with determination to imitate her mother's gestures yet she will never be capable of achieving a perfect replica, just as one can never step twice into the same river. However, through this attempt to copy, the apprentice learns to sense and to adapt to the situation. In this way, after repeated trials, gestures can be adjusted to adapt to a multisensory monitoring of the task as it unfolds. Learning through practice, even when it involves imitating or copying, is a creative process, "a guided rediscovery" as Ingold (2000: 356) calls it.

That creativity lies not in innovation but in improvisation. The apprentice does not wish to invent or to innovate, but to understand the cooking tricks he/she is able to observe in his/her master's practice. In this perspective, "every step of problem-solving is itself an exploratory movement within that world" (Ingold 1997). Thus, when copying, the apprentice develops his/her own voice, own style, own personality. As a consequence, rediscovered traditions are translated and transformed according to the apprentice and the environment. These are transformed not only when the apprentice is in his/her learning phase, but every time he/she carries out the recipe, every time he/she changes environment and must adapt to the new tools available and prove his/her ingenuity by finding or replacing unavailable ingredients.

Conclusion

To assume that protecting food traditions stems from a well-intended desire to counter-balance the power of giant corporations is both simplistic and erroneous. A close look at the definition of tradition offers a greater understanding of the current trend towards 'protecting' traditional produce. The meaning of tradition is often based on a linear time line and a fragmented history. Cut-off points in time, such as the Second World War, have been artificially created but they quickly reveal their arbitrariness. On the contrary, one can argue that traditions should be taken not as a tool of study, but as the objects of study. This chapter has offered examples[17] where the duality tradition/modernity takes on different meanings in different social contexts. The way people use this dichotomy reveals a lot about their vision of themselves in the world (as in a peripheral nation such as Malta), and can be especially useful in post-colonial studies. One cannot, however, condemn the use of the word tradition as it is still crucial to the understanding of both continuity and change in societies and the transmission processes. The definition, in this case, must be completely reformulated and kept free of any time or space limitations as this would inevitably insert traditions into a political discourse. Traditions are living skills that are rediscovered by every apprentice in his/her practice with a master. Learning through practice engages the body, the senses, the environment and the mind together. Because mental representations cannot be transmitted, it becomes evident that books, computers or any artefact that intends to extract tradition from its practice are bound to fail. What needs to be insisted upon is that traditions, as rediscovered skills, relocate the individual in his/her society, because the apprentice shares emotions with his/her masters, immersed in a unique sensual and moral environment. It therefore becomes clear that traditions are a thing of the present and not a whimsical vestige of the past.

Notes

1 The product or practice in question is required to be certified as authentically traditional by authorities such as UNESCO or the French INAO (Institut National des Appellations d'Origine). These institutions are moral judges deciding whether a tradition is worth keeping. For instance the tradition of female circumcision is not part of the protection programme of UNESCO.
2 Lewis H. Morgan wrote (1871: 165): "Among the traditions of the Senecas there is one to the effect that they had a distinct and independent history anterior to the epoch of their confederation with the other Iroquois nations."
3 I conducted fieldwork in Malta from 2004 to 2008.
4 In 1964, Malta was granted independence, thus becoming a sovereign nation. Ten years later Malta became a Republic, the nation remaining within the British Commonwealth.
5 This is why I have argued elsewhere (2006) that the repertoire of recipes commonly named 'Traditional Maltese Food' can be called an 'invented tradition' following Eric Hobsbawm's famous definition (1992: 1): "a set of practices, normally governed by overtly or tacitly accepted rules and of a ritual or symbolic nature, which seek to inculcate certain values and norms of behaviour by repetition, which automatically implies continuity with the past." Hobsbawm insists that if invented traditions look old, their relation with the past is tenuous at best. It is more accurate to see invented tradition as "responses to novel situations which take the form of reference to old situations, or which establish their own past by quasi-obligatory repetition." (*ibid.*: 2).
6 Some characteristics of Maltese society are commonly misconceived as backward, for instance: the high percentage of women as housewives, the strong adherence to religious faith and rituals, the absence of divorce laws (until 2011), the deplorable state of the roads, etc.
7 Some have even argued that this obsession with documenting the past makes us more traditionalist than the so-called traditional societies usually associated with 'oral society' or societies which have a limited use of writing (Lenclud 1987).
8 This introduction of wine and olive oil production has been helped by foreign experts from France, Italy and Spain who have contributed by setting up an up-to-date savoir-faire.
9 The Phoenicians brought olive trees to Malta and the Romans maintained the practice of olive pressing. Village names like Zejtun, Ħaz-Zebbug and Birzebbuga reflect the connection of these localities with this crop and its oil as, in Maltese, *zejt* means oil and *zebbug* olive. However, during the Arab period, olive cultivation was replaced with cotton. It seems that even during the sixteenth century, olive oil continued to be exported from Malta, but the quantities were small, and possibly the oil was imported from Tunisia, Malta being just a transit port. However, historians like Simon Mercieca (2001) insist that this 'liquid of gold' (as it was called), was too

expensive to be used in everyday cooking. It is more likely that the oil was sold as fuel for oil lamps.

10 "La tradition est un processus de reconnaissance en paternité."

11 I am quoting an extract from an unpublished communication "Negotiating Maltese Identity between Italy and Britain" given during the conference entitled Islands and Britishness, held in June 2009 and organized by the University of Huddersfield, Scotland.

12 *Trifle* is a dessert that originated in England. It is made of custard, fruit, sponge cake, fruit juice or gelatine, and whipped cream. The layers of ingredients give the typical appearance of the trifle.

13 In Malta, bread pudding is referred as '*puddina tal-hobz*'. Like *trifle*, pudding is a truly English dessert. Christmas, rice and bread puddings illustrate the versatility of the recipe, always based on starchy ingredients and milk.

14 Bovril is a British meat extract introduced in Malta in 1870s. It can be consumed as a warm drink when diluted with hot water. It can also be used for flavouring soups, stews or porridge, or for spreading on bread, like Marmite and Vegemite.

15 In the hamlet of Manikata, inhabitants decided to convert their tiny terraced plots of lands into olive groves for oil. Cultivation of these dry and rocky fields had been abandoned and the land was used for bird trapping. Farmer-hunters told me that the decision to plant olive trees was based on three reasons: the 700 trees came free (they were mostly given by private enterprises), the project was part of a wider project for the enhancement of the local environmental heritage (Koperattiva Rurali Manikata), and finally, bird trapping was increasingly prejudiced and restricted because of the decreasing number of migratory birds. Therefore the change to olive production does not stem from a straightforward concern for preserving local traditions.

16 "An agricultural product intended for human consumption or foodstuff with a traditional composition, or produced according to a traditional production method may obtain the label Traditional Speciality Guaranteed (TSG). This possibility encourages the diversification of agricultural production and has positive consequences in several areas." (Council Regulation (EC), No 5009.2006 of 20 March 2006 on agricultural products and foodstuffs as traditional specialities guaranteed).

17 In Malta, tradition and modernity are reflected in the opposition between Italian and British cultures; in Trinidad, Miller tells us, red soft drinks represent tradition while black soft drinks stand for modernity (Miller 2005). We saw that nostalgia is, ironically, becoming the ultimate modern stance, where slow cooking, a practice symbolising the good old days, is being reintroduced to fight back against modern 'loss of culture'.

References

Appadurai, A. (1996). *Modernity At Large: Cultural Dimensions of Globalization*, Minneapolis: University of Minnesota Press.

Billiard, E. (2006). "When traditions become trendy", *Anthropological Notebooks*, Vol. 12 (1): 113–126.

Billiard, E. (2010). "Searching for a national cuisine", *Journal of Maltese History*, Vol. 2 (1): 47–57.

Bourdieu, P. (1984). *Distinction, A Social Critic of the Judgment of Taste,* Cambridge, MA: Harvard University Press.

Bourdieu, P. (1977). *Outline of a Theory of Practice*, Cambridge: Cambridge University Press.

Bourdieu, P. (1990). *The Logic of Practice*, Cambridge: Polity Press, 1st publication 1980.

Braudel, F. (1996). *The Mediterranean and the Mediterranean World in the Age of Philip II*, Vol. 1, Berkeley, CA: University of California Press.

Descartes, R. (1996). *Meditations on First Philosophy*, Cambridge: Cambridge University Press, 1st publication 1651.

Dickie, J. (2007). *Delizia!: The Epic History of the Italians and their Food*, Great Britain: Hodder & Stoughton.

Fabian, J. (2003). *Time and the Other: How Anthropology Makes its Object*, New York: Columbia University Press.

Hobsbawm, E. (1992). "Introduction", in E. Hobsbawm and T. Ranger (eds.), *The Invention of Tradition*, pp. 1–14. Cambridge: Cambridge University Press, 1st publication 1983.

Ingold, T. (1997). *From the Transmission of Representations to the Education of Attention*. http://lchc.ucsd.edu/mca/Paper/ingold/ingold1.htm (retrieved on 12.09.2011).

Ingold, T. (2000). *The Perception of the Environment. Essay in Livelihood, Dwelling and Skill*, London & New York: Routledge.

Ingold, T. (2001). "Capacity, competence and skill", in. H. Whitehouse (ed.), *The Debated Mind: Evolutionary Psychology Versus Ethnography*, pp. 113–153. Oxford: Berg Publishers.

Ingold, T. (2010). *To learn Is To Improvise A Movement Along A Way Of Life*, Seminar given at the London School of Economics 27 April 2010.

Latour, B. (1993). *We Have Never Been Modern*, Harvard, MA: Harvard University Press.

Lenclud, G. (1987). "La tradition n'est plus ce qu'elle était…", *Terrain*, Vol. 9 : 110–123.

Leudar, I. and Costall, A. (2009). *Against Theory of Mind*, New York: Palgrave Macmillan.

Mauss, M. (1990). *Gift: The Form and Reason for Exchange in Archaic Societies*, New York: Norton, 1st publication 1924.

Méchin, C. (2000). "Le four à micro-ondes, usages et représentations", *Revue des Sciences Sociales*, Vol. 27: 117–125, 'La révolution des cuisines', ed. by I. Bianquis.

Mercieca, S. (2001). "'Il-Kultura ta' l-Ikel fl-Epoka Moderna", in D. Massa (ed.) *Malta: Esplorazzjoni Dghajsa Karti*, pp. 73–110. Malta: Universita of Malta.

Miller, D. (2005). "Coca-Cola; A black sweet drink from Trinidad", in J.L.Watson and M.L. Cadwell (eds.). *The Cultural Politics of Food and Eating: A Reader*, pp. 54–69. Malde, MA: Wiley-Blackwell Publishers.

Miller, D. (2012). *Worlds Apart: Modernity Through the Prism of the Local*, London: Routledge

Morgan, L.H. (1871). *Systems of Consanguinity and Affinity of the Human Family*, Lincoln: University of Nebraska Press.

Nietzsche, F. (2005). *The Use and Abuse of History*, New York: Cosimo.

Pouillon, J. (1975). "Tradition : transmission ou reconstruction", in J. Pouillon (ed.), *Fétiches sans fétichisme*, pp.155–173. Paris: Maspero.

Sanchez, S. (2007). *Pizza connexion. Une séduction transculturelle*, Paris: Editions du CNRS.

Sanchez, S. (2008). "Frontières alimentaires et mets transfrontaliers : la pizza, questionnement d'un paradoxe", *Anthropologie et Société*, Vol. 32(3) : 197–212.

Sperber, D. (1996). *Explaining Culture: A Naturalistic Approach*, Oxford: Blackwell Publishers.

Sutton, D. (2001). *Remembrance of Repasts: An Anthropology of Food and Memory*, New York: Berg Publishers.

Tannahill, R. (1988). *Food in History*, New York: Penguin Books.

Trichopoulos, A., Vasilopoulou, E., Georga, K., Soukara, S. and Dilis, V. (2006). "Traditional foods: why and how to sustain them", *Trends in Food Science and Technology*, Vol. 17: 498–504.

Wacquant, L. (2011). "Habitus as topic and tool: reflections on becoming a prizefighter", *Qualitative Research in Psychology*, Vol. 8: 81–92.

Warnier, J.-P. (2002). *La mondialisation de la culture*, Paris: La Découverte.

Weichselbaum, E., Benelam, B., and Costa, H.S. (2009). "Traditional foods in Europe". Synthesis report no. 6, *European Food Information resource EuroFir*. Under the sixth Framework Food Quality and Safety thematic Priority. www.EuroFir.net (retrieved on 12.09.2011).

4 The protection of traditional local foods through geographical indications in India

Delphine Marie-Vivien

Introduction

Traditional foods products are often from a specific place which means that, besides their roots in history and tradition, they have quality, characteristics or reputation due to their geographical origin. Compared to products in the same category, they usually benefit from an added value in the market. However, as one goes back in history, one finds numerous products differing widely from each other that have gained in reputation thanks to their geographical origin. It might be minerals (marble), art objects (bronze or terracotta), cloth (silk), perfume (incense) or agricultural products (honey). Such a reputation results from the specific know-how, skills and practices of local communities, usually but not necessarily, combined with elements of the natural environment such as climate, soil, water etc., what is called the '*terroir*' (Barham 2003). They reflect 'historical echoes and collective practices' grounded in a specific milieu (Bérard and Marchenay 2007). The geographical names used to designate those origin-based products may be protected as geographical indications (GIs).

The very old concept of GIs was first legalised in France and Europe through the protection of appellations of origin. For example, since the fifteenth century, Roquefort cheese has been the subject of a royal charter, granted to the inhabitants of Roquefort, conferring on them a monopoly over the maturing process which was carried out in well-guarded cellars. In the Middle Ages, guild trademarks were normally used to indicate the geographical origin of products. Many of these GIs are still used today, such as Murano glass named after the island near Venice where it was manufactured (O'Connor 2004). In 1905, following massive frauds in the wine industry, France implemented a legal framework to protect appellations of origin. This system was extended at the European level within the common market in 1992, and after tumultuous negotiations between the Old and the New Worlds (Addor and Grazzioli 2002), internationalised within the World Trade Organization (WTO) in 1995, as a trade regulation in the era of globalisation.

Products which gain a reputation thanks to their geographical origin are increasingly becoming desirable objects, perceived as 'local symbols', even though current globalisation might lead us to believe that they are going to disappear. On the other hand, this desire results from globalisation which does not entail the disappearance of 'local and regional products' but rather their emergence or reconstitution. Traditional origin-based products reflect cultural identity and, while economic growth is on the rise and populations are migrating beyond cultural frontiers, populations display a tendency to use their cultural identity as a rampart against globalisation (Bowen 2010). Indeed globalisation represents a threat to cultural identity. Local traditional products are vulnerable to the opening of frontiers for two reasons: first, the delocalisation of production which dilutes or refutes the close link between products and their origin; second, the waning of life styles which supported these traditional products due to the arrival of new products. Local traditional products are therefore the expression of the right to be different, "allowing the preservation of localization in the context of globalization".[1] Open to underprivileged producers, the objective of GIs is to boost the earnings of those producers by adding value to their products, making them remunerative enough to cover the cost involved in respecting traditional production methods (Van de Kop *et al.* 2004).

In this context, GIs were included in the Trade Related Aspects of Intellectual Property Rights (TRIPS) Agreement of the WTO. GIs are defined in article 23 as indications which "identify a good as originating in a region where a given quality, reputation or other characteristics of the good is essentially attributable to its geographical origin". It may be a geographical term, such as Champagne, Roquefort, Parmigianino Reggiano, Porto or any other sign which refers to a place, for example Feta for cheese in Greece or Basmati for rice in India/Pakistan. The TRIPS Agreement being part of the WTO package, all members must provide means for the protection of GIs in their own legal framework.

The example of India is particularly significant as it has a strong cultural identity founded on the thousands of years of its past and offers numerous products which are locally rooted such as, Basmati and Navara rice, Darjeeling tea, Malabar pepper, Coorg oranges, Dharwad *peḍha* (sweet) and *Feni* (liquor from Goa). According to Marie-Claude Mahias (1997), India defends the idea that the Indian tradition, in the area of 'material know-how', is as legitimate as any other tradition and can play a major role in nation building. India is therefore searching to protect GIs, legally and with commitment, for products reflecting its cultural identity and liable to be threatened by globalisation.

The practice consisting of naming products based on the place of production is well established in India. But the need to protect those names emerged mainly in 1990s with the Basmati case when India contested an American multinational company which had applied for patents for new Basmati rice varieties cultivated in the US and for trademarks evoking the indication, Basmati. Finally, the long legal battle won by India ended at the same time as the deadline for WTO to implement TRIPS obligations with the adoption of the Geographical Indications of Origin of Goods (Registration and Protection) Act, 1999, hereinafter called the GI Act, 1999 and later the Geographical Indications of Origin of Goods (Registration and Protection) Rules, 2002, hereinafter called the GI Rules, 2002 (Balganesh 2003). India may thus qualify as a new country in the Old World. Since then, India has manifested a strong interest in registering GIs at the national level, and also in Europe, and this dynamism is the best example among developing world countries. The GI Act, 1999 is actively implemented to protect horticulture products such as banana, mango, jasmine, spices, rice, tea, coffee as well as many handicraft goods in the domains of textile, woodcraft, etc. Agricultural products protected under the GI Act, 1999, are usually obtained from the cultivation of traditional plant varieties in the hope of preserving them and of avoiding any act of 'biopiracy' resulting from globalisation as happened in the case of Basmati. Compared to Europe where only agricultural products and foodstuffs are covered by European regulations, in India, GIs concern mainly the handicraft sector, and till now, few food products have been registered. Each Indian participant feels concerned and proceeds to GI registration, whether government bodies actively involved in the protection of the Indian heritage, intellectual property lawyers whose expertise serve in documenting the products and their regions, or universities convinced of the benefits of intellectual property rights (Soam 2005). For example, many GIs on horticultural products in Karnataka were registered by the Department of Horticulture of the Government of Karnataka, and those on spices by the Spice Board of India. Nevertheless, the producers are often unaware of the existence of GI, although it is a useful tool to protect, and give high value to, their products.

To better understand the challenges behind the protection of GIs in India, this chapter will first describe the GI Act, 1999, and then, give a full set of examples from the agricultural sector which demonstrate the dynamic effort going on in India to promote traditional food.

The Indian Geographical Indication of Origin of Goods: the GI Act, 1999

The GI Act, 1999 sets up a Registry of Geographical Indications,[2] which is a department of the Office of Intellectual Property under the umbrella of the Ministry of Commerce. A GI register has been developed with part A for registration of the GI, and part B for registration of authorised users. All GI applications are advertised in the GI Journal, accessible online at: http://ipindia.nic.in/girindia.

The link with the origin: emphasis on 'uniqueness'

'Uniqueness' is the innovative concept which prevails in India in determining what may be registered as a GI. The concept of 'uniqueness' enables a link to the origin to be expressed that allows for a broader understanding of the GI, which includes handicrafts in India.

The GI-1 form of a GI application includes 13 sections that must be filled out by the applicant. Six sections serve to determine the link between the product and its geographical origin: 'Specification', 'Description of goods', 'Geographical area of production and map', 'Proof of origin (Historical records)', 'Method of Production' and finally 'Uniqueness'. In practice, the data under 'Specification' and 'Description of the goods' provided by applicants are similar, relatively brief, and mention the main characteristics of products, whereas those under the 'Method of production' section are more consistent and detailed, and those under 'Proof of origin (Historical Records)' are entirely devoted to the history of the product and/or of the producers and the place. Indeed, in India, a GI product is, first and foremost, one that has been in existence for a long time; history is thus the main criterion for recognition as a GI. The GI application should also comprise the geographical map of the territory in which the goods are produced, originate or are being manufactured.

The core of the system is that the GI application must describe the particulars of special human skills involved, or the uniqueness of the geographical environment or other inherent characteristics.[3] However, the study of a full range of GIs applications shows that uniqueness is an autonomous concept that may be described as a criterion in its own right in view of the registration of a GI. In Europe, the criterion would be that of 'specificity' or 'typicality'.

The applications are examined by the GI Registry which comprises a consultative group of a maximum of seven members. These members are selected from institutions, such as universities, or from well-known organisations, for their expertise in the field of the application and ability to assess it.[4] Such substantive examination is a characteristic of the Indian system, similar to the European practice but very different from the trademark system used in the US for example. If the application is accepted, it is published in the *Official Journal of Geographical Indications* and becomes liable for potential opposition which may be submitted by any party within 3 months. If there is no opposition, the GI is validated by the Registrar, and then registered in Part A of the register of GIs, unless the Central Government decides otherwise.[5] The protection of the GI is established for 10 years, after that, an application may be filed for renewal.[6]

Applicant and authorised users

The entire requirements of the 'Method of production' and the 'Geographical area of production' described in the GI application have to be respected by the producers who wish to use the GI. But the producers and the users are different from the applicant who is, designated by the term 'registered proprietor', responsible for drafting the content of the GI.[7] GI being in its concept a collective right, the applicants may be any association of persons or producers or any organisation or authority established by or under any law that represents the interest of the producers of the concerned goods.[8] Interestingly, the Act does not explicitly state under what law an authority has to be established, nor what is meant by 'to represent the interest of the producers'. The applicant does not seem to be allowed to use the GI which can only be used by the producers. But, to obtain the right to use the GI, the producers have to register at the GI registry,[9] and for this, they need to get the approval of the applicant. Therefore, the role of the applicant is crucial because, first, it defines the content of the GI application, i.e. the method of production and the geographical area and, second, it gives its consent to producers to be authorised users.

Rights conferred

As any intellectual property right, GI registration confers exclusive rights to the use of the GI on the authorised users. GI registration mainly facilitates actions against misuse of the GI. It gives to both the registered proprietor of the GI and the authorised user the right to obtain relief in respect of infringement. Infringement means any use of the GI that indicates or suggests that goods originate in a geographical area other than the true place of origin in a manner as to mislead people. For example, the mention 'Darjeeling tea produced in Malaysia' is prohibited only if it misleads the public. The mention 'produced in Malaysia' might be enough to inform the public of the true origin of the tea, Malaysia, so that consumers are not misled. It also prevents any use as would constitute an act of unfair competition including copying.[10] According to the possibility offered by the TRIPS Agreement, the Central Government may provide additional protection to certain goods.[11] In that case, the use of any GI for goods which do not originate from the place indicated by the GI is prohibited, even if there is mention of the true origin of such goods, accompanied by expressions such as 'kind', 'style', 'imitation' or the like. For example, the mention 'Darjeeling tea produced in Malaysia' is prohibited even if it does not mislead the public, just because it uses the GI Darjeeling. The effect of such an additional protection is to reduce the burden of proof upon the users/proprietor of the GI regarding the misleading of the public. The registered proprietor together with the registered authorised users of the GI may apply for additional protection once it has been notified by the government.[12] This special protection is granted keeping in mind the reputation of the goods on the global scale.

Relation with trademarks

It is not possible to register a trademark if it contains or consists of a GI for goods that are the same but do not originate from the place indicated by that GI or when such use misleads the public as to the true origin of the good.[13] For example, it might be possible to register a trademark consisting of 'Malaysian Darjeeling Tea'. When the GI is protected under the additional protection scheme, it is not possible to register a trademark containing, or consisting of, such a GI without further justification. Therefore, any trademark comprising Darjeeling shall not be registered. In the case of trademarks registered in good faith before the GI was registered, nothing contained in the GI Act may prejudice the validity of the registration of such a trademark which can thus continue to exist.

Assignment

As GI is a right having some kind of 'public' flavour, the right can only be given to the original applicant, as a GI shall not be the subject matter of assignment, transmission, licensing, pledge, mortgage or any such other agreement. This is to secure the interest of the local producers, considering that the rights are linked to their territory and accessible to all of those located in the area. This point is very important as, by indicating the difference from a trademark, it characterises a GI.[14]

Traditional Indian products benefiting from GI protection

Since the implementation of the GI Act, 1999, in 2003, 272 GIs have been registered. One third of Indian registered GIs belong to the domain of agriculture: cereals, horticultural products, spices and wines. Many GIs have been registered in the area of horticulture, for products commercialised either for the local market or for export markets. Some GIs have been registered for rice varieties, as in the controversial and emblematic case of Basmati rice which is intensively exported, and some for local rice renowned for medicinal values. Finally GIs have also been registered for cash crops such as tea or coffee. Even if there are few GIs on agricultural products, the GI dynamic in this sector reflects the great diversity of the Indian sub-continent, inherited from its long agricultural history and from colonisation, as well as its wish to preserve its pool of genetic resources.

The uniqueness of food products justified by history

As in the case of GIs in the handicrafts domain, history is the glue attaching food products to their origin. Historical data which constitute the 'proof of origin' is primordial. For example, according to the GI application 'Allepey green Cardamom', the existence of cardamom crops in South India since the fourth century BC can be vouched for. Its history is described at length and embellished with much detail. Similarly the cultivation of jasmine is a very old practice in India, dating back, according to different historians, either to fourth century BC or to fourth century AD. Betel leaves, commonly used for mastication, started being cultivated 5000 years ago. The justifications for the GI 'Malda Fazli mango' are based on the Mahābhārata, the Sanskrit epic poem dated fourth century BC, testifying to the antiquity of mango crops. This predominance of history in the process will lead to registering GIs which are also names of traditional plant varieties.

Ancient Indian history will welcome a modern legal tool such as GIs in an original way, at a time of increasing nationalism. Indeed, this law was passed during the government of Bharatiya Janata Party (BJP), an ultra right-wing Hindu party which has built its entire political identity on a political history platform that promotes the Hindutva concept. A section of the BJP Members of Parliament (MP) was delighted that this law allows India to be a global player with its own products in the market. Shri Bikram Keshari Deo, for example, saw it as an awakening of India: "Right from Ghori, Lodi, Moghuls to British, when they were taking away everything, of ours, we were sleeping. It was a sound slumber with loud snoring. We did not wake up. This is an enactment of awakening though it is a belated awakening".[15] This explains the somewhat imperialist behaviour of India, desiring to protect everything through the registration of numerous GIs, and still wary of any risk of piracy, while most of the countries that adopted GI laws after TRIPs have not shown so much fervour. But apart from the BJP vision, all India is awakening. In the last few decades, as the role of India in the world has become increasingly important, its culture is being vindicated with growing pride. The success of the GI legal tool seems inevitable. Contemporary India does not hesitate to point out the superiority of its history[16] and that the perception other countries have of India has changed considerably. This pride is apparent in the speech by the ex-Prime Minister of India, Manmohan Singh, at Oxford in July 2005: 'the resurgence of India resulting in renewed confidence in itself', whose 'new optimism (...) today shapes the vision of the world.'[17] Another testimony is the advertising campaign on the Daily News & Analysis, Bangalore (www.dnaindia.com August 2006): 'We used to export cardamom now we exports CEOs [Chief Executive Officers]'. Nevertheless, GIs will be used to protect cardamom which is still an important product of the Indian heritage.

GIs for protection of traditional varieties: the cases of rice, bananas and mangoes

For traditional food products, GIs are regarded in India as a legal tool allowing for the protection of ancient heritage which is threatened by innovations in the world of agriculture, such as the introduction of new varieties developed by the seed industry. Therefore, a large number of GIs in the domain of agriculture concern local, traditional varieties.

In India, as numerous plant variety appellations include a geographical name eponymous with the geographical indication, these varieties can be qualified as local. But what is a local variety? According to Philippe Marchenay and Marie-France Largarde (1987) most of the varieties have become local because they have been adopted at a certain period, in a zone where they suited the climatic conditions, soil, cultural techniques, and above all, the needs (of populations). It is not rare to come across varieties which are foreign to a region, or even to a country, which have been 'assimilated' locally. They have left traces in cultures of which they have become a part of the collective memory and bear witness to the role they played in regional economy. This tends to prove that the local or traditional status depends less on the origin of a cultivar than the importance it has acquired in a region through the years.'

The importance that a cultivar has acquired in a region is testified by its name, which is that of the region, and this emphasises the strong link with the variety's geographical origin. But the importance and reputation of such varieties may generate misuse as in the case of Basmati. Following this case, the authorities concerned with the protection of genetic resources received a letter from the Ministry of Commerce asking them to identify and protect all traditional plant varieties through the GI Act, 1999, so that they may be protected from 'piracy'. Is this a misunderstanding regarding the aim of the GI Act which does not protect *per se* the genetic resources heritage but only a name? Thanks to the protection of the name and, therefore, of the added value in the market, GI protection may be a way to preserve and maintain the cultivation of traditional local varieties.

Nevertheless, if the name of a plant variety is registered as a GI, it means that only producers located in the area delimited in the GI application may use the name. Therefore, there is a risk of appropriation by a local community of the name of a plant variety for use only by those located in the geographical area delimited by the GI application, to the exclusion of producers located outside the area who cultivate the same variety. This risk does not seem to exist when the varieties are endemic to the area delimited in the GI application and when there are no producers outside such an area. This is the case in the following examples.

Navara rice

A particularly interesting example of plant varieties protected by GI law is 'Navara rice' which, according to the GI application, designates a type of rice resulting from the crossbreeding of two indigenous varieties found in Kerala (a South Indian state): the black-glumed variety and the golden-glumed variety. Both of them are violet in colour. Navara rice, called in Sanskrit *saśitika*, term derived from '*sastika*' in Malayalam (vernacular language of Kerala), is translated into English as 'red rice', a variety that grows to maturity in 60 days (Thomas *et al.* 2006). 'Navara' is not a geographical name but the name of a rice variety which is specific in its very short cultivation cycle and its period of maturation. The GI application mentions that Navara rice is originally from Kerala and has not spread elsewhere, assuming that it is endemic to Kerala. The application mentions the use of this rice for its medicinal properties in traditional medicine, widely practised in Kerala;[18] the rice is mixed with medicinal plants and is used for preparing oil for massage. It is also used in diets during the monsoon, and for treating blood circulation, digestive and osteoarthritis disorders. Considered as auspicious, it is also used in religious ceremonies. The producers of Navara rice call it 'Golden rice with fragrance' in keeping with the high price at which it is sold, or 'the grain of Kerala', as symbolic of cereals consumed in this South Indian region. Nevertheless, Navara rice is slowly becoming extinct due to difficulties in its cultivation and its low yield (Prabhakaran 2004). Indeed, The GI application mentions that it must be cultivated under irrigation because of its delicate nature and its constant need of water.

According to the GI application for Navara rice, its cultivation must be exclusively organic because of its medicinal use. This constraint involves particular expertise and a specific manner of processing. The method of production described in the specification is very precise regarding cultivation requirements: organic fertilisers, little water input, and presence of tree species which repel pathogenic plants. It also demands intensive manual work and care to ward off rats and other pests. It is transplanted at the end of January and harvested at the end of March; only one crop is allowed to be cultivated per year. However, until recently, Navara rice had not been produced using organic farming except on one farm, Ecofarm Navara, which belongs to P. Narayanan Unny,[19] the first applicant for the GI who specifies organic methods of production.[20]

Thanks to the GI, producers are encouraged to cultivate Navara rice as they will then be able to fight against the misuse already existing with certain traders selling 'false' Navara rice. False Navara rice consists of other rice varieties grown in the same geographical zone. GI may also be a tool for marketing a declining variety. In that sense, GI registration helps to promote the biodiversity of varieties. As the variety is not spread throughout Kerala with the name Navara, the registration of the name of the variety as a GI and its exclusive right of use by producers located in the geographical area mentioned in the GI application is legitimate.

GIs for bananas and mangoes

The GIs 'Virupakshi Hill Banana' and 'Sirumalai Hill Banana' are for varieties of 'Vannan' bananas (ecotypes), registered in the name of the Tamil Nadu Hill Banana Growers Federation. These varieties are cultivated in Madurai district (Tamil Nadu, South India) at an altitude of 1200–1500 metres. The plants yield fruits with a special perfume when they are cultivated at higher altitudes. Virupakshi and Sirumalai are geographical names which reinforce the link between the place and the product, and presume that the varieties are endemic and that the reservation of the name to the local producers is legitimate.

The situation has been different for the GIs 'Malda Lakhasman Bhog Mango' and 'Malda Fazli Mango' which designate mangoes cultivated in Malda district (West Bengal, North India). The indications protected as GIs, applied by the National Horticulture Board, were modified following the request of the consultative group. The first GI applications were only on the denomination 'Lakhasman Bhog Mango' and 'Fazli Mango' which designated the varieties without including the geographical names. Malda was added later, probably to avoid the appropriation of the name of the variety or to distinguish the GI product from the variety. The request to add the name was probably a result of the experience gained by the consultative group, as those GIs for mango were filed in October 2007, three years after the GI Act entered into force. As for Navara rice, one may note that GIs have been registered for traditional varieties, but not for export such as Alphonso mangoes, so that the farmers are able to boost the small yield of the former varieties.

These three examples show that GIs can be a useful tool for maintaining the cultivation of traditional varieties, considering that, thanks to the protection of the name and the fight against misuse, the benefit of the consolidated added value of products goes to the producers. GIs are based on history and tradition and, in that sense, they should be a protection against changes that would be prejudicial to the original quality. But market demand may influence the choice of innovations such as evolved varieties against traditional varieties, even for a product as notorious as Basmati.

Traditional variety or evolved variety: the case of Basmati rice

The eventful case of the protection of Basmati rice (Marie-Vivien 2008, 2015) illustrates two issues. The first concerns the replacement of traditional varieties by evolved ones in order to meet the growing demand, with the risk of a loss in terms of traditional food preservation. The second issue is the fact that Basmati has been defined as a list of varieties without specifying the geographical area of production. This legal definition of varieties is risky because it leads to Basmati becoming generic, i.e. no longer designating a rice cultivated in a specific place, but rather a range of rice varieties which may be cultivated anywhere in the world.

Since the beginning of the twentieth century, Basmati rice has been particularly subject to intensive plant breeding programmes in order to increase the yield of traditional varieties considered too low. The different varieties which have been obtained, qualified as traditional, or evolved, were registered in accordance with the Seed Act, 1966, a law regulating the marketing of seeds. Eleven varieties had been notified by 2007.[21] Regarding the exceptional quality of Basmati rice, the European Union has, since 1996, implemented a policy of exempting duty on Basmati from India and Pakistan. The peak in Basmati rice export since 2000 led the Indian government to redefine Basmati rice more precisely in order to avoid fraud. As traditional varieties fetch a better price in the international market, they were distinguished in 2003 from the evolved varieties: "traditional variety shall mean land races or varieties of rice of uniform shape, size and colour traditionally recognized as Basmati and evolved variety shall mean a variety whose one of two parents is a traditional variety and which has been recognized as a Basmati variety".[22] Among the 11 varieties of Basmati rice which have been notified in accordance with the Seed Act, 1966, six varieties are traditional and five are evolved varieties.[23] Consequently the European Union adapted its exemption of duty policy to promote only the six traditional varieties, which are considered of better quality.[24]

The demand for Basmati rice nowadays continues to rise exponentially in a context in which the Indian Research Institute has come out with new varieties. This has given rise to the question of whether the list of varieties qualified as Basmati may be enlarged by the inclusion of new varieties. After debates and controversies, the decision has been to remove from the 2003 definition of Basmati rice the condition of the immediate direct linkage with traditional varieties. The principle is to classify all these varieties as Basmati based on the criteria that the family history (genealogy) includes a Basmati variety (traditional or evolved) notified under the Seed Act, 1966, and that the 'Basmati quality genes' have passed into the newly evolved varieties. The aim is to include more evolved varieties with much higher yield that the varieties initially notified according to the Seed Act.

This new decision favours the risk of delocalisation of the cultivation of Basmati as the evolved, high yielding varieties may be able to adapt to different geographical environments without necessarily having the qualities or characteristics of traditional varieties grown in their place of origin. Concomitantly, the risk is that traditional varieties and traditional cultivation zones might be abandoned. To avoid this, in 2008, the notification of an evolved variety, Basmati Pusa 1121 was accompanied by a statement limiting the geographical area to Delhi, Punjab and Haryana.[25]

The interaction variety/milieu which was at the origin of the quality of Basmati rice is preserved by registering a GI if the specification of varieties and the definition of the geographical area is rigorous, but the GI protection is known for being turbulent. The Ministry of Trade and Industry, through its government body APEDA (Agricultural and Process Food Products Export Development Authority) applied for a GI for Basmati on 26 November 2008, after the first GI application made in August 2004 by the NGO 'Heritage' was rejected. The oppositions to the GI application concerned both the identity of the applicant, a government agency and not a producers' association which is assumed to be more representative, and the delimitation of the geographical area, Madhya Pradesh demanding to be included in the area. Finally, APEDA was considered as a legitimate applicant, representing the stakeholders of the value chain and GI being a tool for traditional food, and Basmati rice GI was registered in February 2016 with a cultivation area restricted to that historically known, formed by the states of Punjab, Haryana, Himachal Pradesh, Uttarkhand, parts of western Uttar Presdesh and Jammu Kashmir, and the territory of Delhi. Lastly, it is essential to remember that India has to come to an agreement with Pakistan, the other Basmati producing country, and use the advantage of the GI tool to find an answer to the issue of conservation of traditional varieties and traditional areas of production.

The uniqueness of GIs based on the combination of the milieu and the know-how: the terroir in the case of Darjeeling tea

For the other GIs of agricultural products, the varieties are neither local nor traditional. They were introduced during British rule and have acquired some specific qualities due to their long tradition of cultivation. Their qualities are inherent in the natural milieu (soil, climate, altitude), selected by foreign travellers and colonialists, and established in India for its capacity to welcome new crops now qualified as traditional. These agricultural products deserve a great deal of attention from the Indian stakeholders.

The perfect example is the GI 'Darjeeling' which refers to a tea which takes its qualities from its exceptional natural environment, notably altitude and climate. Called the 'Champagne of teas' (Das 2006; Rao 2005), Darjeeling tea has distinctive organoleptic characteristics which have won the patronage and recognition of discerning consumers all over the world. It is produced in 87 gardens located in the Darjeeling district over an area of 19,000 hectares which receive an annual rainfall of 320 centimetres. It is cultivated at the altitude of 600 to 2000 metres, on steep slopes, in very specific weather conditions: wet and cool in summer and dry and cold in winter. All the Indian teas are collected from *Camellia sinensis* species. These species, which take four to six years to mature, are hardy, multi-stemmed, slow growing evergreen shrubs which may grow up to 2.5 metres in height. They are able to stand severe winters, droughts and the high altitude of Darjeeling, but their yield there is much lower than in other districts. Leaves are small, leathery, dark, glossy green in colour and often covered with a downy silvery pubescence. The GI application mentions that a set of agricultural practices has been developed to sustain growth of shoots, while maintaining bush heights suitable for manual plucking. Manual plucking begins in March and ends by late November. The population of the tea growing areas of the Darjeeling district is approximately 700,000 out of which 60,000 are workers in the tea gardens.

According to the GI application, the processing of tea leaves is practised in the area of production, following an 'orthodox' traditional manner developed by the British who adapted the Chinese process to India. Once the leaves reach the factory, they are withered by evaporating the moisture. They are rendered limp in order to withstand twisting and rolling under pressure without crumbling. The withered leaves are loaded into rolling machines which, by exerting a pressure on the leaves, twist them, explode the cells and release the natural juice, promoting oxidation and accelerating pigmentation. The leaves are then lightly spread in a cool well ventilated room to favour slow oxidation. This important stage allows for the combination of flavanols with oxygen of the air, and the development of the unique flavour of Darjeeling tea. The tea quality and its perfume are regularly evaluated by experts during the whole process, and fermentation is stopped by drying the leaves at 90°C for 20 to 30 minutes. The leaves are sifted in order to be selected according to sizes or 'grades' which receive different appellations such as Fine Tippy Golden Flowery Orange Pekoe, Tippy Golden Broken Orange Pekoe and Golden Orange Fannings.

Darjeeling tea was the first GI registered in India. The applicant of the GI was the Tea Board of India, founded under the Tea Act, 1953. All the teas produced in India are administered by this Board which is run on a non-profit basis. It is not involved in the manufacture of products: its functions are essentially to regulate cultivation and production of tea, to improve its quality and increase the marketing within India and abroad.

The objective of the Tea Board is to set up a mechanism to ensure the integrity of the supply chain for Darjeeling tea so that this tea, renowned worldwide by its appellation, is genuine Darjeeling tea when it leaves India. While the whole process is located in the area of production, the final packaging is done in the importing countries involving the risk of blending with other varieties and counterfeiting. Nevertheless, the word and logo 'Darjeeling' are broadly protected in importing countries by a very aggressive policy which aims at banning all trademarks using the name 'Darjeeling', even though the products concerned are not tea. Along with the protection of the Darjeeling logo and word via certification marks and GIs, the Tea Board has also introduced a traceability system in 2000. Producers, negotiators and exporters have to sign a license agreement with the Tea Board in order to obtain a certificate of origin authorising them to use the Darjeeling logo.[26]

The misuse of the name 'Darjeeling' justifies such a protection. The tea industry has estimated the sales of Darjeeling tea in the world at 40,000 tons per year while the production does not exceed 10,000 tons (Das 2006). Tea illegally named Darjeeling comes mainly from Sri Lanka, Kenya and Nepal. The high level of fraud has pushed the Tea Board to adopt a more aggressive strategy through the application for certification marks in India and abroad.[27] In 2003, the GI application was filed in India, both for the word Darjeeling and the logo, with the objective of ascertaining a strategy of protection of Darjeeling tea, originally organised through certification marks before the GI Act was passed.[28] In 2008, Darjeeling was registered as a GI in Europe. Subsequently the Tea Board filed lawsuits in courts or in trademark offices against third parties for misappropriating the indication Darjeeling in about 20 countries in the world. Its last action was against France, and was decided in its favour as the validity of Darjeeling GI was recognised. In this case,[29] Jean-Luc Dusong was the owner of a semi-figurative trademark composed of the Darjeeling word and the drawing of a teapot.[30] It designated publications and communication material. The Tea Board demanded that Dusong's registration be cancelled. After an initial refusal from the Court of Paris which declared the trademark to be valid as the products were different, the Court of Appeal cancelled this decision considering that Dusong's products could be taking advantage of the reputation of Darjeeling well known for its association with tea. The Court of Appeal recognised that Dusong's logo for designating products other than tea might be harmful for this prestigious GI, which only the Tea Board had the right to use. To draw its conclusion, the Court of Appeal first qualified Darjeeling as a GI according to the TRIPS agreement. The court was convinced by the product description and the link to its geographical origin, supported by the documents provided by the Tea Board establishing that it was well known in France, particularly in specialised books and articles in the daily press. The court then considered the GI as equivalent to an appellation of origin: appellations of origin having prior rights, the protected terms cannot be registered as a trademark, even if there is no risk of misleading the public, and even when the products are different. In this case, even though there was no risk of misleading the consumer who did not expect the publications and communication material designed by the trademark Darjeeling, decorated with a drawing of a teapot, to come from Darjeeling, the trademark was cancelled because GIs in Europe benefit from a high level of protection. This high level of protection means that GIs are reserved only for the people of the place who are the creators of the reputation of such a place and grants them an intellectual right which goes beyond the simple risk of misleading consumers.

This juridical affair has been a success story of the defence of a famous product of Indian heritage, for which 'uniqueness' reflects the combination of variety, natural environment and processing techniques. Even if tea is not an indigenous plant of India, it is still a traditional drink and may be qualified as a 'terroir product' in India as well as in France, the cradle of protection by appellations of origin.

The uniqueness of the GIs based on traditional processing know-how with little impact by the environment: the case of Feni, Dharwad **peḍhā** *and Tirupati* **laddu**

In the three following examples Feni, Dharwad *peḍhā* and Tirupati *laddu*, the reputation of the products is mainly based on the know-how of local producers with little impact by the environment on the processing, whether through the source of raw material or through the climate/soil/altitude.

Feni: the famous Goanese liquor

The first GI registered for liquor 'Feni', illustrates how the traditional and ancient know-how of fermentation and distillation of the juice of cashew fruits in Goa was enough to justify the registration of a GI applied by the Department of Science, Technology and Environment, Government of Goa, and by the Goa Cashew Feni Distillers and Bottlers Association, given the minor impact of nature. The word '*feni*' comes from the froth that is formed on the surface when the liquor is shaken in a bottle or poured into a glass, called in the local Konkani language as *fen*.

According to the GI application, the cashew tree was introduced to Goa from Latina America by the Portuguese in the sixteenth century. Goa is the only place where cashew fruits are used for the production of *feni*, cashew trees being usually cultivated for nuts. The fruits, fully ripened and fallen to the ground, are collected and crushed to extract the juice. Liquor *feni* is obtained from the fermentation and distillation of this juice without any additive. According to the GI specification, the liquor has to be distilled twice using traditional methods. This method employs a bamboo pipe through which the distillate is collected in an earthenware pot cooled down very carefully by a water circuit. Nevertheless, according to Dwijen Rangnekar (2009), the distillation process described in the GI is rarely practised: the receptacle is quite often aluminium immersed in a large cement tank full of water so that the cooling process is incomplete. This case illustrates the gap between the traditionality of a product accredited by the GI and its actual production which uses modern techniques. Nevertheless, only liquor traditionally processed is entitled to the Feni GI and not that produced by modern means. Therefore, GI might well be a useful tool for maintaining traditional food processing if the control system set up according to the provisions of the GI Act on inspection procedures is properly conducted, but that is unfortunately seldom the case in India.

'Dharwad peḍhā' and 'Tirupati laddu': traditional know-how attached to a single producer

An example of a traditional milk product protected by GI Act is 'Dharwad *peḍhā*', a sweetmeat, brown in colour, made up of milk and sugar, which is unique in its flavour thanks to its processing method. Dharwad *peḍhā* has acquired a valuable reputation and is indicative of quality and uniqueness. It is made daily by a three-hour process. Although its main ingredient is milk, it does not perish easily and its flavour is considered stable for a period of 20 days, thanks to the considerable addition of a specific sugar called *bura* (powdered sugar). The milk is collected from buffaloes reared in and around places in the GI area. For about 2 kilograms of Dharwad *peḍhā*, 4 litres of buffalo milk are required which are converted into 1 kilogram of *khoya* and mixed with1 kilogram of *bura* sugar. These two ingredients are heated uniformly without the addition of preservatives or flavours.

According to the GI application, the historical origin of Dharwad *peḍhā* comes from the Thakur family which migrated from Unnao, in Uttar Pradesh, to Dharwad, in Karnataka, to escape an epidemic of plague in the late eighteenth century. With his meagre funds, Shri Ram Ratan Singh Thakur (first generation of sweetmaker) started making and selling *peḍhā* which gradually became popular. Nevertheless, it was his grandson, Shri Babu Singh Thakur, who built the reputation of the *peḍhā* with missionary zeal. The sweet rapidly gained such a reputation that local people of Dharwad named them 'Babu Singh Thakur' or 'Line Bazaar', according to the street where his shop was located. The method of preparing *peḍhā* is a secret, known only to the family members of Shri Durga Singh Thakur, belonging now to the fifth generation.

Even though the GI application attributes the creation of to the Thakur family, others families like the Mistras are producing similar sweets. With the intention of rooting this product in Dharward, an application for a GI 'Dharwad *peḍhā*' has been filed by the Thakur's Dharwad Manufacturers' Welfare Trust which associates members of the Thakur and Mistra families as well as the Dharwad Sweet and Milk Products Manufacturers' Society. In this case, the link with the origin lies in the tradition of making the product in Dharwad. But, is the production by only one family association sufficient to give the product a traditional and collective qualification and to validate a GI? It seems that any person manufacturing sweets, including Dharwad *peḍhā*, as well as milk products manufacturers, may be a member of the association having fulfilled the GI application, but the issue is whether the product will become an origin product or only a speciality of one or two families.

A rather unusual GI's reputation is based on a product traditionally consumed in the religious sphere, the 'Tirupati laddu', sweets exclusive to Sri Venkateswara temple at Tirumala-Tirupati in Andhra Pradesh. These *laddu* are offered to the divinity, which renders them sacred, and are then consumed by pilgrims or taken home.

The GI has been registered by the Tirumala-Tirupati Devasthanam (TTD), the Hindu religious organisation in charge of the management of the temple complex. Its specifications highlight the holiness of the *laddu* justifying their reputation and indicating their size, method of preparation, and the taste and quality processes followed in the temple kitchen, the consecrated place where they are made.

According to the GI application, the *laddu* are made by about 130 cooks, in vessels called *sīvari pottu*. Around 20,000 *laddu* are produced every day. Some *laddu* are offered to the deity and, having become impregnated by its sacredness, they are mixed with the other *laddu*. The *laddu* are then placed in front of Vakula Devi, the mother goddess, and distributed to devotees. The tradition, in this case, being related to religious belief, it has created a controversy in India regarding whether religious items may be the object of an intellectual property right and be marketable. The action for annulment before the Chennai High Court of the GI is based on the identity of the applicant as the TTD is the only producer and the sole beneficiary of the GI due to the fact that the *laddus* are not prepared by qualified cooks of the temple. The GI should be justified if a specific community of cooks specialising in Tirupati *laddus* were employed by the temple.

Apart from these three examples of food products which are questionable regarding their context, there is no doubt that GI is relevant for products processed traditionally as soon as they gain a reputation by virtue of their historical depth and the implication of a community in their production.

Conclusion

GIs are a valuable tool for encouraging the production of traditional local foods which reputation is well-known in the market, local, national or international. Considered by the members of the Indian parliament as a relevant aid in exporting cash crops such as Darjeeling tea or Basmati rice, the GI Act has been implemented as well to protect local plant varieties in decline, along with other food products such as dairy products and liquors. The use of GIs for horticultural varieties also exists in Europe as, for example, the appellation of origin 'Lentils of the Puy', registered in France in 1936, but in a more marginal way compared to the numerous GIs on wines, spirit, cheese and processed meat. The Indian heritage is rich in old varieties which are still cultivated, but are threatened or in decline; their protection by the GI Act may, thus, be a way to revive them or to avoid their misuse. Europe has, for a long time, been against granting geographical names to grape varieties for wine production in order to avoid confusion with GIs; geographical names are reserved only for origin products and not for varieties. But in the case of India, the GI Act especially protects names which designate local, well-known traditional products, but not the product itself.

Protection of genetic resources is better afforded by the 2001 Protection of Plant Varieties and Farmer's Rights Act (PPVFRA) that came into force on 21 February 2007. This act has been largely influenced by debates on the Convention on Biological Diversity (CBD) signed in Rio, in 1992. The PPVFRA aims at protecting farmers' rights, as participants, by contributing to maintaining diversity of plant varieties in order to counterbalance the restrictions imposed by the intellectual property rights awarded to farmers who develop new plant varieties. The difference of finality between, on the one hand, the protection of plant varieties conferring a temporal exclusivity on innovations, and concomitantly on the sale of seeds and rights on extant varieties to communities, and on the other hand, the *sine die* protection of the name, a competitive advantage justified by the reputation of products, is clearly exposed by S. Nagarajan (2007), the current President of the Indian Office for the protection of plant varieties. However, it is not certain that GI applicants are aware that the protection conferred by a GI concerns only the name, and not the genetic resource, which may be used by a third party if it is identified by another name. Admittedly, GIs may help to promote and encourage the cultivation of traditional varieties and have a positive impact on biodiversity through the protection of added value local products. And India is in the process of actively protecting its heritage, using modern intellectual property tools with dynamism, as a new symbol for the fulfilment of its wish to preserve its traditions in this time of globalisation. For India to succeed, however, its producers have to be more aware of, and informed about, GIs.

Notes

1 Producers from all over the world requested the WTO to proceed on the issue of the extension of protection to all products; see the communication of Origin, www.origin-gi.com. (retrieved January 2007).

2 Section 7 of the GI Act, 1999.

3 The GI Rules, 2002, Rule 32.1(6): The GI application shall comprise: *Rule 32.1(6)b "The benchmark standards for the use of the geographical indication or the industry standard as regards the production, exploitation, making or manufacture of the goods having specific quality, reputation, or other characteristic of such goods that is essentially attributable to its geographical origin with the detailed description of the human creativity involved, if any or other characteristic from the definite territory of the country, region or locality in the country, as the case may be," and *Rule 32.1(6)e: the particulars of special human skill involved or the uniqueness of the geographical environment or other inherent characteristics associated with the geographical indication to which the application relates.

4 The GI Rules, 2002, Rule 33.

5 The GI Act, 1999, Section 14 and 16.

6 The GI Act, 1999, Section 18.

7 The GI Act, 1999, Section 17.

8 The GI Act, 1999, Section 11.

9 The GI Act, 1999, Section 21.

10 The GI Act, 1999, Section 20, 21, 22, 23.

11 TRIPS agreement provides two levels of protection: a standard level for all products where the GI is protected against use that would mislead the public, and an additional level of protection for wine and spirits where the GI is protected *per se*, even without any question of misleading the public. India, together with other developing countries and Europe, is negotiating for the extension of the additional protection to all the products. See F. Addor and A. Grazzioli (2002).

12 The GI Act, 1999, Section 22, the GI Rules, 2002, rules 77 and 78.

13 The GI Act, 1999, Section 24.

14 The GI Act, 1999, Section 25 and 26.

15 Member of the Parliament, Discussion on the Geographical Indications of Goods (Registration and Protection) Bill, 1999; XIII Lok Sabha Debate, *Session II (Winter Session)* Wednesday, December 22, 1999/Pausa 1, 1921 (Saka).

16 See, for example, the comments by B.P Singh (1999) on the art of Ajanta (near Mumbai) having influenced numerous temples in Tibet and Sri Lanka, according to him.

17 For an analysis of the speech of Manmohan Singh at Oxford on 8 July 2005, see Prabhat Patnaik P. (2005).

18 The GI application mentions the Suśruta saṃhita to which it attributes the date of 2500 BC. But, according to experts on traditional medical texts, this text would have been written between second century BC and second century AD.

19 P. Narayanan Unny is an activist farmer who promotes organic cultivation practices and the use of traditional varieties.

20 See the website of the Navara Eco Farm: www.navara.in (retrieved August 2008). This farm, which has applied for the GI, is certified organic by Indocert, an Indian certification body. This certification is in conformity with the National Programme for Organic Production (NPOP) and with European regulation on organic farming EEC 2092/91 and 1788/2001.

21 Basmati 217, Basmati 370, Type 3, Punjab Basmati 1, Pusa Basmati 1, Kasturi Haryana, HKR 228, Mahi Sugunda, Taraori HB 19, Ranbir, Basmati 386. See http://seednet.gov.in/SeedVariety (retrieved November 2007).

22 Notification 68 under the Export (Quality Control and Inspection) Act 1963 named 'The Export of Basmati Rice (Quality Control and Inspection) Rules, 2003', adopted on 23 January 2003.
23 See the notification 68 of the Export Act, 1966: "The Export of Basmati Rice (Quality Control and Inspection) Rules, 2003", 23 January 2003 adopted under the Export Export (Quality Control and Inspection) Act, 1990. Since 1990 the "Export (Quality Control and Inspection) Act", has been monitoring the export of Basmati rice.
24 Regulation (CE) no. 2294/2003, 24 December 2003 amending Regulation (CE) no. 1503/96.
25 Notification no. S.Q.2547 (E) of the Seed Act, 1966, 29 October, 2008.
26 The rules for the use of trademarks are published by the Tea Board of India.
27 In 1998, in UK; in 2002, in US.
28 Certification Trade Mark no. 532240, registered in India since 1986 for the logo consisting of the word Darjeeling and a representation of an Indian woman holding tea leaves, all arranged in a roundel, it has been registered in many foreign countries. See http://www.teauction.com/industry/boards.asp (retrieved December 2009).
29 Court of Appeal of Paris, November 22, 2006; Tribunal of first instance of Paris, 6 July 2005.
30 The application for the trademark was registered under the n° 3.193.817 in November 2002.

References

Addor, F. and Grazzioli, A. (2002). "Geographical indications beyond wine and spirits, a roadmap for a better protection for geographical Indications in WTO/TRIPS Agreement", *The Journal of World Intellectual Property,* Vol. 5(6): 865–897.

Balganesh, S. (2003). "Systems of protection for geographical indications of origin: a review of the India regulatory framework", *The Journal of World Intellectual Property,* Vol. 6(1): 191–205.

Barham, E. (2003). "Translating terroir: the global challenge of French AOC labeling", *Journal of Rural Studies,* Vol. 19(1): 127–138.

Bérard, L. and Marchenay, P. (2007). "Localized products in France: definition, protection and value-adding", *Anthropology of Food,* Vol. 'From local food to localised food', March. http://aof.revues.org/415?lang=fr (retrieved on 03 March 2013).

Bowen, S. (2010). "Embedding local places in global spaces: geographical indications as a territorial development strategy", *Rural Sociology,* Vol. 75(2): 209–243.

Das, K. (2006). "International protection of India's geographical indications with special reference to "Darjeeling" tea", *The Journal of World Intellectual Property,* Vol. 9(5): 459-495.

Mahias, M.-C. (1997). "Les sciences et les techniques traditionnelles en Inde", *L'Homme,* Vol. 37(142): 105–114.

Marchenay, P. and Lagarde, M.-F. (eds.) (1987). *A la recherche des variétés locales de plantes cultivées,* Paris: Page PACA, Bureau des ressources génétiques, Muséum national d'histoire naturelle.

Marie-Vivien, D. (2008). "From plant variety definition to geographical indication protection: a search for the link between basmati rice and India/Pakistan", *The Journal of World Intellectual Property,* Vol. 11(4): 321–344.

Marie-Vivien, D. (2015). *Geographical Indications in India, a new perspective on the French and European experiences,* New Delhi: Sage Publications, 'Sage Law'.

Nagarajan, S. (2007). "Geographical indications and agriculture related intellectual property rights issues", *Current Sciences*, Vol. 92: 167–171.

O'Connor, B. (ed.) (2004). *The Law of Geographical Indications*, London: Cameron May.

Patnaik, P.P. (2005). "Manmohan Singh and colonialism", *People's Democracy*, July 17.

Prabhakaran, G. (2004). "Njavara facing extinction", *The Hindu*, June 07.

Rangnekar, D. (2009). "Geographical indications and localisation: a case study of feni", CSGR Report 2009, *Social Science Research Network*. http://papers.ssrn.com/sol3/papers.cfm?abstract_id=1564624&http://search.avg.com/route/?d=4c69fc58&v=7.007.026.001&i=23&tp=chrome&q=Rangnekar%2C+Dwijen+%282009%29+%27Geographical+Indications+and+Localisation%3A+A+Case+Study+of+Feni%27%2C+CSGR+Report.&lng=fr&iy=&ychte=us (retrieved on 10 July 2011).

Rao, C. N. (2005). "Geographical indications in Indian context: a case study of Darjeeling tea", *Economic and Political Weekly*, October 15: 4545–4550.

Singh, B.P. (ed.) (1999). *L'Etat et les arts en Inde*. Pour une culture citoyenne, Paris: Editions Karthala.

Soam, S.K. (2005). "Analysis of prospective geographical indications of India", *The Journal of World Intellectual Property*, Vol. 8(5): 679–704.

Thomas, G., Sreejayan, R. and Dinesh, R. (2006). "Njavara, the single largest used medicinal rice in the world: genetic structure, varietal discrimination and phylogenetic affinity". Paper presented at 2nd International Rice Congress on Science, Technology, and Trade for Peace and Prosperity, New Delhi, India, 9–13 October, 2006.

Van de Kop, P., Sautier, D. and Gerz, A. (eds.) (2004). *Origin-Based Products-Lessons for pro-poor market development*, Amsterdam: Royal Tropical Institute KIT and Montpellier: CIRAD.

5 Are *buuz* and *banš* traditional Mongolian foods?

Strategy of appropriation and identity adjustment in contemporary Mongolia

Sandrine Ruhlmann

Introduction

Mongolian culture and identity remain rooted in its history and in nomadic pastoralism.[1] Mongolians often contend that the diet of nomadic people and the urban population is still mainly based on livestock-derived food: meat and dairy products.

This article draws on fieldwork conducted between 1999 and 2007, and focused on 20 families in the regions of Töv and Hentij.[2] It describes the importance attributed to meat and dairy products in the Mongolian universe; they hold a central place in consumption, in offering rituals, and in symbolic representations. The traditional Mongolian food pattern is a binary system based on a dichotomy of colours of ingredients: dairy products are classified as 'white foods' (*cagaan idee*); meat as 'grey-brown food' (*bor idee*).

A third food category, cereals (*guriltaj hool*), i.e. 'food based on flour', began to appear in domestic food practices in 1970, first in urban areas, and then, in the last decade, in rural areas where nomadic herders used to eat traditional food, meat and dairy products. Flour-based foods, in particular steamed and boiled dumplings, *buuz* and *banš*,[3] although not traditional food, are today highly valued precisely as traditional Mongolian food. For the past three decades, these dumplings, probably borrowed from Chinese cuisine, have increasingly been replacing the mutton dish (*šüüs*), traditionally consumed at the Mongolian lunar New Year.

Taking into account the transformation of food patterns in Mongolia, this study will revolve around three main subjects: firstly, the social practices related to traditional foods; secondly, the place of non-traditional foods in consumption with attention to the specific status of dumplings; and lastly, the political and religious factors at stake in the change in food practices and social rituals. The latter topic will allow for showing how, in the present democratic context, the consumption and offerings of dumplings combine some features of Shamanic and Buddhist beliefs against an historical background of widespread anti-religious and 'egalitarian' Communist politics. Employing Claude Lévi-Strauss's term, those arrangements and readjustments emphasise the '*bricolage*' under which the food sphere of Mongolians is defined. Going into the various influences at work, this article aims to show how these influences are historically contingent and linked to political, ideological and religious processes, as well as to analyse tensions around the consumption of dumplings which are both called for as an aspect of Mongolian identity and exemplify the anti-Chinese movement in Mongolia.

Traditional foods in Mongolia: meat and dairy products as structural foods

Meat: an important hierarchical food in traditional Mongolian society

Depending on the region and local ecosystem, Mongolian nomadic pastoralists rear five animal species: cows or yaks, horses, camels, sheep and goats. Mongolians claim to be meat eaters.[4] When asked what they eat, they responded without hesitation "meat!" Meat does not mean simply flesh, it means flesh and fat, as I had to experience when, at the request of a family of the provincial capital Öndörhaan, I chose to prepare for them a dish of spaghetti Bolognese. Parents and children politely ate the dish and said: "This is good; the taste of tomato is curious, but good." But, immediately the woman added: "Well, now let's eat!" She hurried to cut meat and prepare a soup. The minced meat that I used to prepare Bolognese sauce did not agree with the taste of my hosts: the essential component of the Mongolian food system, fat, was missing. A meal can be composed of a single dish, but it must include meat, i.e. flesh and fat meat. Mongolians favour cooking meat by boiling as this preserves fat. They distinguish two kinds of fat: the 'juice' (*šüüs*)[5] that melts and dissolves into the broth with which eaters grease their face and their hands during the meal; the hard 'fat' (*ööh*) that remains after cooking and crunches between the teeth. For Mongolians, meat (*mah*) is the food that nourishes and provides a feeling of being 'full' (*cadsan*).

Social rules of distribution of meat

In order to preserve their livestock, pastoralists restrict animal slaughter which means that meat is consumed in small quantities, mostly in the form of soup, the sole daily dish, of which it is the main ingredient.

Preparation and consumption of meat is distinguished according to two sorts: meat separated from the bone (*mah*) and meat attached to the bone (*jas*) and named according to the bone. The first is distributed in an egalitarian manner, and the second according to the hierarchy. The bone is the element that lends meat its distinctive character and reflects the social status of the consumers. It reveals the social structure of Mongolian society, both in terms of social relations and degree of kinship. Elders (men and women), men, and some family members such as the maternal uncle, receive the best parts of bone-attached meat (*hündtej* 'with respect') that include head, four upper ribs, scapula, sacrum and tail while 'juniors', i.e. women and children, receive the other parts of the animal (Hamayon 1975).

Eating practices are also dependent on social and family stratification. 'Seniors' have their meal in honorific area of the yurt (*hojmor*), situated in the northern and western part directly opposite the door and devoted to men's work. 'Juniors' eat in the less respected part of the yurt, located in the southern to eastern parts that include the stove[6] and are devoted to the domestic work of women in charge of maintaining the fire and preparing food. It is in this area too that women sit when they receive visitors. Food consumption depends on social situations, ordinary or extraordinary, and the share of meat dishes distinguishes the eaters socially. Commensality rules tend to be more flexible in nuclear families, but they are still strictly observed in hospitality situations: guests who share the best parts of the meal with the 'seniors' are served first, while the 'juniors' eat the parts that are left over by the visitors.

The relationship between bone and meat in the social and family structure

The social stratification of meat sharing is in accordance with the ancient shamanistic beliefs concerning flesh, blood and bone that linger in Mongolian culture. Flesh and blood represent the maternal lineage, while bone embodies the soul of all patrilineal descendants of a common ancestor (Hamayon 1990; *Histoire secrète des Mongols* 1994). Mongolians believe that the soul enters the body at birth and is fixed in the bones at the ritual of the first haircut (three or five years old). This stage is materialised by the first consumption by the child of meat attached to the bone.[7] The bone which is given to the child at this ritual confirms the child's status as a social being. This concept of the bone means that during slaughter, preparation and consumption of the animal, many precautions are taken in order to avoid bones being broken. They have to be intact in order to encourage symbolically the rebirth of the soul in a new animal, and thus perpetuate the species. The carcass is cut up at joints (*üje*), a metaphoric term that designates generation (Hamayon 1990; Even 1999), and by extension, filiation.

Meat with the symbolic function of 'closing'

In the thirteenth century, an entire cooked sheep constituted the festive dish par excellence and held the predominant place on the table at the large banquets to honour Mongol nobles (Ruhlmann 2011). Sheep were also used in sacrifices performed by Mongolians for reaffirming their membership in a clan; through the sacrifice to the ancestors, they received 'ancestral grace'. Over the course of several centuries, the concept of 'ancestral grace' became associated with the Buddhist notion of happiness. Thus today, Mongolians share and consume meat in order to accumulate happiness.

At the lunar New Year in Mongolia, a dialectics of 'closing/opening' is associated with the accumulation of happiness. Mutton is the prominent element in the rites of closing and opening: it is the compulsory food to 'close' (*bitüüleh*) the year and, implicitly, to favour the opening of the lunar New Year (Ruhlmann 2007).[8] The day before this event, Mongolians prepare and eat the traditional dish of the entire sheep (*šüüs*) whose head and tail are the two parts that 'close' the animal, alive as well as dead. As the animal's head needs more time to cook, it is quite often removed nowadays, and the tail thus becomes the 'bone of excellence' that symbolises and materialises the closing of the year. This specific dish is called *bitüüleg*, i.e. the dish of closing (*bitüü* 'closed'). In opposition to the closing function of the mutton dish, the 'opening' of the lunar New Year is realised with another food category, dairy products, which constitute traditional foods regarded by Mongolian herders as socially and symbolically important.

Role of dairy products and the symbolism related to the colour white

Although Mongolians describe themselves as 'meat eaters', their diet consists mostly of various processed dairy products, the 'white foods' (*cagaan idee*).

The large variety of 'white foods' derived from or composed of milk

Mongolian herders have evolved various techniques for processing fresh milk from the five species of animal that they rear. Women, who nowadays do all the milking, are responsible for the preparation of dairy products, with the exception of alcoholic beverages made from fermented or distilled milk which is the men's task.

Boiled, and fermented with old yogurt, milk is transformed into a cream (*öröm*), creamy yogurt (*tarag*), melted rancid butter (*šar tos*), curd (*eedem*), cottage cheese (*bjaslag*) and different dried cheeses (*aaruul*, *huuruud*) that are stored throughout the winter. Fresh milk is used to prepare two drinks. The first, the iconic drink in Mongolia today, is fermented mare's milk (*ajrag*), obtained by churning milk vigorously with a wooden churn in a goatskin bottle, nowadays replaced by a plastic barrel. The second, which tends to be replaced by industrial vodka, is an alcohol produced from the distillation of milk (*arhi*).

The category of 'white foods' includes butters and porridges which may be composed of several dairy products. *Hajlmag* is butter composed of cream (*öröm*) and melted butter (*šar tos*) to give nourishment value and enhance the taste of the cream. Mongolians designate this product as *cagaa* – a generic term for porridges formed from the term *cagaan* which means white. *Cagaan tos* 'white butter' is made from the flour of freshly roasted wheat mixed with heated milk and cream, filaments of dried crumbled cheese (*eezgij*) and sugar. Porridges, prepared specifically to be consumed during the day, are made of rice and/or foxtail millet (*Setaria italica*). They are cooked in a mixture of milk and yogurt, are sweet and often decorated with small raisins. They are of various sorts: some are thick and 'eaten' while others are liquid and 'drunk'; *cagaalag* is enriched with melted butter and flour, while *šingen budaa* (liquid rice) is *cagaalag* liquified with milk. These types of butter and porridge are consumed at specific celebrations, as the symbolism attached to their whiteness is fundamental to the satisfactory performance of the celebration.

The sharing, consumption and distribution of milk and of dairy products, as with meat, are rooted in hierarchical rules: fresh and fat dairy products, socially honorific, are generously offered to visitors during festive occasions, while dried products, considered as less fatty and nutritious and socially depracated, are restricted to family members or camp dwellers. They are also rooted in metaphysical concepts pertaining to the Mongolian symbolic universe.

Milk as propitiatory traditional food

Every morning, women perform a libation (*cacal*) with the 'upper, above' part (*deež*) of the milk tea (*süütej caj*) which they prepare for the whole day in the early morning in a large pot. First, the *deež* is collected by skimming the surface of the tea with a ladle. Then, standing on the threshold of the yurt, the head covered out of respect, women, using the right hand, which is considered 'pure', sprinkle a small part of the *deež* using a large spoon (*cacuur*) into the air 'in the four directions of the universe'. The droplets of liquid fall 'onto the earth', implicitly on the ancestors' earth. They have not to fall on the roof of the yurt, as that would prevent them from reaching the beneficiaries. Women accompany this ritual gesture by whispered prayers – Buddhist blessing formulae. The ritual which involves the sprinkling of white liquid is propitiatory. It aims to 'call' happiness (*duudah*) for all family members (health, success, love) and herds (health, prosperity). Such propitiatory rituals existed as far back as the thirteenth century.

According to the testimony of the thirteenth century Franciscan monk, Jean de Plan Carpin (1965), Mongolians offered the 'first milk of cattle and mares' to the spirits. A few excerpts from *The Secret History of the Mongols* (2004) testify that milk, especially fermented mare's milk, was associated with the idea of abundance and celebration among Mongolian people. During banquets, after the Emperor was served, jugs of *ajrag* (fermented mare's milk) circulated among the guests. Since then, 'white foods' have been associated with the symbolism of beginnings, renewal, i.e. prosperity of herds and abundance of milk. Prior to the thirteenth century, New Year was celebrated in summer and coincided with the period of lactation and the abundance of milk and dairy products (Hamayon 1978). Since the adoption of the Chinese calendar at the end of the thirteenth century, Mongolians have celebrated the lunar New Year in winter so that, to keep the symbolism of this feast intact, they have to store large quantities of milk and fresh dairy products from the end of the autumn.[9]

Milk: the traditional food of hospitality and auspiciousness

The modalities of dairy product consumption, as well as the manner in which these products are offered, reveal the principles of Mongolian culture and associate them with the hospitality of nomadic herders.

The daily life of herders is marked by many unexpected visits. To welcome their visitors, hosts, in reverential fashion, offer them a plate of 'white foods' and a bowl of milk tea. The plate is composed of fresh and fat honorific dairy products put 'above' (*deež*), and of dry and light depracated dairy products put 'below' (*doož*). Visitors have to take only the *deež* food called the 'beginning', while the *doož* will be consumed by household members when the visitors have gone. Food offering is beneficial not only for visitors who receive and ingest the auspiciousness attached to *deež* food but also for hosts, as the offering of food allied with hospitality allows, according to Buddhist principles, for increasing the karmic potential for the future rebirths.

The function of 'white foods' in the act of 'opening'

Dairy products are offered and consumed during celebrations of life course transitions (birth) and calendar celebrations (lunar New Year). As 'white food', they enable Mongolians who offer, share and consume them, to enact and materialise the correct opening of the year. Families prepare and offer a wide variety of dairy products and food made with dairy products, and other foods, also 'white' and assimilated to the whiteness of milk, such as milky porridges, sugar pieces, fried cakes, sweets, and *buuz* and *banš*.

The concept of 'opening', represented by milk products, opposed to that of 'closing' represented by meat, underlies the Mongolian notion of happiness. 'Opening' the New Year consists in propitiatory acts that promote the happiness of oneself and of one's family, and preserve it by rituals for accumulating and redistributing happiness. In other words, the concept of 'opening' aims to multiply and circulate happiness in order to ensure the successful beginning of a new cycle of nature, to propitiate souls and enhance the cycle of births and deaths.

According to the context and rituals, the acts aim to open the body (of a pregnant woman to help her give birth), to open social relationships (sharing food with visitors) and sociability (resumption of greetings and work after a mourning period). These acts are usually accompanied by the offering and consumption of food symbolising the act of opening (*ongojloh*). A particular day that perfectly illustrates this concept of renewal is New Year day, the day that 'opens' (*ongojlo-*) the new year.[10]

Buuz and *banš*: new food endowed with both traditional and Buddhist values

The Mongolian diet is now more varied than previously and includes foods borrowed from the Russian (boiled and fried dishes) and Chinese culinary worlds (*buuz*, *banš*, noodles, etc.) The 'foods [made] with flour' (*guriltaj hool*) have appeared gradually in the Mongolian cuisine. Nowadays, for instance, homemade or industrial noodles give consistency to everyday dishes such as soup. In order to welcome a visitor properly, sweet donuts adorn the top of the plate of hospitality composed of fresh and fat dairy products; slices of bread or manufactured biscuits are put on the bottom of the plate with lean and dry, depracated, dairy products. With the aim of satisfying and honouring the visitor, *buuz* or a soup with *banš* are offered along with a bowl of milk tea. The cooked dumplings (*buuz*, *banš*), the food the Mongolians have most widely adopted, are served in rituals related to Buddhist concepts, to produce 'merits' and to invoke happiness, acts which are correlated with the rebirth of souls and the reproduction of the society.[11]

The Dumpling as a 'closing' and 'opening' metaphor

Mongolians classify the dumplings, *buuz* and *banš*, served for the New Year as either 'grey-brown food' or 'white food'. The duality of *buuz/banš* results from their composition (envelope and filling) the consumption of which illuminates the notion of 'closing' and 'opening' the year.

The dumplings, a new category of foods

Buuz (raviolis; steamed dumplings) and *banš* (raviolis; small boiled dumplings) belong to the category of cereal-related foods, because they are defined according to their envelope made of a wheat flour dough (*gurilyn boodol*) which identifies them as 'enveloped food' (*boohyn hool*). *Buuz* and *banš*, considered analogically as filling the stomach, consist of a dough envelope filled with a mixture of onions, meat and mutton fat. In the most honorific version, meat comes from the thigh of the sheep and fat from the tail.

The Mongolian *buuz* and *banš* are similar to Chinese dumplings. These borrowings have obliged Mongolians to learn and master new techniques of food preparation and cooking, and to use unfamiliar kitchen utensils. The dough is made of a subtle combination of white wheat flour and water with a ductility[12] and compactness that allows it be shaped into various forms.[13]

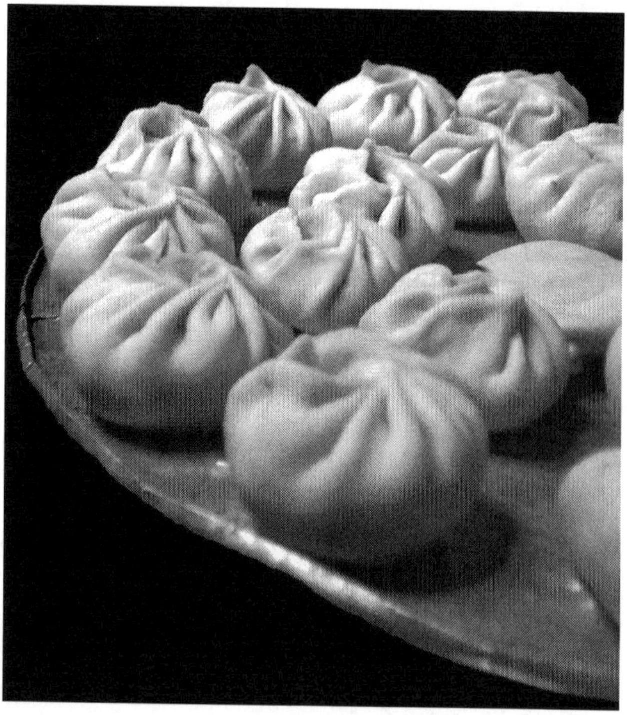

Figure 5.1 Mongolian dumplings *buuz*

Source: © Sandrine Ruhlmann.

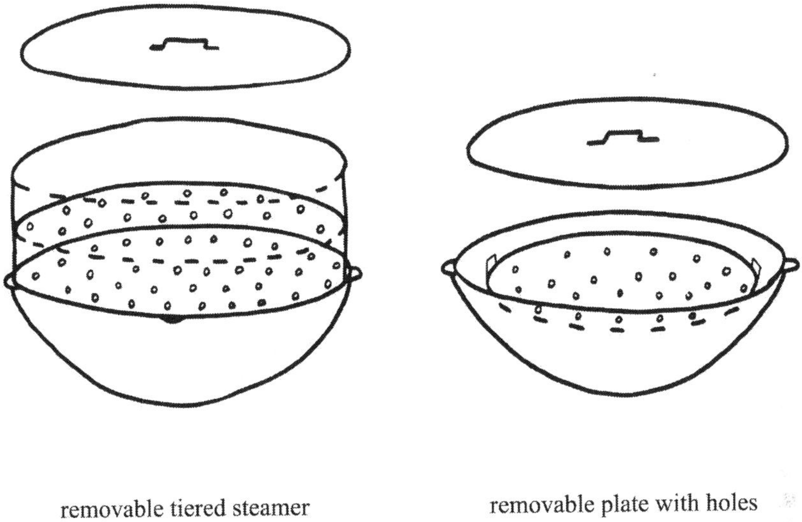

Figure 5.2 Types of steamers used in Mongolia

Source: © Sandrine Ruhlmann.

The *buuz*'s envelope has to be sufficiently thick and elastic to retain the fat of the meat during the steaming process, and not to absorb the meat juice so as the eater can suck the juice when he/she bites the envelope. The *buuz* are cooked in an aluminium steamer made up of layers (one to three) pierced with holes and placed on a large pot of boiling water. *Banš* are small dough balls boiled in the soup of meat or milk tea and eaten with the broth with a large spoon. The dough envelope has to be properly closed to retain the juice of the meat and the fat. The boiled-cooking mode does not preserve the folds and the shape of the envelope, which are, in fact, less precisely prepared than those of the *buuz*.

Conceptual ambivalence: envelope and filling

Beauty and flavour are associated in the cuisine domain but underlying issues of aesthetics and taste, important social and cosmological questions are at stake: for example, the constant concern with doing things 'in good manner'.[14] The actions of 'well closing' (*sajn bitüüleh*) the ending year, and 'well opening' (*sajn ongojlgoh*) the New Year, are two actions that are essential to attracting happiness to oneself, family and herds. To close/open the ending/opening year, families principally use foods that allow for these two actions.

On the evening of the Mongolian lunar New Year, *buuz* and *banš* are considered as 'meat' and served with the whole sheep dish (*šüüs*). Like *šüüs*, their preparation, offering and consumption allow families who offer them and visitors who consume them to 'close' the year. The following day, lunar

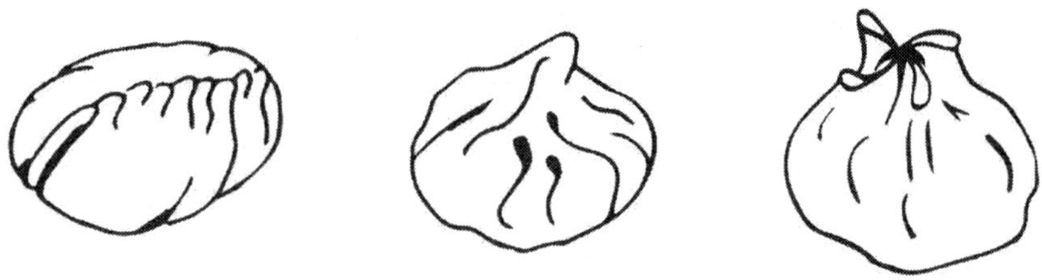

Figure 5.3 Shapes of Mongolian Dumpling

Source: © Sandrine Ruhlmann.

New Year's Day, dumplings are considered as 'white food' with regard to their white envelope and they are consumed with several dairy products, the 'white foods' associated with feasts and used for their auspiciousness and abundance. With reference to the Mongolian metaphysical system of closing/opening, the evening before lunar New Year, on 'the closed night' (*bitüün oroj*), when the 'sky is closed' (*tenger bitüü*le-), only members of the camp share the 'closed foods' (*bitüü hool*), which constitute the dish of closing (*bitüüleg*) and consist of steamed and boiled, tightly closed dumplings. On lunar New Year Day, literally 'the first new day' (*šine negen ödör*), in a symmetrical and opposite way, Mongolians perform rituals of enacting opening, implicitly, to open the year properly and set social relationships on the right course. Once the sky is open, i.e. when the sun is above the horizon, they open up their home to a 'multitude' of visitors. The lunar New Year takes the form of an open and extended sharing of foods which symbolises and materialises the beginning of a new year, expected to be prosperous and happy. Dishes eaten to celebrate an opening are considered auspicious; there are white dishes that symbolise renewal such as 'foods with flour' (pasta, dumplings, salted and fried pancakes, cakes, donuts, etc.) and sweets. These are termed 'white merits' (*cagaan bujan*).

Merits and purification: association of Buddhist notions

Offering and consuming merits is correlated to the Buddhist concept of the accumulation of merits (*bujan*, from Sanskrit *punya* 'good action, good deed'). Like dairy products, dumplings represent merits, precisely 'white merits', because they have white envelopes and are offered and consumed in 'multitude' (*zöndöö*). In Buddhist philosophy, accumulation represents the multiplication of the elements that are the basis of the life principle, as for instance, a seed, which produces an infinite number of grains. Concretely, dumplings are accumulated and shared: *buuz* are served in multiples of three (an auspicious Buddhist number) and *banš* with the broth in large numbers. The *banš* can also be boiled in milk tea to which a 'multitude' of foxtail millet grains has been added. Mongolians argue that these multitudes of 'white foods' ensure a safe return and a good life to the visitors at the lunar New Year's celebration. The custom of good auspices is to ask a person if they "have greeted a multitude multitude [*zöndöö zöndöö*] of people?" Visitors by the hundred have to answer that they "have greeted a multitude multitude" [*zöndöö zöndöö*] of people." For hosts, the main challenge is to receive the greatest number of visitors in order to offer the largest number of 'merits'.

From the late sixteenth century, when the Mongol Emperors gradually converted to Buddhism, their beliefs and ritual practices came to be associated with the concepts of auspiciousness and the abundance of dairy products. After 1990, the beginning of the period of political democratisation and religious liberalisation, Buddhism again became the official and dominant religion in Mongolia. Twenty years later, foods made of flour were again being conceptualised, just as traditional foods, as capable of attracting happiness, bringing 'merits' (*bujan hij-*) and promoting the auspicious rebirth of souls.

The Buddhist concept of merit (*bujan*) is correlated with the notion of purification (*ariutgal*), symbolised by the colour white. Since adopting Buddhism, Mongolians have integrated notions of merit and purification into their daily life and ritual practices to favour the auspicious rebirth of souls. By producing 'merits', Mongolians consider that they 'purify' (*ariula-*), 'wash' (*uga-*), 'whiten' (*cajlga-*) their polluted soul, through the redemption of negative acts accumulated during their human life. In funeral and birth rituals (Ruhlmann 2008b, 2010), as well as in the celebration of the New Year, milk, dairy products, dishes with milk and hundreds of boiled grains of rice and millet as well as dumplings, are served as 'purification foods'[15] by families to their visitors.

From culinary communism to identity discourse: strategies of appropriation

Concerning Mongolian dumplings, the objective is not to know if they come from China or Tibet but even so it is worth mentioning that Mongolian families oppose their dumplings to those of the Chinese and affirm that, because they favour the auspicious fate of the soul, they cannot belong to the Chinese culinary world. In order to explain why *buuz* and *banš* have been become an integral part of the Mongolian diet, two suggestions may be made. 1) Dumplings are a food borrowing from China as their names are formed from the Chinese word[16] and they have been largely promoted by the Mongolian Communist government in 1950; 2) Dumplings come from China and, at least since 1990, Mongolians have not conceived them explicitly as Chinese dishes and have claimed that they are 'traditional', 'authentically Mongolian'. This is an invitation to make a detour through culinary history, political contexts and identity stakes regarding food, in order to shed light on the mode of propagation, appropriation, consumption and social valorisation of dumplings.

A detour through history

The gradual adoption of *buuz* and *banš*, whether voluntary or encouraged, and their integration into the Mongolian diet as well as into the food taxonomic system, is a reflection of Mongolian history and politics in a specific period.

Before 1975, there is no mention in texts of dumplings and *buuz* or *banš* (Hamayon 1975). Indeed, travellers such as de Plan Carpin, Guillaume de Rubrouck and Marco Polo, who visited Mongolia in the second half of the thirteenth century as well as missionaries such as Antoine Mostaert who lived in the Inner Mongolia region of Ordos in the early twentieth century, all mention that the Mongolians used to consume cereals (wheat, millet, rice) in the form of grains, flour or alcohol. Like anthropologists present in Mongolia between 1950 and 1970, they never observed *buuz* or *banš* in domestic meals, but rather a great consumption of *tsampa*, a Tibetan dish composed of barley flour. Nowadays *tsampa* is made with grilled wheat flour, diluted in hot milk tea with salt and rancid butter added.[17]

Chinese and Mongolian people have been in contact since the eighth century and had many social, cultural and economic exchanges at the Yuan court of Khubilai Khan (1279–1294).[18] At this Mongol court, Turkish, Chinese and Tibetan dishes were mixed together with Mongolian dishes; the taste, because of the meat, mutton and fat, is Mongolian even if the dishes are not.[19] It is difficult to be sure when dumplings were introduced into Mongolia.[20] According to my informants, including monks from the Gandan Monastery, the principal Buddhist learning centre in Mongolia, it seems that the dumplings appeared first in the capital,[21] specifically in monasteries and Chinese canteens, and then, more recently, in Mongolian canteens, and then, in camps on the routes of jeeps and postal convoys linking various provincial capitals to Ulaanbaatar. As one informant told me, “in temples, monks have always eaten *buuz* and *banš* […] and also porridges (*budaataj cagaa*). Monks eat a lot of cereals, rice or millet, in soups, porridges, and milk tea with *banš* and sometimes with millet.”

The change of lifestyle has facilitated the adoption of dumplings. Their introduction is considered by sedentary urban families of Ulaanbaatar as a practical simplification of festive meals. Some women even mention that they can today buy frozen dumplings; this emphasises their higher economic and social status, as frozen dumplings are more expensive than homemade ones. It is an ostentatious act too because paying more for festive foods and saving time in meal preparation are means to display one’s social and economic status and to distinguish oneself from the tradition which consists of sharing distinctive parts of meat. Therefore, some families distinguish themselves by producing homemade dumplings, valued for their beauty, while other families do it by purchasing expensive frozen dumplings.

Some political foods, two egalitarian dishes

From the end of the 1930s until late in the 1980s, Mongolia’s communist government carried out policies against religion, religious practices and beliefs. It fought Shamanism and Buddhism, and their specialists, shamans and monks, through bloody repressions in the 1930s.[22] This anti-religious movement was part of the communist ideology aimed at eradicating social inequalities.

At the end of the sixteenth century, the Buddhist clergy and the Manchu administration were combating inequalities in social organisation, namely in the shamanic Mongolian society,[23] and acting to impose egalitarian ideology. The Buddhist clergy therefore opposed the clan blood sacrifice of animals at funerals in order to remove food offerings from the souls of deceased clan ancestors,[24] and concomitantly, to impose Buddhist divinities and fix beliefs and practices.

Although foods with flour are egalitarian and traditional foods are hierarchical, Mongolian families understand both as a medium to realise good deeds in a ritual context.

According to Charles Bawden (1968), the 1950s was not a period of destruction of the old order but the beginning of one that saw the construction of communism. This political ideology was imposed on the population with such pressure that even food practices were transformed. The government opposed the meal of whole sheep (*šüüs*), as this famous New Year's dish, shared according to the commensality rules, was considered as 'non egalitarian'.[25] It was replaced by an 'egalitarian' meal, the *buuz* and *banš*,[26] composed of undifferentiated pieces of meat, unattached to a bone. The government did not explicitly introduce dumplings into the daily diet, but rather selected the dish for the New Year's celebration as it would better reflect 'egalitarian' ideology. In addition to its hierarchical characteristics, the traditional mutton dish was strongly rooted in shamanistic beliefs mixed with Buddhist concepts relating to bones and flesh, and implicitly, to soul and body, and was thus incompatible with communist ideology. Dumplings were seen as a means of regulating social and economic inequalities.

With the collapse of the Communist bloc in the early 1990s, the Mongolian government established a democratic republic. It started promoting Buddhism as the official state religion in 1990 and allowed the practice of Shamanism. Thanks to this, new practices combining Buddhism and "shamanic elements"[27] are emerging. One might think that the revival of shamanic beliefs would have revived the non-egalitarian iconic mutton dish of the lunar New Year. However, the *buuz* and *banš* meals have, in urban areas, and partially, in rural areas, replaced the traditional mutton of the lunar New Year celebration, maintaining thereby the Buddhist notion of 'merit' and 'multitude'. Thus, the Mongolians shifted from a Communist imposition of an egalitarian dish to a religious choice to conserve this dish to celebrate the most important of events, the New Year. This invites an analysis of how they came to consider *buuz* and *banš* as an object of an identity claim, specifically, an anti-Chinese claim.

Identity claim foods

In 1962, the communist government condemned 'Qing domination', the dynasty Qing established in 1644 by the Manchu, and prohibited any historical reference to the medieval past, especially, to Genghis Khan. But over the last two decades, the new republic of Mongolia has been developing the conception of the Mongolian nation as one ethnic and cultural unity. The Halh, the descendants of Genghis Khan's ethnic group that forms the majority of the population, became the 'reference' in this national construction. New and reinvented shamanic practices, attributed to Genghiskhanids, were raised to the rank of 'tradition' (*jos zanšil*) and a national folklore was created, legitimised by the return to authentically Mongolian values (Aubin 1993, 1996).[28] Today, the State appoints shamans to perform its major national celebrations. A strong nationalist feeling emerged from this process, reinforced by the Mongolian elites designed as the "holders of knowledge" (Aubin 1996: 306, 311, 315–316). Historians, archaeologists, folklorists, anthropologists and journalists created a history of the Mongol Empire by styling Genghis Khan as the first Emperor who formed a Mongolian nation endowed with a code of laws and ethics.

Since the 1990s, the government has promoted activities and emblematic products that contribute to the economic wealth of the country (nomadic herding, dairy products), in order to create an 'authentic Mongolian nation'. The nomads' lifestyle and culture has become the pride of the Mongolian people.[29] In the 2000s, a discourse began to emerge based on the 'Mongolian purity', using the ideology of a primary and biological ethnicity. The process of 'Mongolisation' has affected Mongolians food practices and perceptions: the majority of families consider dumplings as a Mongolian dish and integrate them into their representation system of traditional food, using terms such as 'authentic' (*žinhene*), 'true' (*jostoj*), 'pure' (*cever*), 'traditional' (*jos zanšiltaj*), to qualify them.

The rise of nationalism has reached a climax in recent years with expressions of 'ultra-nationalism' in Ulaanbaatar, targeting the Chinese in particular. Isolated cases of the lynching of Mongolian–Chinese mixed couples are always widely publicised by Mongolian media. The growing nationalist ideology of 'pure' and 'unmixed' is also at the heart of the Halh Mongolians' discourses when they distinguish themselves from other Mongolian ethnic minorities, by brandishing their iconic founder father, Genghis Khan.

It is nevertheless necessary to note that many parts of the contemporary cooking equipment of nomads are Chinese, such as the central closed stove (*zuuh*) with its three concentric circles which replaced the typical Mongolians open stove (*tulga*) or the tripod used in the thirteenth century. The tiered steamer and its pierced plates are also imported from China. The method of cooking by steaming and the consumption of cereals as well as steamed and boiled dumplings had been in use in China for a long time. The term *buuz*, used to refer to the steamed dumplings in the Mongolian language, in fact derives from the Chinese term *baozi*. However, Mongolians refuse to consider dumplings (*buuz* and *banš*) as a food borrowing from China. In spite of a strong feeling of aversion towards China, Chinese people, Chinese culture and everything made in China, they attribute a high value to dumplings. Their opinion of Chinese-made products as 'poor quality' products,[30] has probably emerged in response to Mongolian–Chinese relations and the conflicted history composed of invasions and dominations accompanied by ideological and religious repressions.

Implicitly, *buuz* and *banš* dishes are understood as inherited from an ancient past, as several Mongolians expressed it: "our *buuz*, our Mongolian *buuz* (*mongol buuz*) have nothing to do with Chinese *buuz* (*hjatad buuz*). *Buuz* are an authentic (*žinhene*) Mongolian food."

Conclusion

Food is arguably the most resistant link with the land of the ancestors. The claim to the authentic Mongolian nature of *buuz* and *banš* is found in the terms used to naturalise Chinese dumplings as Mongolian traditional foods. In this type of identity construct Mongolians re-appropriate culinary elements: cooking utensils, recipes, techniques, gestures and knowledge. In addition, they develop discourses justifying these particular dishes as not borrowed, but strictly native. This process is a kind of *bricolage* that combines different elements of discourse and practice, and readjusts them depending on situations, questions and ritual requirements. Mongolians prepare, offer, share and consume dumplings, and confer upon them a place of excellence in their system of valorisation of foods because they refuse to recognise their Chinese origin. Identifying their dumplings as a Mongolian food, they give them the capacity to promote the beneficial fate of the soul after death and an auspicious rebirth in a human body. Mongolians are appropriating exogenous culinary elements by creating a link with their ancient beliefs, in their domestic practices and traditions.

Dumplings assume an indispensable position within a culinary system of meanings and are the basis of a dichotomy of colours (white envelope/grey-brown filling). This dichotomy takes place in a religious and philosophical context and the dumplings are thus considered as opening/closing foods and 'merits' that accumulate and guarantee happiness (individual and collective happiness). Moreover, by their symbolism, they allow for the revival of an ancient order of beliefs, mixing reinvented shamanic elements with Buddhism, in a contemporary context of political democracy, religious tolerance and openness to the global market economy. When it comes to the question of cooking, there is always something to say about religion and politics!

Notes

1 See: *Histoire secrète des Mongols* 1994; Paul Pelliot 1949 and *The Secret Story of the Mongols* (2004).

2 During fieldwork I participated in Mongolian women's activities and shared the daily lives of 20 families: 10 families in the national capital Ulaanbaatar located in the region of Töv and six in the provincial capital of Öndörhaan in Hentij, as well as four nomadic pastoralist families in Mörön, a commune of the Hentij region. All these families are linked by marriage alliances or by relationships of mutual aid and service exchange (commercial and non-commercial) of food exchange (vegetables), fuel (wood, coal), water (blocks of ice), fodder, or other goods.

3 *Buuz* and *banš* are neither ravioli nor dumplings. However, I use *dumplings* when referring jointly to *buuz* and *banš*, in order to simplify my remarks.

4 According to their place of residence (grassy steppe, forest, desert), nomadic pastoralists breed, and draw their subsistence from herds of one or two species.
5 The term *šüüs* refers to the broth of meat soup, the sheep that is slaughtered for consumption, as well as the traditional dish of whole mutton.
6 The opening of the stove through which women introduce dried cow dung faces the southeast.
7 Meat is in line with a 'rite of passage' (Van Gennep 1960).
8 Similarly, in France and other European countries, the period between Christmas and Epiphany is 'time out' during which the quality of the new coming year calls for some opening acts (Perrot 2000). This is a period of passage and initiation for children and adolescents (Van Gennep 1987, 1988), a propitious period of communication between the living and the dead (Lévi-Strauss 1952). During this period, many prophylactic practices are used to "ensure the success of the coming year" (Perrot 2000: 17–18).
9 Milk and dairy products are frozen by exposure to winter temperatures and stored in external warehouses.
10 While families that I surveyed mentioned the word 'close' in terms of what the lunar New Year celebration allows them to do, a few of them never evoked the symmetrical verb of 'open' for the day that opens the new year.
11 The notion of 'merit' merges with a deeper critical issue, that of the soul's life in general, and of its future after death, in particular. Auspicious acts performed during life by the individual and his/her family are counted at the time of death to define the soul's future. The threat inherent to a bad rebirth of the soul in Buddhist philosophy has entered into Mongolian popular shamanistic beliefs. More specifically, the Buddhist notions of sin, the moral judgment of the soul and individual *karma* (Chabros 1992) are mingled with shamanistic concepts of 'soul' (*süns*) and 'rebirth' (*dahin töröl*), resulting in syncretic conceptions of the soul and its fate after death. Mongolians believe that the soul leaves the body at death and is reborn either in the body of an animal – a bad rebirth that does not allow reproduction of the kin-group, or in the body of a newborn baby – a good rebirth allowing for the perpetuation of the lineage or clan.
12 On the importance of the ductility of dough, see Françoise Sabban (2000).
13 On technical gestures and details of preparation of *buuz* and *banš*, see Sandrine Ruhlmann (2008a).
14 A concern that is inculcated from an early age through a domestic training process using imitation and improvement (Ruhlmann 2008a).
15 Alimentary purification consists not only of ingesting purifying foods, but also of purification acts, such as sprinkling liquid or raw foods on objects (milk, raw rice or millet), or anointing body parts with specific foods or liquids (milk, milk tea or holy water mixed with milk) (Ruhlmann 2008b, 2010).
16 The Mongolian ethnographic references concerning food practices do not mention dumplings as a dish (Ongoodoj 1991).
17 This dish seems to have become less common, and I am not aware of any families that still consume it today. This being said, the 'white butter' (*cagaan tos*) dish still prepared today resembles the grilled flour dough of the *tsampa*.
18 The Yuan dynasty is a Mongol dynasty founded by Khubilai Khan and reigned over China from 1279 to 1368.
19 See Herbert Franke 1970, Françoise Sabban 1983, Paul D. Buell 1990, Eugene N. Anderson 1994, Paul D. Buell and Eugene N. Anderson 1997.
20 I have not found any indication of this in English, French or Mongolian sources, but perhaps some might be found in Russian, Tibetan or Chinese texts, and it would certainly be relevant to differentiate dumplings prepared and eaten at home from those served in Chinese or Mongolian canteens in Ulaanbaatar. My informants attempted to evaluate the period of the introduction of the dumplings and the

beginning of the domestic consumption of *buuz* and *banš* by identifying the different generations of their family who did not possess a steamer, did not know how to use a steamer or to prepare dumplings. But their responses revealed their ignorance.

21 My informants do not specify if it concerns the medieval capital, Har Horijn (thirteenth century), or Ih Hüree or Öörgö (seventeenth century) renamed Ulaanbataar in 1924, that could indicate a period.

22 For further information on the religious and political history of Mongolia, and the waves of repression against Shamanism by the Buddhist clergy from the late sixteenth century, or against Shamanism and Buddhism by the Communist government, see Charles Bawden (1968), Walter Heissig (1953), Valentin A. Riazanovski (1965) and Chris Kaplonski (2004).

23 Edmund Weber discusses the egalitarian and anti-caste aspect of Buddhism (in ancient Indian) which distinguishes it from Hinduism (2001). In another article (1999), he explains how, in India from the 1950s, neo-Buddhists have been forming a movement that spreads Buddhism as a higher form of the Indian religions and philosophies, encouraging Dalits (untouchables) to convert to Buddhism. Thus, in India and other countries of South and East Asia where Hinduism is prominent, the egalitarian aspect of Buddhism is reflected in its opposition to the Hindu caste system. From ancient India to modern Mongolia, Buddhism was adopted in different Asian countries and syncretic practices and beliefs emerged in these Asian countries through a process of integrating local beliefs; but arguably in Tibet and Mongolia egalitarian claims were not developed.

24 Regarding this Buddhist prohibition of the ritual of animal sacrifice, see Riazanovski (1965), Heissig (1953) and Ruhlmann (2008c).

25 Personal communication from Françoise Aubin and Roberte Hamayon. I could find no precise information on the government's process.

26 I am grateful to Françoise Aubin, orientalist and specialist in Mongolian and Chinese worlds, for drawing my attention to this distinction between the status of different dishes which makes sense in this political context.

27 Expression borrowed from Hamayon (1990: 706).

28 According to Alain Babadzan (1999), in contemporary societies, traditions are created or invented when a strong nationalistic sentiment emerges from a context of long political, economic and historical conflicts. Concerning the invention of traditions, see Eric Hobsbawm and Terence Ranger (1983). Regarding the nationalism as social artefacts and political constructions, see Hobsbawm (1990). Concerning the creation of a national identity in communist Mongolia and the role given to Genghis Khan, see Chris Kaplonski (1998).

29 For further reading on the exaltation of the nomadic lifestyle by the government since the 1990s, see Uradyn E. Bulag (1998). He explains how, after having been looked down upon by the communist government, the herder is now erected as a reference figure replacing the emblematic figure of the proletarian from the communist epoch.

30 Local and Russian vodkas are preferred to the cheaper Chinese ones. Mongolians, nevertheless, prefer the Čingis vodka, named for the eponymous emperor; the name in Mongolian classic writing enhances the emperor's portrait on the bottle's label.

References

Anderson, E.N. (1994). "Food and health at the mongol court", in E.H. Kaplan and W. Whisenhunt (eds.), *Opuscula Altaica, Essays Presented in Honor of Henry Schwarz*, pp. 17–43. Bellingham: Washington, Center for East Asian Studies 19.

Aubin, F. (1993). "Renouveau gengiskhanide et nationalisme dans la Mongolie postcommuniste", *Cahiers d'Etudes sur la Méditerranée Orientale et le Monde Turco-Iranien*, Vol. 16: 137–207.

Aubin, F. (1996). "La Mongolie des premières années de l'après-communisme: La popularisation du passé dans les mass media mongols (1990–1995)", *Etudes Mongoles et Sibériennes*, Vol. 27: 305–326.

Babadzan, A. (1999). "L'invention des traditions et le nationalisme", *Journal de la Société des Océanistes*, Vol. 109(2): 13–35.

Bawden, C. (1968). *The Modern History of Mongolia*, London: Weidenfeld and Nicolson, 'Asia and Africa Series'.

Buell, P.D. (1990). "Pleasing the palate of the Qan: changing foodways of the imperial Mongols", *Mongolian Studies, Journal of the Mongolia Society*, Vol. 13: 57–81.

Buell, P.D. and Anderson, E.N. (1997). *A Soup for the Qan. Introduction, Translation, Commentary and Chinese Text*, London, New York: Kegan Paul International.

Bulag, U.E. (1998). *Nationalism and Hybridity in Mongolia*, Oxford: Clarendon Press.

Chabros, K. (1992). *Beckoning Fortune: A Study of the Mongol* Dalalga *Ritual*, Wiesbaden: Otto Harrassowitz.

Even, M.-D. (1999). "L'au-delà dans les représentations religieuses des Mongols", in P. Servais (ed.), *La mort et l'au-delà: Une rencontre de l'Orient et de l'Occident*, pp. 149–196. Louvain-la-Neuve: Academia Bruylant.

Franke, H. (1970). "Additional notes on non-Chinese terms in the Yüan imperial dietary compendium Yin-Shan Cheng-Yao", *Zentral Asiatische Studien*, Vol. 4: 7-16.

Hamayon, R. (1975). "L'os distinctif et la chair indifférente", *Études Mongoles*, Vol. 6: 99–122.

Hamayon, R. (1978). "Marchandage d'âme entre vivants et morts", *Le sacrifice II. Système de pensée en Afrique Noire*, Cahier 3: 151–179.

Hamayon, R. (1990). *La Chasse à l'âme. Esquisse d'une théorie du chamanisme Sibérien*, Nanterre: Société d'Ethnologie, Mémoires de la Société 1.

Heissig, W. (1953). "A Mongolian source to the lamaist suppression of shamanism in the seventeenth century ", *Anthropos*, Vol. 48(4–5): 493–533.

Histoire secrète des Mongols. Chronique mongole du XIIIe siècle (1994). Translated and annotated by M. D. Even and R. Pop, preface by R. Hamayon, Paris: Gallimard.

Hobsbawm, E. and Ranger, T. (eds.) (1983). *The Invention of Tradition*, Cambridge: Cambridge University Press.

Hobsbawm, E.J. (1990). *Nations and Nationalism since 1780: Programme, Myth, Reality*. Cambridge: Cambridge University Press.

Kaplonski, C. (1998). "Creating national identity in socialist Mongolia", *Central Asian Survey*, Vol. 17(1): 35–37.

Kaplonski, C. (2004). *Truth, History and Politics in Mongolia: The Memory of Heroes*, London: Routledge Curzon.

Lévi-Strauss, C. (1952). "Le père Noël supplicié", *Les Temps modernes*, Vol. 77: 1572–1590.

Ongoodoj, Č. (1991). *Mongol ideen tovčoo (Abrégé des aliments mongols)*, Oulan-Bator: Ulsyn hevlelijn gazar.

Pelliot, P. (1949). *Histoire secrète des Mongols. Restitution du texte mongol et traduction des chapitres I à VI*, Paris: Adrien-Maisonneuve.

Perrot, M. (2000). *Ethnologie de Noël. Une fête paradoxale*, Paris: Grasset.

Plan Carpin, J. de (1965). *Histoire des Mongols*, translated and annotated by J. Becquet and L. Hambis, Paris : Adrien-Maisonneuve.

Riazanovski, V.A. (1965). *Fundamental Principles of Mongol Law*, Bloomington: Indiana University Publications, Uralic and Altaic Series, 43, 1st publication 1937.

Ruhlmann, S. (2007). "Les 'nourritures enveloppées' du Mois blanc: nourritures de fête du nouvel an lunaire en Mongolie", *OCHA*, article online *www.lemangeur-ocha.com*.

Ruhlmann, S. (2008a). "La beauté des farineux. Une approche anthropologique de la notion mongole d'esthétique", in *Perceptions esthétiques en contexte mongol et sibérien*, Communication du 3e Congrès du Réseau Asie-IMASIE, www.reseau-asie.com.

Ruhlmann, S. (2008b). "Les pratiques alimentaires funéraires chez les Mongols Xalx. Purifications, offrandes et repas", in G. Boëtsch, M. Signoli and S. Tzortzis (eds.), *La mort en montagne – Perceptions, représentations, rituels*, pp. 243–256. Gap: Éditions des Hautes Alpes.

Ruhlmann, S. (2008c). "Une soupe peu ordinaire. Analyse du repas des funérailles chez les Mongols", *Techniques et Culture*, Vol. 51: 246–271.

Ruhlmann, S. (2010). "Les rites de naissance chez les Mongols Halh: la fermeture/ouverture des corps, des nourritures et du social", in I. Aigle, D. Charleux, V. Goossaert and R. Hamayon (eds.), Mélanges en l'honneur de Françoise Aubin, pp. 225–247. Monumenta Serica Monographs Series LXI, Miscellanea Asiatica.

Ruhlmann, S. (2011). "Festins claniques ou repas de fête des foyers domestiques. Étude des pratiques mongoles du banquet, XIII/XXIe siècles", *Journal Asiatique*, Vol. 299(2): 601–613, 'La fête au Palais: banquets, musique et parures en Orient'.

Sabban, F. (1983). "Cuisine à la cour de l'empereur de Chine: les aspects culinaires de Yinshan Zhengyao de Hu Sihui", *Médiévales*, Vol. 5: 32–56.

Sabban, F. (2000). "Quand la forme transcende l'objet. Histoire des pâtes alimentaires en Chine (IIIe siècle av. J.-C. – IIIe siècle ap. J.-C.)", *Annales HSS*, 'Histoire de l'alimentation', Vol. 4: 791–824.

The Secret Story of the Mongols (2004). *A Mongolian Epic Chronicle of the Thirteenth Century*. Translated with a Historical and Philological Commentary by Igor de Rachewiltz, Vol. 2, Leiden: Brill.

Van Gennep, A. (1960). *The Rites of Passage*, London: Routledge, 1st publication1909.

Van Gennep, A. (1987). *Manuel de folklore français contemporain*, tome I, volume VII, *Cycle des douze jours: Noël*, par B. Guichard, Paris: Picard.

Van Gennep, A. (1988). *Manuel de folklore français contemporain*, tome I, volume VIII, *Cycle des douze jours: de Noël aux Rois*, Paris: Picard.

Weber, E. (1999). "Ambedkar and the Hindu Culture", *Journal of Religious Culture*, Vol. 18b. http://web.uni-frankfurt.de/irenik/religionskultur.htm (retrieved on 03 March 2012).

Weber, E. (2001). "Buddhism: an Atheistic and Anti-Caste Religion ? ", *Journal of Religious Culture*, Vol. 50. http://web.uni-frankfurt.de/irenik/religionskultur.htm (retrieved on 03 March 2012).

6 "Beef is our secret of life"

Controversial consumption of beef in Andhra Pradesh, India

Brigitte Sébastia

Introduction

Indian food culture is unique in its elaborated taxonomy of ingredients which is strongly determined by interwoven social, philosophical, religious and medical rules (Khare 1976). The Indian diet is seen today as facing changes in consumption with the introduction of new products, either imported or developed by agro-industry, and in eating habits which increasingly include eating-out (Dittrich 2009; Nandy 2004; Pingali and Khwaja 2004). However, it remains largely 'traditional', based on cereals accompanied by sauces made of pulses and/or vegetables, curd, pickles and side dishes prepared with green leaves, vegetables and/or meat, fish, eggs whose composition is very much conditioned by religion, socio-cultural milieu and economic resources.[1] In this food pattern, consumption of animal products is especially governed by strict rules, and thus represents an important cultural marker on which the whole of Indian society is structured. Beef and buffalo meat has a particular status that may be qualified as peripheral: Indians, except Jains, consume it but only according to location, and caste (for Hindus and Christians) or community affiliation (for Muslims and Buddhists). Due to western influence and the development of catering that today offers a wide variety of regional and international cuisines, well-off urban upper castes, notably the younger generation, may be attracted to experience the taste of bovine meat. Nonetheless, apart from Kerala where its consumption is common – though not among upper castes – beef remains strongly associated with marginalised people: Hindu and Christian Dalits,[2] Muslims and tribal people.

This was not always so. Studies on food consumption in ancient India show that cow's meat was the most valued of foods and served during festivals and rituals and to welcome important guests (Jhā 2009; Prakash 1961). Its gradual proscription by Hindu upper castes results from a long movement of 'sacralisation' of the cow that emerged with a revival of Brahmanism aimed at thwarting influential movements by Buddhists and Jains against animal sacrifice (Jhā *ibid.*; Shah 1967). This prohibition grew stricter during the nineteenth century when Hindu nationalists struggled to protect cows from being slaughtered. Brandished as the symbol of Hindu identity, or according to Shraddha Chigateri (2011: 141) as "a potent symbol of religious difference", the cow was used overtly as a tool for stirring up religious hatred against Muslims, and less openly against the British, both regarded as consumers of beef, and as anti-Hindus. Although the Hindu lower castes were not directly targeted by Hindu nationalists, they were blamed for their undesirable food habits and exhorted to give them up (Abbasayulu 1980).

The cow-related emotional charge means that the subject continues to be instrumental in unleashing inter-communal dissension. Although more frequent in the north, altercations sometimes erupt in southern states, as in April 2012 at Hyderabad where two conflicts occurred. The first was provoked by Hindus who, in line with a well-established strategy, introduced legs of beef into a temple in order to trigger Hindu reprisals against Muslims during the festival of Hanuman's birthday (Hanuman Jayanthi).[3] The second, more innovative, was sparked off by students of Osmania University (OU), Hyderabad, mostly Dalits, when they organised a 'beef festival' on 15th April 2012, during which they distributed beef *biriyāni*. Based on this event which I attended, and where I conducted interviews with diverse actors: organisers, students, professors, journalists, supporters of, as well as opponents of the festival, the present chapter aims to analyse the discourses legitimising the right to consume beef. Compared to the previous debates on cow protection between nationalists, politicians, jurists, and academics the students' arguments present a counterweight, fuelled by knowledge of nutrition sciences, valorisation of cultural diversity and human rights. It is this richness of debate that the chapter aims to demonstrate. It will consist of three parts. The first will trace the main movements to have supported cow protection, thus elucidating the Dalit students' choice of beef as a symbol of their food culture, and why debates on cow protection continue to occupy the political scene with an increasing number of states enacting bills forbidding cow slaughter, transport, eating and export. The second part will analyse the values that the students attributed to the cow to justify its flesh appearing in university messes. It will discuss the choice of beef *biriyāni* to symbolise their 'food culture' or 'traditional food', as this dish, created by Mughals, has not been consumed much at all by lower caste people. Lastly, the third part will analyse the values attributed to the cow which have fuelled the debates on the relevance of protecting it. These borrow from three paradigms: materialism, symbolism and ethics. As the analysis of the plurality of discourses on beef consumption in India addresses materialism, commensality, identity, culturalism and symbolism, it is, undoubtedly, the food which best fits Claude Levy-Strauss' formula: "good to think about".[4]

Historical context of cow protection

Examples of communal riots based on cow issues abound in studies on Hindu nationalist movements which were the instigators and supporters of cow protection. Compared to the context which will be explored at OU, the conflicts revolving around the cow were based primarily on religious affiliation: Hindus/cow-protectors *versus* Muslims/cow-killers. Ian Copland (2005), from his analysis of Arab and Persian commentaries and accounts of European travellers, argues that Muslim–Hindu conflicts over the cow are certainly old but difficult to apprehend in terms of frequency and intensity due to scarcity of documentation. Some facts suggest that cow consumption was a controversial subject in India before the emergence of Hindu nationalist movements. In some regions, Muslim rulers such as Akbar, Al-Biruni, Babur, Jahanjir and Aurangzeb, had banned cow slaughter so as to maintain harmonious relationships with Hindus and Jains (Al-Biruni 1971; Jhā *ibid*.; Krishna 1985; van der Veer 1994), and the British imposed the same policy in sensitive places such as Madura in 1805 (Copland *ibid*.). Two decades before that, the Arya Samaj, a nationalist movement founded in 1875 by Dayananda Saraswati, led actions for cow protection in Punjab; this region had been affected by serious riots instigated by Sikhs who attacked Muslims butchers in reprisals for the British victory over them (Jhā *ibid*.; O'Toole 2003).

The ideology of Arya Samaj was to purify Hinduism of 'evil habits' such as child-marriage or widow-burning, and to revitalise and unify the Hindu community in order "to resist attacks by Muslims and British invaders" (O'Toole *ibid*.: 86). In this perspective, Arya Samajists strongly encouraged low castes to cease consuming beef and alcohol that they presented as being the root of discrimination against them. Preaching the 'true' Hinduism – that of the Vedas –, founding cow protection societies (*gaurakshini sabha*) and *gaushala* (cowshed)[5] and taking actions against cow slaughter by Muslims, Arya Samajists spread the cow protection movement over a large part of North India. In his treatise *Gokarunanidhi* (Ocean of Mercy to the cow), Dayananda Saraswati firmly opposed to slaughtering cows, his justification being that, as the cow is the symbol of the nation, killing was an anti-Hindu act (van der Veer 1994; O' Toole *ibid*.). This movement, widely publicised through pamphlets, meetings, tracts etc., inevitably stirred up Hindu hatred for Muslims, notably during the festival of Bakr-Id.[6] Numerous riots broke out between the two religious communities, such as at Azambarh in 1893, Ayodhya in 1912–1913 and Shabalad in 1917, to name the most violent and best known ones (Pandey 1983).

To put an end to communal riots, a regulation on slaughterhouses and protection of cattle was introduced into the Indian constitution in 1958, in the form of Article 48 emanating from a judgment of the Supreme Court.[7] It stipulates: "The State shall endeavour to organise agriculture and animal husbandry on modern and scientific lines and shall, in particular, take steps for preserving and improving the breeds, and prohibiting the slaughter of cows and calves and other milch and draught cattle". This article, still effective, belongs to the 'Directive Principles' that aim to guide the states of the Indian Union to enact their regulations which might be appealed or challenged in courts (Raj 1979). Christophe Jaffrelot (1996) interprets the inclusion of this article into a Directive Principles of State Policy as the intention of Jawaharlal Nehru, like Mohandas Karamchand Gandhi,[8] not to pass a law which could be used against Muslims. Chigateri (*ibid*.) gives a different interpretation: considering the fundamental rights dealing with human rights, the protection of animal rights might not be considered "in the same veins as human rights" (*ibid*.: 143).

Elevating the cow to the symbol of the Hindu nation has been for Arya Samaj, and then, for Hindu nationalist parties such as Bharatiya Jana Sangh, founded in 1951, and Rashtriya Swayamsevak Sangh (RSS), Vishva Hindu Parishad (VHP) and Bharatiya Janata Party (BJP) which emerged after 1980, a highly effective instrument for unifying and mobilising Hindus against Muslims. On 31st October 1952, the RSS launched an anti-cow slaughter movement and a procession of petitioners, seen by Jaffrelot as "clearly an attempt at ethno-religious mobilization" (*ibid.*: 113), that collected hundreds of thousands of signatures. In the next decade, a huge *satyāgraha*[9] to demand a total ban on cow slaughter was organised by the Sarvadaliya Goraksha Maha Abhiyan Samitri. Put into operation largely by *sadhus*,[10] among them the Shankaracharya of Puri who embarked on an unlimited fast when police arrested demonstrators, it gathered between 125,000 and 700,000 demonstrators (Jaffrelot *ibid.*; Shah *ibid.*). The agitation culminated in a massive demonstration outside Sansad Bhavan in New Delhi on 7 November 1966. The death of eight demonstrators caused the resignation of the Home Minister of the Indira Gandhi government, Gulzarilal Nanda, followed by the Shankaracharya of Puri suspending his fast. Once again, in April 1979, a demand for the strict prohibition of cow slaughter applied to the whole country was presented to the central government by Achaya Vinoba Bhave, the spiritual successor to Gandhi, who also undertook a hunger strike (Raj 1979). After obtaining an assurance from Morarji Desai, he broke his strike (Jha *ibid.*). Nonetheless, no uniform law on cow slaughter was enacted by the central government, neither at this time nor later. The fact that the regulation against cattle slaughter depends on the authority of the state/territory governments has two consequences: first, a lack of uniformity between states/territories; secondly, the temptation for nationalist political parties to harden the law in states/territories where they are powerful. The states of Kerala, Arunachal Pradesh, Manipur, Mizoram, Nagaland, Tripura and Meghalaya and the union territory of Lakshadweep have no such legislation. The other states and union territories have enacted regulations, more and less prohibitive, ranging from a moderate ban on slaughtering cows and bullocks under ten years old to a total ban on slaughtering, transporting, storing and consuming bovine meat, including buffalo meat, whatever be the age, gender, biological stage and health condition of animals, violators to be severely punished by fines and imprisonment. Under the impetus of the BJP, which won the national election in 1998 and in 2014, and plays an increasing political role at the local level, several states have reinforced their regulations on cow protection. Gujarat, Rajasthan, Maharashtra and Haryana are the last states to have strengthened their laws in 2015 (Venkatesan 2015); the state of Kerala, famous for its cow slaughter, faces regular pressure to stop this activity. The new legislation of the state of Maharashtra, even though it excludes buffalos, has been the most contested by opponents of the ban. As the state hosts, at Deonar (suburb of Mumbai), the largest abattoir in the country, providing 25% of the beef and buffalo meat on the Indian market (Saglio-Yatzimirsky 2010), the law endangers the livelihood of numerous low caste people who work in abattoirs, industries transforming cow products (meat, carcasses, hide, blood, fat, etc.) and in the transportation of cattle.[11] It affects the livelihood of farmers who are constrained to feed unproductive cattle, increases the risk of cattle abandonment and weakens the meat trade in Kerala and Goa which imported cattle from Maharashtra. Moreover, it deprives poor people of cheap protein-rich resources as the price of this meat is increasing.[12] Compared to these states, the regulations on cow protection enacted by Andhra Pradesh are very moderate, but this does not mean that consumption of cow flesh is not an issue there.

The beef festival: a highly controversial subject

A glance at the beef festival

We resemble black lotus	We have been eating tasty beef
We have been shining like a black sun	We have been fighting for social justice
We have been standing very healthy	We have been struggling against the state
We have been singing very beauty	We hate hierarchy in the world
We have been learning more very easy	We hate casteism in the soul
Reason for all these things is	We hate patriarchy – we love democracy
Beef secret of my energy	Every quality got from *shiyya* [beef]
Beef secret of our knowledge	

(Song composed and written by Sharat Naliganti, Student at OU on the occasion of the beef festival organised in the University 15 April 2012)

While I was passing the EFLU (English and Foreign Languages University) on my way to the library of the National Institute of Nutrition (NIN) where I was documenting food-related diseases in Indian history, I was attracted by a banner at the gate announcing a workshop entitled 'Food culture and democracy'. The workshop had already taken place but, interested in information about the topics and participants, given that food is hardly studied in India in social sciences,[13] I contacted a professor mentioned on the banner. He informed me that this workshop concerned beef consumption and invited me to contact a food scientist of the NIN who had participated in the workshop. After I had explained my interest in food culture to this scientist, she suggested that I attend the beef festival organised by students at OU on 15th April 2012 that she expected to attend herself. Intrigued by the reasons for such a festival which seemed to me highly sensitive given the recent communal conflict at Hyderabad, I went to the Department of Political Sciences where a professor introduced the organisers, mostly Dalit students of political science, to me. They explained that they were planning to cook and distribute a beef *biriyāni* on the campus in order to promote consideration of beef: "Beef belongs to our food culture and we want beef to be served in the university messes." They speculated that, after tasting beef, students would accept it on the menu of OU. They also argued that studies conducted by the NIN show that beef is the most nutritious food. Mentioning the recent brawl between Hindus and Muslims during the Hanuman Jayanthi, I asked if they did not fear that beef distribution inside the campus, i.e. in the public sphere, might lead to violence. They reassured me, saying that no objection to this issue was heard during the workshop 'Food culture and Democracy' that they had organised on 9th April in order to win opponents over to their cause. Nevertheless, the day before the celebration, the organisers of the beef festival received a pamphlet from Akhila Bharatya Vidyarthi Parishad (ABVP), a student nationalist association with close links to the BJP and RSS, denouncing the festival as an attempt to 'degrade Indian culture', and threatening reprisals.

The day of the festival arrived. Accompanied by my husband, I went in the morning to the Narmada Hostel, also called Ambedkar Hostel[14] where we joined a group of 30 students gathered around a 'beef festival' banner. On the banner were portrayed politicians, philosophers, social activists and reformers: Karl Marx, Jyothi Rao Phule, Periyar E.V. Ramaswamy, B.R. Ambedkar, Narayana Guru, Komaram Bheem, Chakali Ilamma and Jagjivam Ram.[15] The students explained that they chose 15th April for the beef festival in memory of Jyothi Rao Phule, B.R. Ambedkar, Jagjivam Ram and Kormaram Bheem.[16] Among these, Komaram Bheem and Chakali Ilamma were particularly effective in rallying participants to celebrate the 'beef festival' as they fought for Telangana independence,[17] a cause supported by many student associations of Hyderabad universities. The inclusion of Karl Marx among Indian figures was with regard to his works on colonial imperialism, Indian society and peasantry, etc. (Iqbal 2008; Basu 2007), which fed the students' struggle against caste discrimination, inequality in education and political imperialism, and for democracy. It was also in accordance with his political affiliation. Andhra Pradesh is one of the Indian states where the Communist party (Marxist) is powerful, notably in Telangana as, before independence, it fought the power of the Nizam and the ostracism of low castes, tribes and women. This link was obviously attractive to Dalit students who envisaged Telangana as a territory in which everybody would be treated with respect and without discrimination (*Anveshi* 2012).

The organisers had planned to cook beef *biriyāni* in front of the Narmada Hostel at 3 o'clock, but they received a notification from the police ordering them to arrange the meal off campus so as not to offend the sensibility of beef non-eaters. Around 6 o'clock, the organisers took their positions on the podium erected in front of the Narmada Hostel, on which ten professors and/or activists, among them several who had participated in the workshop 'Democracy and Food Culture', sat facing the crowd of participants and the serried rows of media cameras.[18] Among the best known were Kancha Ilaiah, professor of politics and director of the Centre for the Study of Social Exclusion and Inclusive Policy at Maulana Azad National Urdu University, and also a Bahujan[19] activist, author of *Why I am not a Hindu* and *Buffalo Nationalism: A Critique of Spiritual Fascism*; P.L. Visweswara Rao, retired professor of communication and journalism at OU and an activist; Sambaiah Gundimeda, an assistant professor of political sociology at the Council for Social Development, Hyderabad; Gali Vinod Kumar, professor of law, OU; and Bhangya Bhukya, head and associate professor at the department of Social Exclusion Studies, EFLU, and a specialist in the Lambada community (Schedule Tribe ST).

Police, who had been standing by since the start of the afternoon and were later joined by a large deployment of paramilitary forces, moved closer to the podium. The organisers and some of the professors and activists gave talks about the benefits of eating beef and, after singing the song 'Beef is our secret of life', they invited participants to share beef *biriyāni*. While the meal was being distributed, shouted slogans such as *Bharat Mata ki Jai* (Glory to Mother India) were heard from the neighbouring student hostel. Immediately, paramilitary forces rushed at a large group of students determined to destroy the material related to food distribution; *lathi* charges and teargas were use to contain the violence. The meal which began in a joyous atmosphere ended in desolation with several students injured; a university bus and a media car were set on fire.

The next day, the opposing students, mostly from ABVP, insisted on being received by the vice-chancellor of the university to lodge a complaint against the organisers and professors who dared to defy the rules by imposing beef eating in the public sphere. They submitted a memorandum demanding that action be initiated against the three professors of OU who attended the beef festival. The vice-chancellor reassured them as regards the total ban on beef in messes. With the support of right-wing members of Vishwa Hindu Parishad and Bajrang Dal, they organised a provocative cow ritual (*Gau puja*) in the temple adjacent to the Art College to clean the campus of pollution. A few days later, the three denounced professors were arrested. The defeat of the organisers may be explained by their failure to approach the OU vice-chancellor for permission to hold the beef festival, a step necessary to ensure the security of the event. According to the information posted on a nationalist website, the Andhra Pradesh Goshala Federation would have demanded that the vice-chancellor ban the beef festival.[20]

The use of controversial beef as a food offering raises two questions: what are the reasons promoting this initiative, and what are the qualities attributed to beef that justify its introduction into the menu of university messes?

Beef consumption as a political strategy

The organisation of a beef festival (*Pedda kōra panduga*) inside a university campus was not a novelty, two other universities in Hyderabad had already experienced distribution of beef meals: the University of Hyderabad (UoH) in 2006, and since 2008, and EFLU in 2011.[21] These two universities depend on the central government and their students maintain close relationships with those of OU through their associations.

At UoH, the first beef stall to be set up was at *Sukoon* 2006. *Sukoon* is a three-day festival peculiar to UoH, organised by students at the end of the university year

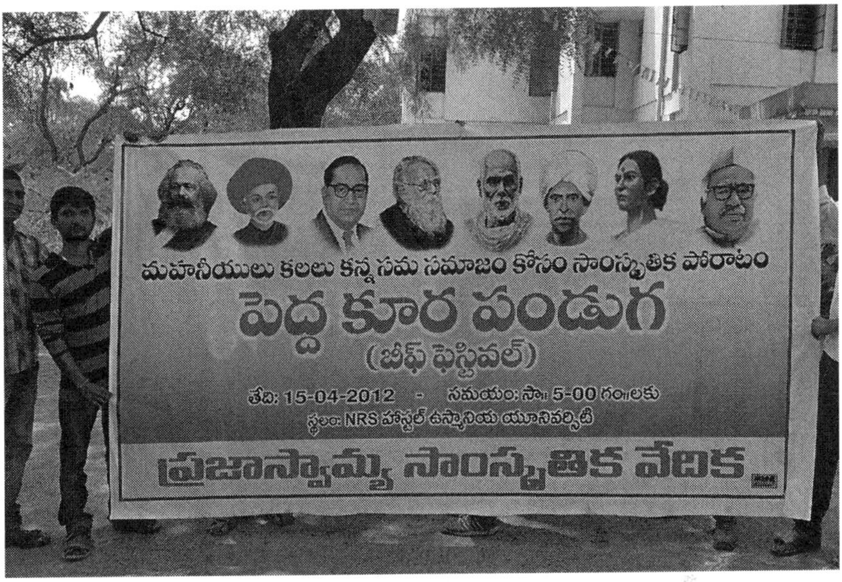
మహనీయులు కలలు కన్న సమ సమాజం కోసం సాంస్కృతిక పోరాటం
పెద్ద కూర పండుగ
(బీఫ్ ఫెస్టివల్)
తేది: 15-04-2012 - సమయం: సా॥ 5-00 గం॥లకు
స్థలం: NRS హాస్టల్ ఉస్మానియ యూనివర్సిటీ
ప్రజాస్వామ్య సాంస్కృతిక వేదిక

Figure 6.1 Banner of the beef festival

Source: © Christian Sebastia.

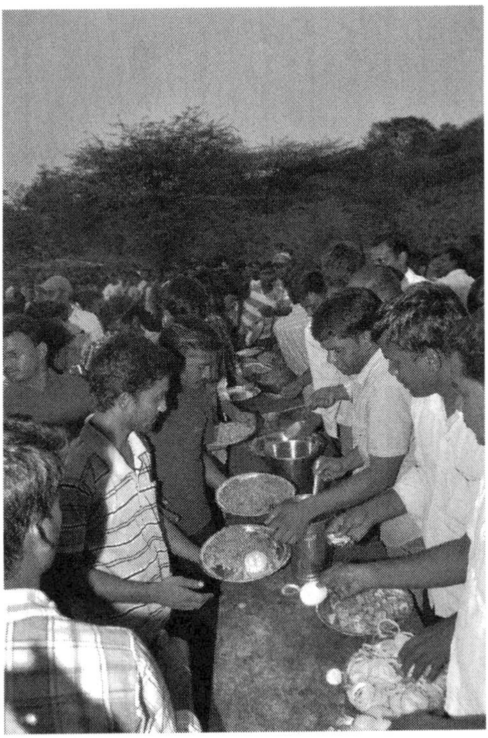

Figure 6.2 Distribution of beef *biriyāni*

Source: © Christian Sebastia.

and open to all: the festival includes sports competitions, concerts and exhibitions of books and cloth; some stalls sell food and drink. A beef stall was launched by the Dalit Students' Union (DSU), despite the university administration's refusal on the grounds that the initiative might create communal tensions. Students publicised their action by clapping, dancing and shouting slogans in praise of Ambedkar. Irritated, opponents demanded intervention from the administration which, after "taking cognizance of the prevailing local as well as national laws on the issue of beef consumption", gave permission (Gundimeda 2009: 132). Since *Sukoon* 2008, a stall, among others which sell vegetarian and chicken *biriyāni*, is authorised to serve beef *biriyāni*, and no trouble has disrupted the festive atmosphere. The choice between three sorts of *biriyāni* allows for the sharing of meals. As Sambaiah Gundimeda comments: "Democratisation is fully actualised when there is evidence of mutual respect among members for each other's culture" (*ibid.*: 143). Nonetheless, beef remains a peripheral meal at UoH as the Dalit students have not succeeded in introducing it into the messes' menu.

The beef festival at EFLU, in contrast, ended in violence when opponents attacked organisers and spoiled the food which had been prepared on campus by throwing dust and urinating on it. The assailants were members of the ABVP supported by various organisations: Telangana Rashtra Samiti, Telangana Joint Action Committee and National Students Union of India (allied to the Indian National Congress), while the beef festival was organised by the Prajasvamya Samskruthika Vedika (Union for Democratic Culture) in alliance with Telangana Students Association, Progressive Democratic Student Union, Student Federation of India, Ambedkar Students' Association and the DSU. The multiplicity of associations reflects the rivalry and division between students over two major issues at this period: the reservation quota based on caste, and leadership for conducting actions for or against the creation of the Telangana state. The sensitivity about beef was obviously an excellent ploy in this game of power between student associations, on which Gundimeda (*ibid.*) casts some light, particularly, on those at UoH for the period 2006–2008. He argues that the competition between student associations echoed that of Indian politics in general. The co-existence of multi-caste/ethnic/cultural organisations in universities encourages the battle to capture power in the University Student Union, in which one organisation manages to defeat the others, and then forms an alliance with contesting parties, the aim being to share the power according to the model of coalition in Indian politics. The author argues that the central issue for Dalits is their extreme heterogeneity: they are divided between those, namely Malas and Adi-andhras, who benefit from the most seats reserved to scheduled castes (SC) in universities and hold the dominant position among Dalits, and those, mostly Madigas, who compose the bottom of the Telugu society, with scheduled tribes (ST). Madigas constitute the student group that demands the right to eat beef, claiming it as their food culture. They are supported by tribes, some middle castes (Other Backward Castes, OBCs), and by progressive members of upper castes. In contrast, Dalits such as Malas and Adi-andhras, do not share this view as they prefer to throw off all untouchability-related stigmata in order to accomplish their social uplift. This process of 'de-untouchabilisation' is in accordance with the recommendations of Gandhi who invited Harijans to change their 'evil habits' in order to gain more recognition in Hindu society. Lower Dalits, on the other hand, oppose this change, interpreting it as a way to 'enculture' all Indians, whatever their status, taste, culture, feeling etc. in the brahmanical mould.

Value of beef: 'Beef is our culture'

Stratification of foodstuffs in India: a taxonomy with regard to caste status and religion

Claude Fischler, in his classic book *L'homnivore* (2001), points out that, while meat is the most desirable and sought-after food category, it is also the most abhorred. Compared to other food categories, he argues, the consumption of meat and animal products is the most subject to strict rules of consumption and proscriptions of a religious nature. The prohibition of pork by Muslims and Jews is well known, as is that of all meat by Jains or Hindu upper castes. The classification of animal products in brahmanical ideology is based on the concept of *prakṛti* (physical manifestation of everything in the universe), developed in Saṃkhya philosophy, which attributes to each ingredient one of three qualities (*guṇa*): *sāttvika*, *rajastika* and *tāmasika*, these qualities shaping the body and mind of the person. Dairy products are classified as *sāttvika* and confer perfection, discernment and intelligence. The egg-fish-meat category is classified as either *rajastika,* favouring vitality and force, or *tāmasika*, causing obscurantism, wildness and darkness, and is stratified from the most acceptable (*rajastika*), namely egg-fish-goat/sheep-chicken, to the most polluting (*tāmasika*), namely pork, buffalo/beef and wild animals. This tripartite classification illustrates the principle of incorporation by which the eater acquires the quality of what he eats (Fischler 1988). Dairy products by their softness and whiteness are associated with the purity which is the inherent quality of Jains, and higher castes not involved in warrior functions (Brahmaṇa and Vaiśya), while meat is associated with energy, violence, aggressiveness and/or impurity. Meat is necessary for warrior castes (Kṣatriya) who need forceful energy for fighting and ruling; it is also associated with the violence of sacrifice to which warrior castes contributed as donors. Meat is also necessary for lower castes involved in hard manual work (Śudra and Avarṇa).[22] Nevertheless, with the increase of sanctity attributed to the cow in the brahmanical ideology, consumption of beef (and of buffalo) has become taboo. Therefore, the evolution of meat food habits in India has resulted in divisions on two levels: a division of society between vegetarians and non-vegetarians and a division of non-vegetarians between beef/(buffalo)-eaters and non-beef/(buffalo)-eaters. In this stratification, low castes (Dalits) are strongly associated with beef-eating and dead cows.

Students' discourses on beef for the promotion of Dalits' identity

One of most degrading functions of some Dalit castes has been, and still is, to remove the carcasses of dead cows from places where higher castes reside. The relationship between beef-eating/dead cows and untouchability is pointed out by Ambedkar, quoted by D.N. Jhā (*ibid*.: 184), who referred to the Census Returns of 1910: "No Hindu community, however low, will touch cow's flesh. On the other hand, there is no community which is really an Untouchable community which has not something to do with the dead cow. Some eat her flesh, some remove the skin, some manufacture articles out of skin and bones." Ambedkar emphasised that the state of untouchability intrinsic to beef consumption was ancient, attested by the Veda Vyas Sṃṛiti (Kane 1946). The excerpt from Veda Vyas Sṃṛiti mentions that contact with untouchables demanded purification rites.[23] Ambedkar interpreted this relationship as a strategy of Brahmins and upper castes to compete with Buddhists who denounced them for their sacrifices of animals, especially of cows, and their discriminative social system. So, the students' demand for beef to be recognized as their 'food culture' and their denunciation of Hinduism as being "hegemonic", "fascist" and "anti-democratic" are in tune with Ambedkar's thought. Although the society is constituted by culturally, socially, economically and politically diversified communities, they claim that only the culture of the dominant group, that of Brahmins and people who have adopted Brahmins' habits and concepts, is recognised as normative. As explained by the leader of the beef festival, a PhD research scholar in political sciences:

> Our action is an ideological fight. In democracy, everyone has the right to eat what they want. Beef eating is part of the identity of several communities in the country. It was eaten by Bahujans and also by certain sections of the society for centuries. This should continue as beef consumption is a fundamental right which needs to be recognized by all and integrate into Indian consciousness. It is a political act to conduct a beef festival. In excluding beef from the menu, the university is guilty of showing an unjustifiable predilection for the religious sensitivity of high-caste Hindus. We want to remove the dirty image associated with beef, as spread by the brahminical culture.

Beef has to be cleared of its negative image which is a purely brahmanical ideological construction. As another student told me: "All over the world, people eat beef and do not consider it as impure. So we have to fight this taboo and affirm that beef is a part of our culture, of our identity."

Such an appropriation of a cultural feature that has greatly stigmatised the Dalits is made possible thanks to the new opportunities they have progressively acquired in the society. Even though Dalits do not benefit massively from higher education, some do have access to university through the reservation quota defined for them at 15 percent. They are thus in a position to compete with higher castes and to demand more participation in the political life of the university. Moreover, the internationalisation of the university that promotes the presence of foreign students and exchange through international conferences helps them to acquire better self-esteem, and to realise that beef consumption is not regarded as a sign of inferiority in other cultures. As mentioned by James Staples (2008) in his article on Christian Dalits in Andhra Pradesh, their predilection for beef consumption is in accordance with their Christian identity that they claim is modern compared to Hindu culture, regarded by them as rooted in old-fashioned taboos and prejudices.

The students' claim for beef as their own food culture is, however, debatable. Among the Dalit students I met at OU, rare are those who eat beef at home. Because of its condemnation by Hindu higher castes and its 'famine food' identity, bovine meat is no longer prepared in many families. As a Madiga professor of political sciences at OU confided: "beef, notably from animals that died of natural causes, constituted our staple food when grains (cereals, pulses, dry fruits) were not available during parts of the year." (see Sukumar 2015) Thus, the opportunity for Dalit students to join universities and to live in towns where they can taste many kinds of cheap food, opens their eyes to the discrimination that affected their families, obliging them to shift from their 'traditional food habits'.

Beef: the nutritious food

The second reason to denounce the rejection of beef consumption by Hindu nationalists is that it deprives the poor of the cheapest food, rich in proteins and micronutrients. Dalits are those who do the hardest physical work, and this deprivation adds a layer to their difficult lives as it can lead to weakness and health problems. This aspect is brandished by students to justify the introduction of beef into messes. They have had support from Veena Shatrugna, the retired nutritionist of the NIN. [24] Quoted in Ilaiah's article (1996b), she points out that beef contains 21% proteins whereas rice contains only 6–8%, and is richer in protein than other meat, and thus appropriate for fighting micronutrient deficiencies and diseases such as tuberculosis, a disease very widespread among Dalits because of mal- and under-nourishment. Shatrugna's standpoint is consistent with scientific knowledge about nutrition, which considers that proteins and vitamins play a fundamental role in the prevention of diseases and in the management of physical and mental health, and that the quality of animal proteins is higher than those of food plants thanks to their direct assimilation into the body. Nevertheless, not all Shatrugna's peers share her point of view. From my observations of dietetic consultations, presentations in conferences or discussions with professionals, I have noticed how Indian dieticians, who belong mostly to higher castes, are often unable to distance themselves from their own food pattern, so that their food prescriptions tend to focus on vegetable and dairy products and to recommend chemical supplements to compensate for nutritional deficiencies. They do not openly discourage consumption of fish, egg and meat, but advise patients with metabolic disorders not to eat 'red meat' (beef, buffalo, mutton) relying on western epidemiological studies which show its high consumption as responsible for cardiovascular diseases (Sébastia 2010). Such advice does not take into account the Indian context in which, according to the National Sample Survey Organisation, the average consumption of meat, red as well as white, is no higher than 160 g per capita per month (Gandhi and Zhou 2010), or 210 g if we consider that around 75% of Indians are not vegetarians.

The difference in approach between Shatrugna and her colleagues refers implicitly to the Indian conceptual dichotomy between *satvika* and *tamasika*, food highly valued *versus* highly condemned. Such a dichotomy echoes statements on the nutritive values of the cow emphasised since the nineteenth century by some nationalists for whom milk production is more necessary to improve the diet of Indians than meat. Compared to this statement and to recurrent discourses based on utilitarianism, economics, religion, ethics, etc., the Ilaiah-inspired justification by students of the nutritional values of beef in their promotion of its consumption represents a novelty. It draws from scientific discourses on food that have, in recent years, been notably developing in the Indian media with a view to fighting the sharp increase in metabolic diseases and high prevalence of anaemia. However, the students' justification for introducing beef into the messes in order to improve the nutritional value of the meals is debatable. According to my observations and discussions with students, meals served at Narmada Hostel are rich and well balanced, and include, along with rice, thick dhal puree, vegetables, curd and fruit, as well as mutton, chicken or fish three times a week and eggs once a week. So, the intrumentalisation of the nutritional value of beef is essentially political: it serves as a 'scientific argument' to which people may be receptive.

Beef biriyāni: a Hindu Dalit culture food?

The selection of *biriyāni*' to symbolise the Dalit 'food culture' is also a moot point. Although *biriyāni* is a very well known in India, it is a composite Mughlai dish, born from the encounter between Mughal and Indian foodstuffs and cuisine. The synthesis of *biriyāni* in the Mughal kitchens is described by Lizzie Collingham (2006: 27) as: "the delicately flavoured Persian pilau met the pungent and spicy rice dishes of Hindusthan to create the classic Mughlai dish, biryani". The pungent taste of the dish was contributed to by asafoetida, the use of which for flavouring meat in North India is attested in the Mahābhārata (Achaya 1998) and the Gautama Dharmasutra (Prakash *ibid*.). Its spiced taste came from numerous spices and herbs that the Mughals discovered in Indian cuisine. That *biriyāni* was a dish evolved from *pilau* is supported by K.T. Achaya (1998: 174) who reports that the world *pilau* is found in the Yāgñavalkya Sṃṛiti (fourth or fifth century AD) and early Tamil literature (third to sixth century AD). *Biriyāni* benefits, nevertheless, from a better reputation than *pilau*: it is, par excellence, the favourite dish for celebrating religious and biographical festivals in India. This results from the fact that it requires costly rice (Basmati), numerous spices, dried nuts and fruits and, in principle, marinated meat with curd and spices. *Biriyāni* is available in various versions, differing according to the identity of the people who developed the recipes: *vaniyambati biriyāni* (from Nawabs of Arcot, Tamil Nadu); *kutchi biriyāni* (from Nizams of Hyderabad); *pukka biriyāni* (from Mughals of Luchnow); *sindhi biriyāni* (from Pakistan), etc. It is named according to the animal products (mutton, chicken, beef, fish, prawn and egg), or their absence (vegetarian *biriyāni*). It is served in restaurants all over the country, but its quality and taste differ greatly from place to place, the lowest quality – oily and poor in ingredients – being sold in the numerous fast food outlets in towns.

Hyderabad is especially renowned for *biriyāni* which, when it is traditionally prepared, differs from other versions by the fact that the raw meat and rice are cooked together in a pot. This recipe, called *kutchi* (raw), was evolved by Iranians who came to the Deccan in the medieval period, during the Mughal reign. Eaten, accompanied by curd spiced with onions and herbs, it was considered healthy by *hakims* (*unani* medicine practitioners) and prescribed according to season, individual and age (Nalini 1994). The choice of *biriyāni* by students is in line with its excellent reputation, but it gives rise to two problems: the use of beef in *biriyāni* is far from being widespread in Hyderabad, and if beef may be considered the traditional foodstuff of Dalits, its association with *biriyāni* is anything but part of their culture, not only because of its Mughal origin,[25] but also because the price of its ingredients is out of reach of poor families. Most Dalit students have discovered the taste of beef *biriyāni* in a cheap restaurant or a fast food outlet in the city. This dish stands out as the best vehicle for promoting beef inside the Hindu community, and thanks to its predominant place in festivals and celebrations, its distribution allows Dalits to elevate their position and to acquire more consideration.

Sharing beef biriyāni: a political strategy for raising status

In India, food offerings hold an essential place in transactions and communication between deities and their devotees. Feeding gods/goddesses is a way to express one's love and devotion and 'receiving' food from them (as leftovers) is a way to absorb their power and essence. It is also an expression of gratitude as gods/goddesses are supposed to be the providers of food. In principle, food transactions are performed within the field of relationship between castes and deities sharing the same status. The offering of food is rooted in the concept of hospitality which is fundamental to accumulating 'good acts' (*karma*) for future rebirth. Individuals who offer food are venerated for their religious or ethical qualities that lift them to a higher position. Whatever gods or persons food is dedicated to, its offering means that it has to be accepted, and its quality and quantity properly appreciated. This is the *sine qua non* for strengthening the link of dependence between the donor and the receiver: by accepting food from the donor, the receiver integrates the donor's qualities according to the principle of incorporation (Fischler 1988) and recognises and legitimates the donor (Staples

2008). By attributing to themselves the position of food givers and selecting the highly valued *biriyāni* as a food offering, the students expect to gain recognition from the Hindu community. In this context, the sharing of their identity, that of untouchability, is obviously not expected of the recipients. The context is different than that presented by C. Joe Arun (2007) where, in some Paṟaiyar villages (large Dalit community in Tamil Nadu), beef is prepared and eaten at the Sunday communal meal. Mechanism and ideology, both at stake in the sharing of this specific food, have identical roles: raising a negative symbol, 'beef', to a positive one, 'food culture'. Nevertheless, while Paṟaiyars can share beef as a symbol of their untouchability (caste solidarity) and their struggle against discrimination, Dalit students, by distributing beef, expect to rally those who accept their food to their causes: the end of discriminatory attitudes against them and implementation of their rights. All these models borrowed by the Dalit students to legitimise the integration of beef into the mess menus present novelties compared to those which have dominated the discursive field related to cow protection and still continue to fuel this controversial subject.

The three paradigms related to cow protection

The justifications of cow protection rely on three specificities of the cow: wealth (materialist/utilitarian thesis); identity (symbolic thesis); and sacredness (ethical thesis). These aspects have been widely debated not only by opponents to nationalists, but also by historians and anthropologists who have either supported or disclaimed them. The materialist and symbolic theses are those that have fuelled the most prolific discussions: the first because of the predominant importance given to cow products; and the second because of the ambiguity in ancient literature regarding the status of the cow.

Materialist reasons: the cow as economic and ecological resource

Analysing the debates which led the Supreme Court to enact Article 48 of the Constitution, Chigateri (*ibid.*: 138) notes that: "…juridical discourse on cow slaughter, supposedly based on an economic and ecological understanding of the *use* value of cows in a predominantly agrarian economy, is predicated on a fundamental constitutive elision of the religious aspects of cow slaughter." Economic and ecological justifications for banning cow slaughter in India, which focus on milk, cow dung, manure and agricultural work, were considered by Marvin Harris (1966) who used the burning question of cows in India to develop his theory of food taboos. In the domain of food anthropology, Harris has represented the current cultural materialism that explains food preference and avoidance in terms of what is economically and ecologically acceptable or unfavourable. For example, he interprets the proscription of pork in the Middle East as due to deforestation which restricted their production, and considers the thesis of uncleanliness attributed to pigs as being more recent and inherent to their rearing in enclosures (Harris 1985).

Harris's article on the status of cows in India, published in 1966 during the violent demonstrations demanding a total ban on cow slaughter, has given rise to profuse polemics (Azzi 1974; Dandekar 1969; Diener 1980; Harris *et al.* 1966; Heston 1971; Raj 1971; Freed *et al.* 1981; Simoons *et al.* 1979). It was criticised because it denied the symbolic dimensions attributed to the cow and the *ahiṃsa* principle which led to the ban on cow slaughter (Azzi *ibid.*). As mentioned above in Chigateri's excerpt, Article 48 elides the symbolic dimension of the cow, not from the viewpoint of an epistemological orientation, but rather to maintain the secular spirit of the Constitution. Secondly, it was contested on the basis of economic and ecological considerations that supported preservation of bovine livestock to ensure milk availability, progeny, fuel and a work force. Harris' opponents demonstrated that, to enhance cattle production and quality, and to avoid useless and starving bovines wandering around, it was appropriate to slaughter unproductive animals (Heston *ibid.*). Harris' thesis was denounced for not taking into account the fact that buffalos were much less affected than cows by the ban on slaughter though their milk production was higher, and also, that the prohibition on cow's meat was respected only by Hindu higher castes. The economic aspects of the cow were significantly developed in the book edited by H.K. Lall, Director of Animal Husbandry in Uttar Pradesh, published after the riots of 1966 in order to give "a fair cross-section of public opinion regarding the problem of the Cow in India and an idea as to how wide and deep are the ramifications of this problem, which affects the very vitals of our economy." (1973: xii)[26] Quoting examples from western countries, opponents pointed out that cow slaughter was not the root cause: fodder of higher quality and quantity as well as better care would allow for increasing milk yields and successful cattle breeding.

Symbolic and religious reasons: cow as Gau Mata

In his controversial book on the consumption of cow meat in ancient times, D.N Jhā begins by quoting Gandhi in an excerpt from the journal *Harijan* (*ibid.*: 17):

> Mother cow is in many ways better than the mother who gave us birth. Our mother gives us milk for a couple of years and then expects us to serve her when we grow up. Mother cow expects from us nothing but grass and grain. (…) Our mother when she dies means expenses of burial or cremation. Mother cow is as useful dead as when alive.

Gandhi considered the cow as a valuable resource in the agrarian world but, especially, assimilated it to the maternal icon, superior even to human mothers. Peter van der Veer (*ibid.*) explains that, in brahmanical theology, the cow is perceived as the mother: the cow feeds human beings just as the mother feeds her child; "she is the mother of life, the substance of all things. She is a goddess who fulfills every wish (*kamadhenu*). She is the symbol of wealth and good fortune (*lakshmi*)" (*ibid.*: 87).[27] Not only is her body sacred, but also her products largely used in purification rituals: milk, clarified butter, curd, urine and cow dung. The author mentions the striking relationship between cows and Krishna's life story, in which his thefts of butter and curd from his mother and his love play with the *gopī* (cowherdesses) are metaphors of the maternal and feminine dimension of the cow. Charu Gupta (2001), studying the use of maternal icons to symbolise the Indian nation, claims that the cow as '*Gau Mata*' was propagated in the north during the nineteenth century through handbills, emotional imagery, devotional songs and plays; cow killing was interpreted as matricide and an attack against the Indian Nation. Mahadev Chakravarti (1979) points out that the cow/mother link is ancient and appears in a number of hymns of Ṛg Veda: "(cow is) the mother of Rudras, the daughter of the Vasus, the sister of Adityas, and the centre of nectar."[28] (*ibid.*: 52).

Ethical reasons: ambiguities around sacredness in ancient literature

The third reason concerns the status of the cow in ancient literature, notably in the Vedic literature of the "Aryans" to use Dayananda Saraswati's terminology. In his Satyarth Prakash, as quoted by Therese O'Toole (2003: 87), he argued: "During the rule of the Aryas, no slaughter was allowed of cows or other serviceable animals (…) From the time the flesh-eating foreigners have come to India and begun slaughtering cows, etc., and the rule has passed to wine-drinking officials, the miseries of the Aryas are gradually increasing." This excerpt denies the numerous references in ancient literature to the cow sacrifices widely performed to welcome important guests or honour the ancestors in funeral rituals (*śrāddha*). Many historians and researchers have indeed shown that the flesh of various animals, wild as well as domesticated, was consumed from Vedic times (Achaya *ibid.*; Chakrabarty *ibid.*; Korom 2000; Lal 1967; Prakash *ibid.*; Jhā *ibid.*; Smith 1991). Nevertheless, the economic dimension of the cow was considered and only sterile animals were slaughtered or sacrificed for guests and on special occasions such as *śrāddha*, the rest being classified as *aghnyā* (not to be killed). Chakravarti (*ibid.*) specifies that the Sanskrit word *vasa* defining the sacrificial cow, refers to a sterile cow. The most documented work on the evolution of beef consumption in India is from Dwijendra Narayan Jhā (2009), a former professor of ancient and medieval history at Delhi University. Written in response to the Hindu nationalist discourses, which accused Muslims of having introduced beef-eating habits into India,[29] his book is a compilation of quotations, drawn from Indian literature which demonstrates that while it was eaten in the past, beef consumption declined over the centuries as upper castes banished it from their diet. Works by Dwijendra Narayan Shah, Om Prakash and Chakravarti show that Buddhist as well as Jain texts attest to non-vegetarian people being numerous at the time of Buddha and Mahāvīrā, and that the flesh of game animals, pigs, oxen, cow, fowl, and fish was consumed by all castes including Brahmins. Under the influence of Buddhism and Jainism which have evolved the concept of non violence and non killing, an ambiguity regarding flesh consumption emerged in classic literature: while some texts recommended it during sacrifices, *śrāddha* and worship, others either advised against it for gaining great merit, i.e. improving the *karma*, or condemned it, cow slaughter being considered as a crime equivalent to the murder of a Brahmin (Bodewitz 2007). Buddhists, who did not share the Hindu concept of purity intrinsic to food, did not condemn the consumption of flesh, unless it came from sacrifices (Prakash *ibid.*). The fact that the animals most valued for sacrifice were cows may explain why the ban on killing and consumption concerned this animal specifically. The sacrifice being shared between Brahmins (performers) and higher non-Brahmin castes (donors), cow consumption would have been increasingly avoided by higher Hindu castes and increasingly restricted to lower castes, tribes and other religious members who were excluded from sharing in the sacrifice. Because of the idealisation of beef, and more widely of bovine meat, which pervaded the hierarchy of caste defined according to the concept of purity/pollution, beef-eaters were ostracised, and treated as outsiders. So, according to the social and political environment in which they live, lower castes have ceased to consume beef, and either eat other sorts of flesh much less deprecated (chicken and possibly, according to region, fish, and financial means, mutton) or have adopted vegetarianism, dietary models which are today at the heart of the Dalit contestations for identity recognition.

Conclusion

Emotionally and symbolically charged, bovines, and more specifically, the cow, continue to be a very sensitive subject, sparking off violent communal conflicts between Muslims and Hindus. Elections may be won by the enacting of bills aiming to ban cow slaughter and exportation of its products or to glorify identity. If the cow has long been the identity icon of Hindu nationalists, its use by certain Dalit groups as a marker of their identity, is recent and corresponds to the fresh opportunities that they are acquiring in a changing society. According to period and to the play of power between castes in a particular place, a Dalit group may have shifted from beef eating in a process of recognition if it has benefited from some economic or political support (for example, by conversion to Christianity), or succeeded in abandoning its discriminative function. This is the case of the Mala or Adi-andhra or Madar community cited by Simon Charsley (2010) which stopped eating beef after giving up its function of handling animal carcasses, which function then passed to other, lower Dalits. Conversely, Dalit groups such as the Madiga can demand the right to eat beef if a new situation offers them a means to compete economically and politically with other groups. Beef, in this case, is put forward as a symbol of cultural food heritage, a food testimony to a distant past that only Dalits have been capable of preserving and reviving for its health value (see also Arun *ibid.*).

Compared to Gandhi who spurred Harijans to change their 'habits', and to Ambedkar who encouraged them to convert to Buddhism in order to escape from their marginalisation in Hindu society, the approach of the organisers of beef festivals is the exact opposite. It aims to change the perception of beef and to encourage upper caste Hindus to become more 'democratic' and 'tolerant'. Dalits do not have to blend into the brahmanical mould, but must be recognised for their cultural specificity. Rather than shifting from beef consumption, they invite Hindus to share the taste and the nutritional values of the meat. Their act is not simply convivial or festive but is above all political, rooted in the symbolic functions of *annadāna* (food offering) to provide prestige and recognition to the food donor. Their instrumentalisation of the cow does not differ from that of nationalists: they aim to gain political power and to compete with higher castes at the university level, in the hope of playing a greater political role in civil life later. In other words, students from depressed castes find through associations a means to experience political power, and use all the symbols at their disposal to promote their Dalit identity, an identity redefined on the principles of equality, democracy, science and modernity which, without denying that it belongs to Hinduism, resists and opposes the Hindu concepts of the cow as sacred, and as symbol of the Mother or the Nation.

The first attempt at organising a beef festival at OU which ended in violence has not been beneficial for Dalits. In Delhi, the beef and pork festival which should have taken place on 28th September 2012 was cancelled by an order from the High Court at Delhi stemming from a plea by the Rashtriya Goraksha Sena (associated with the BJP), pointing to the Delhi Agricultural Cattle Prevention Act, 1994, that prohibits cow slaughter, and gives provision for five years of imprisonment and Rs 10,000 fine for storing or serving beef. In this affair, students were presented as Maoist and anti-national forces.[30] At OU and EFLU, no festival was planned for April 2013. However, the Dalit students have not pulled out. In response to a total ban on cow, calves, bull and bullock transportation and slaughtering and on beef trade and consumption ordained by the Government of Maharashtra, the Ambedkar Student Association of the University of Hyderabad organised on 4th March 2015, a distribution of packets of beef dishes in the university's shop, and a rally in the city's restaurants during which they shouted the slogan: "Let's eat Kalyani biryani",[31] Kalyani being a recipe for *biriyāni* introduced in Hyderabad by the Nawabs of Bidar. The attempt by the Dalit students to organise a similar event at OU on 10th December 2015 was stopped by a police raid which resulted in the arrest of 30 of the principal organisers.[32] It seems that the desire for a country free of cattle slaughter and beef eaters as supported by the nationalists in 1966, and by the present BJP Prime Minister,[33] is being realised. According to Jatin Gandhi (2015), "the Bharatya Janata Party will press for stronger anti-cattle slaughter laws in all States and actively pursue the legislative route in the States ruled by it." For how long will Dalits be able to eat and enjoy their 'traditional food'?

Notes

1 India is a multi-cultural country in which many variable parameters have interfered and interfere in habits and practices. Ethnic and religious identity, ecosystems, history of communities with regard to cultural and religious influences, urbanisation, development, migration experience, etc. are the major parameters.

2 Dalit (suppressed; crushed) is a term used for Untouchables, first adopted by Jyothi Rao Phule before being popularised by B.R. Ambedkar.

3 See: http://www.hyderabaddailynews.com/andhra-pradesh-news/crime-news/four-hindu-youths-held-for-desecration-of-temple-hyderabaddailynews-com (retrieved on 13 December 2013).

4 Claude Levi-Strauss' sentence is: "*les espèces naturelles ne sont pas choisies parce que bonnes à manger mais parce que bonnes à penser*" (1962: 128). It has been translated as "natural species are chosen not because they are good to eat but because they are good to think about" (1964: 89).

5 The *gaushalas* were established to shelter and nurture unproductive cows, quite often abandoned or left to starve.

6 This festival commemorates Ibrahim's sacrifice of his son Ismail to Allah. It requires animal sacrifices, in principle, one goat or sheep per family or one cow for seven families, the second option being more common because of the lower cost of the bovine.

7 The article 48 is entitled 'Organisation of agriculture and animal husbandry' http://indiankanoon.org/doc/1452355/ (retrieved on 02 February 2013).

8 A.B. Shah (1967: 14), for example, quotes an excerpt from *Gandhi and communal problems* by M.K. Gandhi: "...Hindu religion prohibits cow-slaughter for the Hindus, not for the world. (...) India is the land not only of Hindus, but also of Muslims, the Sikhs, the Parsis, the Christians, the Jews and all who claim to be Indian and are loyal to the Union. If they can prohibit cow-slaughter in India on the religion grounds, why cannot the Pakistan Government prohibit, say, idol worship in Pakistan on similar grounds?"

9 *Satyāgraha*, literally truth-insistence, was initiated by Gandhi in South Africa, and then, in India, for fighting the colonial power. It refers to a long demonstration rally aiming at diffusing information to the public and promoting adherence to the cause. These rallies, as well as hunger strikes, are based on the principle of non-violence that Gandhi held dear.

10 The *sadhus*, due to their nomadic life, have always played a role in the diffusion of new religious or ideological currents. The British accused them, especially the religious leaders, of spreading the *Gaurakshini* movement and of inciting people to riot (O'Toole 2003).

11 http://www.business-standard.com/article/economy-policy/maharashtra-economy-to-take-rs-10-000-cr-hit-due-to-beef-ban-115031200913_1.html (retrieved on 13 March 2015).

12 The rigid rules on cow protection enacted in some states has translated, since the end of 2015, into repeated deadly attacks of Dalits by gangs (called "vigilante groups" by media and by politicians), accusing the Dalits of keeping beef at home, as in the village of Dadri (Uttar Pradesh) or of Shantipura (Karnataka), or of keeping carcasses of cows they killed, as in the village of Una (Gujarat). Analyses of the alleged beef found at Dadri revealed it to be mutton; the carcasses found at Una came from dead cows that the Dalit families have the task of removing from the streets. In reprisals, the Dalit Manav Adhikar Movement have exhorted Dalits to stop removing the carcasses, thereby creating a critical situation for upper castes who are forced to find another way to rid themselves of such abominable pollution.

13 In India, food is mostly studied in the disciplines of biotechnology and nutrition sciences. There is no faculty specialising in the history, sociology, geography or anthropology of food.

14 This hostel accommodates only PhD students. Despite its 'Ambedkar' appellation, it welcomes not only SC and ST students, but also OBC students.

15 Jyothi Rao Phule (11 April 1827–1890) of Phulmali caste (OBC; flower gardener) was, with his wife Savitribai, the most preeminent social activist of the Social

Reform Movement in Maharashtra (education, woman empowerment, abolition of untouchability). Periyar E.V. Ramaswamy (1879–1973) of Naicker caste (OBC; populous caste in South India) was a politician and instigator of the Dravidian Movement; he fought for women and against caste discrimination. B.R. Ambedkar (14 April 1891–1956) of Mahar caste (SC; removers of animal's carcasses) was a jurist and a political leader; he was chairman of the drafting committee for the Indian constitution in which he abolished untouchability and all forms of discrimination. Narayana Guru (1856–1928) of E̲lava caste (SC, toddy tappers) was a social activist and the founder of the Reform Movement in Kerala promoting equality and religious freedom. Komaram Bheem (?-1940) of the Gond tribe (ST) worked for the uplift of tribals and waged a relentless struggle against the rule of the Nizam for the liberation of Hyderabad. Chakali Ilamma (1919–1985) of Rajaka or Chakali caste (OBC; washermen) was an activist who opposed the Nizam's government and feudal lords in Telangana. Jagjivam Ram (5 April 1908–1979) of the Chamar caste (SC; tanners) was a politician and a member of the Constituent Assembly of India; this allowed him to ensure that social justice was enshrined in the Constitution.

16 Kormaram Bheem's death anniversary is officially celebrated in October, but some supporters considered it to be 8th April 1940.

17 Telangana was a part of Hyderabad state ruled by the Nizams (Moghul princes) until 1956 when it was merged with Andhra state to form Andhra Pradesh state, despite violent agitations demanding a separate Telangana state which have continued to break out periodically. The creation of the state of Telangana was finally approved by the union cabinet 3 October 2013.

18 The festival was extensively covered by journalists from TV, state and national journals, as well as by freelancers. Some media personalities were present, such as Meena Kandaswamy, a Dalit poet born of an intellectual inter-caste family, and called by journalists the 'firebrand poet'. Her participation in the festival elicited streams of abuse to her e-mail address. (*Reddif.New*, May 21, 2012)

19 Bahujan means 'majority', the term chosen by Kancha Ilaiah to qualify low castes because it includes SC, ST and OBC, i.e. "people and castes who form the exploited and suppressed majority" (Ilaiah 1996a: ix). Ilaiah's definition implicitly excludes the group of OBC which is far from being statutorily homogenous in South India. While some OBC groups are close to Dalits (Bahujan) in terms of discrimination, economic and political power, others are economically rich and influential at the level of villages, districts, states etc. Ilaiah himself belongs to the Kumarā caste traditionally involved in sheep herding and breeding.The term Bahujan is used in North India while in the South it is the term Dalit which dominates. The former's popularity in the north come from the Bahujan Samaj Party (BSP) which emerged in 1984 and took power in Uttar Pradesh in 1995, 1997, 2002–2003 (in coalition), 2007–2012 (as a single party) through the emblematic figure of Mayawati, the first Dalit woman Chief Minister in India.

20 See:http://forumforhinduawakening.org/dharma/news/2012/04/16/goshala-federation-demands-to-drop-beef-festival-at-osmania-university/ (retrieved on 20 April 2012).

21 In 1997, the mess secretary had introduced beef into the hostel of the EFLU. His initiative was welcomed by a significant group of students (Bengali, Malayali, Muslims, Christians, Dalits, tribal, progressive upper-castes), but strongly opposed by other students, staff organisations and the head cook. Beef dishes, which were prepared by students and served for one month, were forbidden when a new mess committee was appointed.

22 Brahmaṇa, Vaiśya, Kṣatriya and Śudra form the four *varṇa* or categories which classify the brahmanical society; a fifth category, *avarṇa* comprises those who do not belong to brahmanical society, that is to say, indigenous people. The contemporary

caste system results from this classification, which has become increasingly complex over centuries.

23 The excerpt quoted by B.R. Ambedkar from Pandurang Vaman Kane's book is from the Veda Vyas Smṛiti (I. 12–13): "Carmakāra, Bhaṭa, Bhilla, Rajaka, Puṣkara, Naṭa, Virāṭa, Meda, Cāṇḍāla, Dāśa, Svapaca, Kolika – these lower categories and even those who eat beef (*gavāsanā*) are *antyajā*. If you talk with them, you have to take bath. If you see them, you have to look at the sun." (Kane 1946: 71, note 173); trad. by Anandavardhan S., Indology dept of the French Institute of Pondicherry.

24 See: http://www.youtube.com/watch?v=6ZRtMpveKfY&feature=relmfu (retrieved on 14 December 2013).

25 It is worth noting that although many students of the universities of Hyderabad are Muslims, they are hardly mentioned by organisers who appropriate beef, and implicitly beef *biriyāni,* to their own 'food culture'. They hope to distinguish themselves thereby from Muslims who are accused by nationalists of influencing the food culture of Dalits (Ilaiah 1996b).

26 H.K. Lall's book (1973) comprises one part presenting a collection of articles written by officials on the occasion of *Gopāṣṭamī* festival in 1960s, and a second part compiling press articles, among them 30 letters published in the National Herald of Lucknow from October 27, 1966 to December 19, 1966. *Gopāṣṭamī* is a one-day festival celebrating Krishna as the cow protector (*Govardhan puja*), and the cows (*Go puja*). This festival had been established in 1952 under the auspices of the Central Council of Gosamvardhana that replaced the Central Gaushala Development Board funded in 1949 (*ibid.*: 7). This council, become the Gosamvardhan Advisory Council in 1991, has the specific functions of organising, implementing and coordinating activities relating to the preservation and development of cattle.

27 lakṣmīr yā loka-pālānāṁ dhenu-rūpeṇa saṁsthitā |
ghṛtaṁ vahati yajñārthe yama-pāśaṁ vyapohatu ||
agrataḥ santu me gāvaḥ gāvo me santu pṛṣṭhataḥ |
gāvo me pārśvataḥ santu gavāṁ madhye vasāmy aham ||
"May the goddess Lakshmi who is situated amongst the gods in the form of the cow to provide ghee for the sacrifices free us from the bonds of death. May I always live amongst the cows: may be before me, behind me and to my every side." (Skanda Purana)
http://www.news.vrindavantoday.org/2010/11/gopashtami-the-day-krishna-was-named-govinda

28 In the Ṛg Veda, Rudras are the sons of Rudra, the god associated with wind, storm and the hunt; Vasus are attendant deities of Indra, one of the major gods; **Ā**dityas are solar deities.

29 The first version of Dwijendra Narayan Jhā's book, called *Holy Cow: Beef in Indian Dietary Traditions*, was taken out of circulation on its release in 2001. The author received death threats from BJP leaders who burnt copies of his book and forbade its sale. The book was republished in London by Verso.

30 See: http://archive.asianage.com/india/no-beef-pork-festival-jnu-campus-delhi-high-court-060 and http://news.outlookindia.com/items.aspx?artid=774932 (retrieved on 25 September 2012).

31 http://timesofindia.indiatimes.com/india/Maharashtra-beef-ban-sparks-outrage-in-Hyderabad-varsities/articleshow/46463014.cms (retrieved on 5 March 2015).

32 A Dalit student with a master in Arabic studies, has been denied admission to the EFLU in 2006, despite having passed the entrance test for a PhD programme. The reason given by the administration was that he had participated in the beef festival. http://gulfnews.com/news/asia/india/student-denied-admission-in-university-for-eating-beef-1.1869891 (retrieved on 29 July 2016).

33 http://articles.economictimes.indiatimes.com/2014-04-03/news/48834667_1_cow-slaughter-cow-meat-slaughter-houses (retrieved on 15 March 2015).

References

Abbasayulu, Y.B (1980). *Emergence of Political Leadership Among Scheduled Castes,* Hyderabad: Centre for Harijan Studies, Osmania University.

Achaya, K.T. (1998). *A Historical Dictionary of Indian Food*, Delhi: Oxford University Press.

Al-Biruni (1971). *Alberuni's India*. Translated by Edward C. Sachau; edited by Ainslee Embree. New York: Norton.

Anveshi (2012). What's the menu? Food politics and hegemony, *Broadsheet on Contemporary Politics*, Vol. 1(4).

Arun, C.J. (2007). *Constructing Dalit Identity*, New Delhi: Rawat Publications.

Azzi, C. (1974). "More on India's sacred cattle", *Current Anthropology*, Vol. 15(3): 317–324.

Basu, D. (2007). "CPI(M) and Karl Marx". *Ivarta.com*, February 28. http://www.ivarta.com/columns/OL_070228.htm (retrieved on 30 March 2012).

Bodewitz, H.W. (2007). "Sins and vices: their enumerations and specifications in the Veda", *Indo-Iran Journal*, Vol. 50: 317–339.

Chakravarti, M. (1979). "Beef-eating in Ancient India", *Social Scientist*, Vol. 7(11): 51–55.

Charsley, S. (2010), "Untouchable identity and its reconstruction", in M. Aktor and R. Deliège (eds.) *From Stigma to Assertion. Untouchability, Identity and Politics in Early and Modern India*, pp. 147–177. Copenhagen: Museum Tusculanum Press.

Chigateri, S. (2011). "Negotiating the 'sacred cow': cow slaughter and the regulation of difference in India", in M. Mookherjee, *Democracy, Religious and the Liberal Dilemma of Accommodation*, pp. 137–159. Netherlands: Springer, Studies in Global Justice, Vol. 7.

Collingham, L. (2006). *Curry. A Tale of Cooks and Conquerors*, London: Vintage, 1st publication 2005.

Copland, I. (2005). "What to do about cows? Princely versus British approaches to a South Asian dilemma", *Bulletin of the School of Oriental and African Studies*, Vol. 68(1): 59–76.

Dandekar, V.M. (1969). "India's sacred cattle and cultural ecology", *Economic and Political Weekly*, Vol. 4(39): 1561–1566.

Diener, P. (1980). "On the use of sources in the sacred-cow controversy", *Current Anthropology*, Vol. 21(3): 408–409.

Dittrich, C. (2009). "The changing food scenario and the middle classes in the emerging megacity of Hyderabad, India", in H. Lange and L. Meier (eds.), *The New Middle Classes. Globalizing Lifestyles, Consumerism and Environmental Concern*, pp. 269–280. Netherlands: Springer.

Fischler, C. (1988). "Food, self and identity", *Social Science Information*, Vol. 27(2): 275–292.

Fischler, C. (2001). *L'Homnivore. Le gout, la cuisine et le corps*, Paris: Odile Jacob.

Freed, S.A., Freed, R.S., Ballard, R., Chattopadhyay, K., Diener, P., *et al.* (1981). "Sacred cows and water buffalo in India: the uses of ethnography [and comments and reply]", *Current Anthropology*, Vol. 22(5): 483–502.

Gandhi, J. (2015). "BJP for law against cattle slaughter in all States", *The Hindu*, 16 March. http://www.thehindu.com/news/national/bjp-for-law-against-cattle-slaughter-in-all-states/article6996349.ece (retrieved on 16 March 2015).

Gandhi, V.P. and Zhou Z.-Y. (2010). "Rising demand for livestock products in India: nature, patterns and implications", *Australasian Agribusiness Review*, Vol. 18, Paper 7: 103–135.

Gundimeda, S. (2009). "Democratisation of the public sphere", *South Asia Research,* Vol. 29: 127–149.

Gupta, C. (2001). "The icon of mother in late colonial North India: 'Bharat Mata', 'Matri Bhasha' and 'Gau Mata'", *Economic and Political Weekly*, Vol. 36(45): 4291–4296.

Harris, M. (1985). *Good to Eat: Riddles of Food and Culture,* New York: Simon & Schuster.

Harris, M. (1966). "The cultural ecology of India's sacred cattle", *Current Anthropology*, Vol. 7(1): 51–59.

Harris, M., Bose, N.K., Klass, M., Mencher, J.P., Oberg, K., *et al.* (1966). "The cultural ecology of India's sacred cattle [and comments and replies]", *Current Anthropology*, Vol. 7(1): 60–66.

Heston, A. (1971). "An approach to the sacred cow of India", *Current Anthropology*, Vol. 12(2): 191–209.

Ilaiah, K. (1996a). *Why I am not a Hindu. A Sudra Critique of Hindutwva Philosophy, Culture and Political Economy*, Calcutta: Samya.

Ilaiah, K. (1996b). "Beef, BJP and food rights of people", *Economic and Political Weekly*, Vol. 31(24): 1444–1445.

Iqbal, H. (ed.) (2008). *Karl Marx on India*, New Delhi: Tulika Books.

Jaffrelot, C. (1996). *The Hindu Nationalist Movement and Indian Politics 1925 to the 1990s. Strategies of Identity-Building, Implantation and Mobilisation*, New Delhi: Viking Penguin India.

Jhā, D.N. (2009). *The Myth of the Holy Cow*, New Delhi: Navayana.

Kane, P. V. (1946). *History of Dharmaśāstra. Ancient and Mediaeval Religious and Civil Law in India*, Vol. II, Part. II, Poona: Bhandarkar Oriental Research Institute, Government Oriental Series Class-B, No.6.

Khare, R.S. (1976). *Culture and Reality. Essays on the Hindu System of Managing Foods*, Simla: Indian Institute of Advanced Study.

Korom, F.J. (2000). "Holy Cow! The apotheosis of zebu, or why the cow is sacred in Hinduism", *Asian Folklore Studies*, Vol. 59: 181–203.

Krishna, G. (1985). "Communal violence in India. a study of communal disturbance in Delhi", *Economic and Political Weekly*, Vol. 20(2): 61–74.

Lal, M. (1967). "Cow cult in India", in A.B. Shah (ed.), *Cow-Slaughter. Horn of a Dilemma*, pp. 15–34. Bombay: Lalvani Publishing House, 'Indian Renaissance Institute'.

Lall, H.K. (1973). *The Resurrection of Cow in India*, Hoshiarpur: Vishveshvaranand Institute.

Lévy-Strauss, C. (1962). *Le totémisme d'aujourd'hui*, Paris : PUF; Trad. *Totemism*, London: Merlin Press (1964)

Nalini, F.D. (1994). *Confluence of Culture. French Contributions to Indo-Persian Studies*, Delhi: Manohar.

Nandy, A. (2004). "The changing popular culture of Indian food: preliminary notes", *South Asia Research*, Vol. 24 (1): 9–19.

O' Toole, T. (2003). "Secularizing the sacred cow. The relationship between religious reform and Hindu nationalism", in A. Copley (ed.) *Hinduism in Public and Private. Reform, Hindutva, Gender, and Sampraday*, pp. 84–109. New Delhi: Oxford University Press.

Pandey, G. (1983). "Rallying round the cow. sectarian strife in the Bhojpuri Region c. 1888–1917", in R. Guha, *Subaltern Studies II, Writings on South Asian History and Society*, pp. 60–129. Delhi: Oxford University Press.

Pingali, P. and Khwaja, Y. (2004). *Globalisation of Indian Diets and the Transformation of Food Supply Systems, Inaugural Keynote Address 17th Annual Conference. Indian Society of Agricultural Marketing, Hyderabad, 5–7 February, 2004*. ESA Working Paper No. 04-05, Agricultural and Development Economics Division, FAO, pp. 1–30 (www.fao.org/es/esa).

Prakash, O. (1961). *Food and Drinks in Ancient India: from Earliest Times to 1200 A.D.*, Delhi: Munshiram Manoharlal Publishers.

Raj, K.N. (1971). "India's sacred cattle: theories and empirical findings", *Economic and Political Weekly*, Vol. 16(13): 717; 719–722.

Raj, K.N. (1979). "Demand for total ban on cow slaughter in Kerala and West Bengal: some observations", *Economic and Political Weekly*, Vol. 14(18): 821–824.

Saglio-Yatzimirsky, M.-C. (2010). "Caste as a political tool. The case of the Camakars of Dharavi (Mumbai)", in M. Aktor and R. Deliège (eds.), *From the Stigma to Assertion. Untouchability, Identity and Politics in Early and Modern India*, pp. 201–230. Copenhagen: Museum Tusculanum Press.

Sébastia, B. (2010), "'Be a vegetarian'. Discours en Inde sur les bienfaits du Végétarisme pour un corps pur et sain". Lemangeur-ocha.com (exclusive text published online August 2, 2010) http://www.lemangeur-ocha.com/sciences-humaines/textes-exclusifs/detail/auteur-texte/0/be-a-vegetarian-discours-en-inde-sur-les-bienfaits-du-vegetarisme-pour-un-corps-pur-et-sain/disp/

Shah, A.B. (1967). *Cow-Slaughter. Horns of a Dilemma*, Bombay: Lalvani Publishing House, Indian Renaissance Institute.

Simoons, F.J., Batra, S. M., Chakravarti, A. K., Diener, P., Ferro-Luzzi, G.E., *et al.* (1979). "Questions in the sacred-cow controversy [and comments and reply]", *Current Anthropology*, Vol. 20(3): 467–493.

Smith, B.K. (1991). "Classifying animals and humans in Ancient India", *Man*, Vol. 26(3): 527–548.

Staple, J. (2008). "'Go on, just try some!': meat and meaning-making among South Indian Christians", in C. Osella and F. Osella (eds), *Food: Memory, Pleasure and Politics*, pp. 36–55. *South Asia: Journal of South Asian Studies*, Vol. 31(1).

Sukumar, N. (2015). "Why beef was banished from my kitchen", *Economic and Political Weekly*, Vol. 50(17) (online version) http://www.epw.in/journal/2015/17/web-exclusives/why-beef-was-banished-my-kitchen.html (retrieved on 21 January 2016).

Van der Veer, P. (1994). *Religious Nationalism. Hindus and Muslims in India*, Berkeley-Los Angeles-London: University of California.

Venkatesan, V. (2015). "Legal farce", *Frontline*, Vol. 32 (21): 29–31.

7 Modernity, traditionalism and the silent protest

The Palestinian food narrative in Israeli reality television

Liora Gvion

Introduction

Palestinian cuisine in Israel is usually perceived by Jews as a limited reservoir of culinary knowledge that has undergone little change and as having, therefore, little potential for entering the domain of upscale dining. Although Palestinian domestic kitchens have become modern, incorporating new food stuffs and technologies, this change has only slightly affected Palestinian food in the public sphere. State agencies, and the public in general, still see Palestinians as a group which modernisation has skipped. Palestinian restaurants offer a limited variety of dishes consisting of what Palestinians consider as restaurant food, and Jews as typical Palestinian food. Many women have ceased to prepare traditional and laborious dishes, some of which symbolise a period of scarcity,[1] due to lack of knowledge and/or time, or necessity. However, inclusion of these dishes on restaurant menus is still considered as an offence to Palestinian women as they raise doubts about their domestic knowledge and ability (Gvion 2006, 2009, 2014; Stein 1998).

In light of the above, this chapter aims at looking at the ways in which the Palestinian food narrative is presented in MasterChef Israel (MCI), a highly popular reality television cooking contest borrowed from the British show, MasterChef. MCI consists of 24 episodes during which the contestants have to prepare dishes which are evaluated by four judges. In most of the episodes, the contestants work on their own, but in some of them, they are grouped in pairs competing with each other, or are divided into pairs in which one contestant competes against the other. The episodes end with the dismissal of the contestant whose dishes have not met the necessary standards. Ms Anski, the founder and owner of the largest farmer's market in Israel, Chefs Cohen, Shani and Adar replaced by Chef Roschfeld, act as judges. All the four are major figures on the Israeli culinary scene, and are known for their contribution to the emergence of Israeli cuisine.

Applicants are recruited either after registering on the programme's website, or directly by the producers, after being recommended by alumni or people from the food industry. A unique life story or personality increases the chances of appearing on the show. The programme is filmed for around 22 hours, twice a week, over three months. In each episode, contestants are given a certain amount of time to prepare one or several dishes. While cooking, they are expected to share their difficulties, thoughts and feelings with the audience. Once the time is up, they are confined in a small room that they leave only if they are called for the shooting of their testimonials, of which some parts are selected by the editor to be included in the episode. Upon returning to the studio, contestants are called before the judges who assess the dishes. Although each of the four judges is given five minutes to comment on the dish of each candidate, only a minute and half of the 20-minute evaluation is integrated into the episode. Each episode is a result of excessive editing which allows the production to select and promote certain ideologies stemming from the narratives. None of the episodes, except for the final episode of the fourth season, has been shown live.

Several authors have argued that reality shows are informal means of excluding minorities from the public sphere, and preventing them from challenging dominant narratives of the society in which they reside (Amal *et al.* 2011; Elias *et al.* 2009). But the role these shows play in addressing the interplay between modernity, ethnicity, identity and social marginality has rarely been investigated. A narrative analysis of five seasons of MCI fills this theoretical gap. MCI, which officially presents a neo-liberal story, granting to Palestinians equal opportunity to win the contest, channels Palestinian contestants into a representation of their traditional cuisine that needs to be upgraded and modernised. This chapter shows that the heterogeneity in the Palestinian community in Israel, and its differential reactions to modernity, is concealed by the production with the aim of presenting Palestinian contestants as traditional and devoid of the ability to participate in a modern culinary discourse. These participants, all well-educated and modern individuals, are expected to admit the limitations of their cuisine, to explore foreign kitchens in order to realise and recognise how restricted is their capacity to incorporate them into their cooking, and to return to their native kitchen equipped with the necessary knowledge to modernise it. Although they negotiate their right to present alternatives to the hegemonic narrative on their people and its food, and use various means of protesting against the Palestinian stereotypical image, their voice is heard only if it confirms the hegemonic narrative.

Food, identities and visibility

Reality television programmes are social fields in which institutions, ideologies and groups compete over the definition and construction of reality, and the viewers' consciousness. They use subtle mechanisms, designed to reinforce ethnic, racial, gender and other stereotypes, that facilitate the exclusion of minorities from participation in the society they live in, and their presentation as cultural 'others' (Andrejevic and Colby 2006; Hasinoff 2008). Although all the participants of reality television programmes have, officially, an equal opportunity to win the competition, each episode ruling out past merits, they realise rapidly that there is no one but themselves to thank for success or to blame for failure. The minimal script, put together during the shooting, enables the participants to express their feelings and thoughts rather than to quote what the production has written for them. In other words, they are given some control over their self-presentation (Bauman 2002; Browne 1996; Cottle 2000; Gross 1998; Holmes and Jermyn 2004; Kirby 2013; Newcomb 2007; Orbe 2008; Pozner 2010; Smith and Wood 2003). However, minorities hardly have the opportunity to shape the programme's script, and to have their distinctive identities recognised and respected. Their voices are channelled to echo hegemonic representations, and their 'otherness' is displayed in order to present the society they live in as multicultural and open to minorities (Andrejevic and Colby *ibid.*; Cottle *ibid.*; Downing and Husband 2005; Elias *et al. ibid.*; Goddard 2003; Hasinoff *ibid.*). Their protests, when failing to succeed, are silenced.

An analysis of two Israeli TV reality shows, "The Ambassador", and "Wanted: A Leader", has pointed to the ethno-cultural differences between the contestants, arguing that the judges turn the differences between Palestinian and Jewish citizens of Israel into a meta-narrative of the programmes (Amal 2007; Caspi and Elias 2011; Elias *et al. ibid.*). The winners embody the hegemonic narrative according to which Israel is a Jewish modern state. Seniority in Israel, and the extent to which Palestinian and immigrant contestants resemble native Israelis have, therefore, become essential for staying in the show. Palestinian participants often disguise or mask their distinctive features when they realise that their attempts to protest are fruitless, by conforming to the hegemonic voice in the hope of increasing the chances of winning the show. Both shows, largely unscripted in advance, are edited in order to enable the construction of the meta-narrative and, further, the cultivation of the dominant ideology.

In order to mask the ideology of the production, and to sell products to viewers, cooking shows are presented as lessons given by an experienced cook. Some shows expose the audience to new ingredients, cooking devices and dishes from all over the world (Collins 2012). With time, chefs, some of them having become celebrities, have started monitoring cooking shows that mix cooking with leisure and lifestyle (Johnston *et al.* 2014; Scholes 2011; Smith 2012). Jamie Oliver's show is the most famous programme in this genre. Oliver has been chosen as a presenter because of his ability to appropriate cooking once inherent to the female territory, and to bring it into the kitchens of the urban, middle-class and of hedonistic male bachelors who have escaped the trap of marriage and cook as part of their leisure time activities, cooking providing them with an alternative to hegemonic masculinity. These cooking shows not only turn into a means of fulfilling a fantasy, but show marginal social groups how they can use cooking to position themselves in the society in which they live (Hollows 2002, 2003; Smith *ibid.*; Smith and Wilson 2004).

Very few studies have focused on the connection between cooking contests, reality television and the reproduction of ethnic and national narratives. The article by Mark Gallagher (2004) on the "Iron Chef", for example, states that the programme aims to enhance the feeling of Japanese nationalism. Kaga, a Japanese millionaire, invited the best Japanese chefs to his castle to compete with each other through the preparation of dishes based on a particular ingredient. The show, which was a great success in Japan, has been sold to television channels around the world and adjusted to the local cultures. Its popularity in the United States is attributed to the attractiveness of Asian cartoons and Somo fighters, all subjects of ridicule, ensuring American viewers that the Japanese economy is not going to overtake the American economy, and positioning the American economy and culture above that of the Japanese.

Although often perceived as ideologically free and politically neutral, food-related activities take place in the political sphere (Appadurai 1988; Mintz 1996). One's ability to make a living off his/her cuisine, the food choices made in daily life, and attribution of exoticism or prestige to certain cuisines, all evolve out of the social positioning, inclusion, access to power and social resemblance to, or differentiation from, the groups among which minorities live. "Eating the Other", a concept introduced in the context of ethnic relationship by bel hooks (1992), refers to the process of commodification of the "Other". In the case of food, this concept points to the adjustment of ethnic dishes to the taste of westerners, by detaching them from the historical and social context in which they are usually consumed. Hence, consumers feel they are liberal and free of prejudices against ethnic groups, even though their eating patterns reproduce relations of power (Ferrero 2002; Hirsch 2011). The consumption of hummus in Israel is a good example of these relations. The 'de-Palestinisation' of hummus and its appropriation by Jews, most of them not having been familiar with this dish in their countries of origin, are means of dispossessing Palestinians of their culinary assets, and of manifesting superiority over them. Hummus became common among Israelis who consume it in manners different from the Palestinians. The growing number of *humusiot*,[2] in the last ten years, attests not only to an increasing interest in high quality hummus that is consumed the way Palestinians eat it, but also to the gourmatisation of the dish and to the re-Palestinisation and commodification of Palestinian food in Israel (Gvion 2012; Hirsch 2011; Ranta 2014).

The detachment of the food from the contexts in which it is consumed is not the only consequence of its commodification. Commodification often changes the social relationships embedded in food production and the meanings attached to certain dishes, food items and eating patterns. In her study of rural ethnic tourism in the Palestinian sector in Israel, Rebecca Stein (1998) argues that rural tourism enables Palestinians to reinsert their history in articulation with Jewish history. Palestinian villages and towns are presented as rural communities, and commodified as representing "authentic" Arab ethnicity. Palestinian population centres and rural sites have been reevaluated by state agencies as potential markets and commodified as places of ethnic tourism and as symbols of hospitality. The emphasis on these two themes allows the Jews to experience the Arab village as a touristic site offering a touch of history, culture and traditional forms of hospitality, all these ingredients being incorporated as components of the Israeli national narrative and culture. At the same time, the commodification of rural settings presents the Palestinian citizens of Israel as a traditional community that remains in the background as regards modernisation.

Although both Palestinian homes and cookery have become modernised by the incorporation of new ingredients, dishes and cooking technologies, the traditional image of the Palestinian community is reinforced by the way their restaurants and eateries are represented and the kind of foods they serve. Most restaurants refrain from serving dishes that have been traditionally consumed at home and prepared by women. In preserving a limited menu, Palestinian restaurateurs maintain the traditional division between restaurant and domestic food, but at the same time, contribute to the Jewish vision of Palestinian cuisine as restricted (Gvion 2006, 2009, 2014). The exposure of contemporary Palestinian cooking to changes is surprising as a new generation of well-educated Palestinian, both women and men, are fully engaged in promoting Palestinian national rights, and see Israel as their place of residence rather than their native state. Some have even mobilised hegemonic narratives with the aim of promoting their personal and political interests (Jabarin 2001; Rabinowits and Abu-Baker 2002).

Does MCI promote the image of Palestinians in Israel as traditional? Are Palestinian contestants, presented as lacking the necessary habitus and cultural capital, allowing for full participation in the Israeli culinary scene? Are they given the opportunity to embody the heterogeneous social make-up of their community, or are they assigned particular roles? What strategies do they use for protesting against their social positioning? Participation in MCI, I argue, requires that Palestinian contestants conform to the Israeli hegemonic representation of the Palestinian who is attached to his/her traditional culinary knowledge. They are expected to recognise that their native knowledge limits their ability to cook dishes exogenous to their know-how or to succeed in the upscale dining market. MCI is expected to be an opportunity for them to internalise the principles of modern cooking and to mobilise them in order to modernise traditional Palestinian food. Simultaneously, the upgraded version of Palestinian cookery has to be marketed by using the traditional image of Palestinians and their food. Attempts to negotiate their right to deliver a different message fail.

Palestinian contestants of MasterChef in Israel: some case studies

This chapter benefits from the analysis of the episodes covering five seasons of MCI as well as from interviews conducted with three contestants in each season. Interviews, which lasted on average three hours, started by questioning the circumstances that led the contestants to the auditions, their experience during the shooting, difficulties they were facing, their relations to other participants and their feelings upon leaving the show. Apart from two contestants, all confirmed that they discovered from the start that they had hardly any control over the way they appeared on the screen. They realised that, if they wanted to stay in the show, they had to play the role assigned to them by the production, and that their cooking skills were second to their life story and personality. They, however, enjoyed their time in MCI and kept in touch with other contestants.

In the five seasons of MCI, four Palestinians competed. Musa Abu-Saris, a youth counsellor from Jaffa, entered the competition with the aim of gaining the necessary skills for opening a restaurant that would employ Palestinian school dropouts, in order to prevent them from turning to criminal activity. He was dismissed from the show before the quarter-finals. Salma Fayumi, an observant Muslim and a registered nurse with a master's degree in public health, came out second in the third season; she presented herself as a professional woman who loves to cook. Nof Atamneh, belonging to what Danni Rabinowitz and Khawla Abu-Baker (2002 47–79) called the "stand tall generation" of young Palestinians, won the fourth season. She is a microbiologist, and a secular and independent woman. She did feel her vocation for cooking as a means of modernising Palestinian cuisine and planned to open a culinary institute for training Palestinian chefs. Lama Shhade, a 31-year-old college graduate who came to the show with the perspective of improving her cooking skills came out third in the fifth season. She grew up in Nazareth and learned to cook from her mother, an assistant school principal, who converted to Islam from Christianity after marrying a Muslim man but had lived in Tel Aviv with Jewish roommates since she was 18. Shhade identified herself as a liberal and educated woman who worked in an investment company; the production staged her as a rebellious and courageous woman because she has been living between the Arab and Jewish worlds.

The silent protestors: Musa and Salma

Musa grew up in Germany until he was seven years old. He presented himself as a Palestinian social activist, and frequently mentioned his background, unusually for Palestinians in Israel. Unlike the contestants who had immigrated to Israel, and were encouraged by the chefs to incorporate their natal culinary knowledge and memories into their cooking, the reflections of Musa on his childhood memories on food were perceived as irrelevant by them. For instance, after hesitating between the preparation of *knafeh*[3] and a nut pie, he said:

> You have brought me back to my childhood in Germany, and to the pie I used to eat every Friday with my father, on our way home from the weekly prayer at the mosque.

Chef Shani replied:

> Musa, you belong to the Arab people. That comes with certain culinary obligations. You know what a *baklava*[4] is, and I would expect that part of this native knowledge surfaced in this simple pie you used to eat every Friday while coming back from the mosque.

Musa, according to Chef Shani, does not have the right to mix his genuine childhood memories with his cooking. As a Palestinian, his native culinary knowledge has to be reflected in all his dishes. It is worth mentioning that Musa's reaction was hidden from the audience and his protest was silenced. A few episodes later, when the contestants were instructed to work in pairs that competed with each other, Musa was given the role of a Palestinian cook working under the supervision of a Jewish employer, Eddy, a small-scale Jewish manufacturer of women's clothes who, grew up in Jaffa, lived in an upper-middle class town at the outskirts of Tel Aviv. In contrast, the conversation between Eddy and Musa was broadcasted during the episode.

> Eddy: Musa shows his respect towards me. I didn't have to request it. He was waiting for me to take the lead. Musa, show me what you're doing.
>
> Musa: Everything is under control. I'm starting the *malabi*.[5] I have already taken care of the *qataif*.[6]
>
> Eddy: Is everything working according to the schedule? Is everything under control?
>
> Musa: Yes.
>
> Eddy: I imagine Musa as a fisherman, and myself as a Chef who visits the fish harbour. Musa gets off his boat and I ask him: "Musa, how was the sea today?" Musa replies: "Walla Eddy, I have an 11 kilos white *grouper* (a local fish) for you." I care for Musa. I make sure he will make a living and Musa provides me with fish for my restaurant.

The dialogue's excerpt between Musa and Eddy illustrates the extent to which Jews conceive the employer–employee relationship as an inherent and unchangeable aspect of Jewish–Arab relations. Although Musa and Eddy have been selected by the production to work in partnership, instead of treating Musa as a peer contestant, Eddy, supported by the production, places Musa in the position of a Palestinian working in the restaurant industry under the supervision of a Jew. Musa internalised the message: he no longer recalled the reasons that brought him to MCI. Rather, as mirrored by his exchange with Chefs Cohen and Anski when he presented one dish to the judges, poor connoisseurs of Palestinian cookery, he adopted the role of the Palestinian cook who had prepared a Palestinian dish he had rarely cooked before.

> Musa: I have prepared *kusa makhshi*[7] that I had never cooked before.
>
> Chef Cohen: Does *makhshi* mean squash or any stuffed vegetable?
>
> Musa: Any stuffed vegetable.
>
> Cohen: We have learned something new. Usually the squash is well cooked, and here, it's half raw. I like it.
>
> Ms Anski: The raw squash shows your respect for the vegetables you have used.

The judges complimented Musa on upgrading a traditional Palestinian dish, despite the squash being half raw because Musa ran out of time. Musa was dismissed soon afterwards for failing to prepare a meal that should have been inspired by German cookery. The production cast him in the role of an Arab cook, with limited cooking knowledge and skills and inability to expand his culinary horizon.

Unlike Musa, who expected to use MCI to promote his professional ambition and share his life story, Salma, recently married, had discovered the joy of cooking and wished to improve her culinary knowledge. Although she is an observant Muslim, whose 'Arabness' was visible through her dress code, Chef Cohen casted her as "an unconventional woman who does not think that being an observant Muslim should prevent her from doing whatever she loves to do". Interestingly, she was not instructed to cook Palestinian dishes, maybe because her 'Arabness' was sufficiently obvious or because her participation was too brief as she was dismissed after the first episode. She returned to the show at a later stage. Her first mission being to prepare both a main course and dessert using lemon as flavour, she stuffed a local fish with lemon and herbs which received the felicitations of Chef Cohen: "It is a wonderful typical Israeli dish".

The culinary preparation of Salma, qualified "Israeli" by Chef Cohen, was in fact a Palestinian dish which has inspired many Jewish restaurateurs. Cohen's compliments mask the fact that Salma had prepared a Palestinian dish that Israeli culinary agents had appropriated, and turn Salma into a cook who feeds Jewish Israelis with dishes they see as Israeli. As in the case of Musa, her protest was not revealed to the spectators who saw a contestant preparing a genuine Palestinian dish that she linked to her personal biography rather than to a geo-socio-political context. When she cooked *ftier*,[8] she used an upside down wok as a replacement for the traditional *tabun* (clay oven) to give the *pita* a taste as similar as possible to the original dish. Hiding the fact that the produce and cooking method were used in Arab rural areas, she explained to the chefs:

> Salma: For me, this dish signifies a return to good olden days, when my mother was baking and the smell of fresh bread welcomed me upon my return from school.
>
> Chef Shani: I know this pita. You have added cheese that symbolises time of plenty. It's very good and keeps up with the original taste. If you were born hundred years ago, you would have invented the pizza!
>
> Chef Cohen: It's common in your kitchen to add *za'atar* and cheese to pastries. What is new here, is the dough. Unlike the *ftier*, it has a texture of a crepe. It is your signature dish.

Although Salma was characterised by the judges as an unconventional observant Muslim woman who dared challenging the traditional roles attributed to women, her journey on MCI was mostly centred to channel her into the role of a traditional Palestinian cook who contributed to the local repertoire of native Palestinian dishes whose origins were unknown to Israelis consumers. Like other Palestinian contestants, she chose to play the role of the silent Palestinian cook, and revealed little of her culinary knowledge to the spectators, an attitude expressing dissatisfaction towards the lack of respect of the production for Palestinian culinary heritage (Gvion 2012, 2014).

The proud Palestinian: Nof Atamne

Salma and Musa have expressed their dissatisfaction by seldom communicating their culinary knowledge. Nof Atamne, in contrast, chose to use MCI as a means to win recognition for Palestinians, and to position them as active culinary agents entitled to compete with Israelis in the culinary field. She employed various strategies. She claimed, for instance, that the Palestinian contestants were as distanced from the world cuisines as the Jewish contestants. However, when she and Larry, a Jewish immigrant from South Africa could chose to compete with each other by preparing either Asian or Mediterranean dishes and chose the former, the judges emphasised that she needed to travel a longer distance than Larry before being able to make a good *jiaozi*.[9]

> Nof: I have decided to change the stigmas (sic) people have about Arabs.[10] For instance, [people will say] Nof, from Bakaa-El-Garbia, prepares a good *jiaozi*. Asian dishes are as distanced from me as they are from Larry.
>
> Chef Roschfeld: It's in a shape of a *jiaozi*, but it's not a *jiaozi*. An Arab dim-sum won't get you to go to the next stage.
>
> Nof: It is my stuffing.
>
> Chef Cohen (to Roschfeld): She should have chosen to compete on Mediterranean dishes.
>
> Roschfeld: I agree. At such an early stage of the competition, she shouldn't have taken chances by cooking Asian food.

Chef Roschfeld criticised Nof for her attempt to improvise on a recipe that did not belong to her native culinary knowledge and undermined her chances of staying in the competition. Like Musa and Salma, she learned that she was expected to cook Palestinian dishes with the proposed ingredients. Whereas Musa and Salma chose to cook traditional Palestinian dishes, but refrained from communicating on the origin of their recipes, Nof challenged the judges' image of Palestinian cookery by deconstructing and reconstructing Palestinian classics such as, for example, the *baklava* to which she gave the shape of a flower:

> Ms Ansky: There's a mixture of flavours that creates something new. This is amazing.

> Chef Shani: In your interpretation, you have deconstructed and reconstructed the dish. You have modelled the dough in shape of a circle, in which you have put a ball of nuts, and then, you have turned the circle into petals. It is a piece of art.

By the reconstruction of a dish, Nof won recognition as a modern Palestinian who undertook to modernise her cuisine. Playing according to the production's expectation also granted her the opportunity to bring Arab cooking into primetime television, and to interweave the culinary with the political discourse without directly challenging the Israeli hegemonic perceptions of Palestinian cookery. Moreover, by instrumentalising stereotypical and traditional images of Arabs, she was able to voice her protest against the way in which Palestinians are seen and received in Israel. She adopted the position of a proud and knowledgeable Palestinian who has decided which parts of her knowledge she wanted to display and in which form. Thus, rather than preparing dishes which had been appropriated by Jews, she chose to mobilise the well-established image of the traditional generous Arab hospitality to her benefit, as a manner of offering a present from the Arab people to the Jewish people, a dairy-free dessert:

> Nof: This dish signifies a journey to the Arab world: *qataif* stuffed with pistachio nuts, dates filled with chocolate and cardamom and a *tahini* twill. It's a gift from the Arabs to the Jews.
>
> Chef Shani: The dish is beautiful; you have played beautifully with the colours.
>
> Chef Roschfeld: The tastes aren't balanced. It's sticky and heavy. You should have added something refreshing.
>
> Chef Shani: It's heavy, but very good. It is in line with all the principles of Arab cooking.
>
> Chef Cohen: When you eat it, you feel as if you're sitting in a tent. It needs something refreshing to go with it.
>
> Chef Roschfeld: It should have been easy for you to prepare such a dish. And yet, it is not a good enough job.
>
> Nof: I am a well-educated and articulate Muslim woman who lives in Israel. My identity is not clear, and therefore, my dishes are sometimes odd. You don't meet so many women like me. I dare doing things that most people will not do. Sometimes, it is the price to pay.

In response to the reference to the judges' perception of the Arabs as living in tents in the desert, like Bedouins, Nof claimed, on primetime television, that she saw Israel as a place of residence, but not as her nation-state. She used the culinary discourse to deliver her message and combined it with images the judges associated with the Palestinian community. The culinary discourse, through which she delivered her messages, enabled her to protest against Palestinians' social positioning in Israel. Her decision to offer the Jews a gift was not an expression of generosity, but a way of protesting against the ongoing appropriation of Arab dishes. The quality of the product she chose to prepare was criticised, but the act of giving was both appreciated and taken for granted. But when Nof chose to upgrade the *fatat-el-hummus*, an old dish symbolising poverty and abandoned by Palestinians, she initiated a discussion on the kind of dishes that call for upgrading and the appropriate means of modernising them:

> Nof: I added agar to tomato juice to make tomato caviar. I connected a traditional dish to the world of molecular biology. It is as if I am saying it is time Palestinian kitchen changes.
>
> Chef Shani: I understand the idea of preparing tomato caviar but your *fatat-el-hummus* has no connection to it. You'll have to learn a lot about food to realise that there is nothing like a good tomato to accompany the dish.
>
> Chef Roschfeld: When you'll start serving it with tomato again, you'll do it because you'll understand all this caviar business, which people make nowadays, is bullshit.
>
> Nof: For you, it is bullshit, but for me agar is something with which I work in the lab. It is fun to combine my 'Arabness' with my doctorate study. Each one of you has his own signature. Why can't I have mine?
>
> Chef Shani: We know from our own experience that you need to go through the entire process. Your mode of thinking is revolutionary, and it will dissolve the boundaries of your cuisine.
>
> Nof: The judges undermine my confidence. All I think about is what do they want me to do? What do they want? Food is something very intimate, and when I share my food with others and they say unpleasant things about it, it hurts.

While the judges evaluated the dishes according to culinary standards, and referred to the learning process which professional chefs have to go through, Nof interpreted their comments as a critique on her entitlement to use scientific knowledge for upgrading her native dishes, and preventing Palestinians from marrying their tradition with modernity. The judges, however, pointed out a gap between her mode of thinking and her culinary skills, claiming "there is a lot for you to learn before you upgrade traditional Palestinian dishes". However, her mode of thinking played in her favour when she prepared a contemporary version of the *helzale* (stuffed turkey throat), a traditional eastern European

Jewish dish. She used her familiarity with Arab cooking and its staples to change the *helzale*'s shape, taste and texture:

> Chef Roschfeld: You have turned the *helzale* into a historical classic: an Israeli dish.
>
> Chef Shani: Your version of the *helzale* which you have prepared by using the language of the Palestinian cuisine, makes me think about the beginning of the Jewish people, the time Moses walked with his people in the desert.
>
> Chef Cohen: The use of cracked wheat and smoked goose gives a unique flavour and makes the dish perfect.
>
> Nof (laughing): It is a great achievement for the Palestinian people to have figured out the essence of the *helzale*.

Nof's *helzale* is contextualized in a geo-socio-political context that mixes ancient Judaism and Eastern European Jewry with Israeli and Arab cooking cultures. She mobilized Palestinian food items that help eastern European Jews to update their traditional dishes and adjust them to the time and place where they live. Through her humorous reaction, Nof voices her protest against the judges' perception of Palestinians as lacking of sophistication, and regarding dishes as Israeli when they have, in fact, been borrowed from Palestinians. However, after this episode, Nof no longer attempted to innovate, but prepared only traditional Palestinian dishes, conforming to what the judges expected. This tactic paid off:

> Nof: I made *kaek-el-id*,[11] the most famous Palestinian cookies we prepare for holidays, according to the original recipe. They are classics and not to be changed. Prior to major holidays, my mother and I go to my grandmother's house to prepare them while talking and gossiping.
>
> Chef Roschfeld: It is wonderful and reflects the culture you come from. It is the best dish we have tasted today.
>
> Nof: Today is the peak of my life. It is more exciting than getting a PhD. It is an indication that my food is good and I am qualified to go on.

Nof finally succumbed to the role of the traditional Palestinian woman whose schooling and scientific achievements were considered as secondary to her culinary know-how. When the production invited the contestants' mothers to come in the studio to taste their children's dishes so as the present them as traditional, Nof's mother, a professional and secular woman, was not invited. It was her grandmother, an observant Muslim dressed in a *hijab*, who came. Nof used her presence to get her approval of the *kubbe*, a Palestinian classic, that she upgraded by stuffing it with fish instead of lamb meat. She interpreted her grandmother's consent as a sign that the Palestinian community was ready to modernise its cuisine. In the semi-finals, she modernised another classic, the *kubbienieh*, an Arab tartar made of ground *burghul*,[12] raw meat, parsley and sweet red pepper, that she stuffed with nuts, scallions and mint. She explained:

> Originally we serve a mixture that looks like a dough in a bowl from which diners take their share. By sticking to the original ingredients yet creating a ball stuffed with nuts, scallions and meat, I turn it into a gourmet dish."

Modernising Palestinian classics, by deconstructing and reconstructing them while preserving their original essence resulted in Nof being seen by the judges, as certainly a talented and excellent candidate who had gained the permission of Jewish culinary agents to upgrade her native cuisine. Nof played along:

> Nof: I wanted to modernise my cuisine. In MCI, I learned how to do it. If I win, my life is going to change.
>
> Chef Shani: Nof is the woman who will take Palestinian cuisine one step further.
>
> Chef Cohen: She is in charge of Palestinian cooking culture.
>
> Ms Ansky: She is at her best when she upgrades one of her grandmother's dishes. If she prepares one of her native dishes with the tools she has acquired here, she will win.

The fact that Nof did not choose to challenge the hegemonic narratives of Israelis on Palestinians and their cuisine, and provided the judges with dishes they associated with Palestinian classics, gained her the title of MasterChef. Simultaneously, this limits her culinary options, and if she was positioned as a good Palestinian cook, because she attempted to modernise Palestinian cookery, she was not a labelled as a good cook per se. Cooking modern versions of Palestinian classics was not only a strategy for staying in the show; it was also a means of repositioning Palestinians in Israeli society, by bringing onto primetime television the distinctive features of Palestinian culture, and claiming acknowledgement of Palestinians as a distinct national minority.

The modern Palestinian woman and her home: Lama Shhade

The participation of Lama Shhade, the fourth contestant, was directed neither by the desire to play the role of the traditional Palestinian woman nor by the attempt to use MCI to modernise the Palestinian kitchen. Her narrative revolved around the interplay between modernity and tradition, as experienced in the lives of young, educated and modern Palestinian women. Although the production casted her as "a fighter who lived neither in the Arab nor in the Jewish world" (Chef Cohen), with a lifestyle similar to that of Jewish women of her age, she was expected to play the role of the traditional Palestinian. Lama accepted this assumption of Palestinian identity, but negotiated the right to introduce contemporary Palestinian domestic cookery. Consequently, her dishes, mostly adapted from world cuisine to the Palestinian palate, displayed her as a woman who was familiar neither with traditional Palestinian cookery nor with modern cooking as practised by Jews.

Contemporary Palestinian cooking, according to Lama, consists of three distinctive features. First, it comprises world dishes adapted to the Palestinian taste, incorporating ingredients exogenous to the Palestinian cuisine. Secondly, it is done by women who know little about Palestinian culinary classics. Third, it has to be characterised by abundance which is expressed by the use of expensive ingredients, such as fillet of beef, even though the recipe does not require it. Whereas the primary goal of Nof was to modernise Palestinian cuisine, Lama considered her cuisine as modern already.

Contemporary domestic Palestinian cookery, as practised by Lama and women of her generation, still retains some characteristics of traditional Palestinian cooking. First, her inability to think out of the Palestinian culinary framework turned to her disadvantage, and she was qualified as unfamiliar with the Israeli culinary scene, and lacking the necessary skills to become a chef. Secondly, she used traditional principles of Arab cookery in order to prepare either modern Palestinian dishes or foods that were external to Palestinian cuisine. She cooked, notably, by feeling rather than by using precise measurement. Her dishes were often cooked in layers, and she served them, even those which were not Palestinian, with yogurt sauce or cheese, on the side, a traditional Palestinian method for providing protein.

Lama used the show to expose the viewers to a different 'type' of Palestinian woman, whose life experience was similar to that of her Jewish peers, even when it applied to norms and behavioural codes not accepted in Palestinian society. For instance, when Ms Anski instructed the contestants to cook a dish they had previously prepared to express their feelings toward their lovers, Lama chose to tell the spectators she visited her lover who was sick and prepared him a chicken soup. This gesture, familiar to Jewish women in Israel or in Western societies, is interpreted in the Palestinian community as an offence to the woman's virtue, and therefore, neither acceptable nor to be reported in public. Lama shared her story knowing it might embarrass the Palestinian spectators.

> Lama: When I prepared the soup for my sick fiancé,[13] I even deboned the chicken so that it was easier to eat.
>
> Ms Ansky: It's very comforting when someone cuts chicken meat with his/her hands and feeds you. I can feel your love through the soup.

In exposing the spectators to the context in which she first prepared the soup, Lama informed them about the lifestyle of young and modern Palestinian women who neither concealed their romantic relationships nor worried about their reputation. Moreover, living a life similar to that of Jewish women of her age entitled her, she felt, to participate in public activities as a Palestinian, and to commodify domestic Palestinian food. When she and her MCI partner, Massimiliano, an Italian immigrant and the winner of the fifth season, had to prepare lunch for 100 visitors in a shopping centre at Tel Aviv, she suggested cooking Bolognese, but diverging from the original recipe:

> Lama: Trust me. I am an Israeli. I know what people here like. We need to avoid conflicts over the recipes. I'm going to cook the meat in the sauce and add *ras-el-hanut*,[14] cinnamon, cardamom and pepper. This is my place and I know what I am doing.
>
> Massimiliano: It is going to be an Italian dish with an Israeli sauce.

By defining herself as Israeli, Lama claimed her right to communicate her culture in the public sphere and present Palestinian versions of dishes from all over the world, according to the method by which they are cooked in Palestinian domestic kitchens (Gvion 2012), to both Jews and Palestinians who visit the shopping centre. As many Palestinian women do, she added vegetables and traditional Palestinian spices to the sauce, and served it, topped with *labane*.[15] She demonstrated to Massimiliano that he was less of an Israeli than her, and unfamiliar with the local culture. The judges defined the dish as being an adaptation to Palestinian taste, and called it "an Arab Bolognese".

Cooking in the way modern Palestinian young women often do, prevented Lama from serving good classic Palestinian dishes, but also masked her lack of knowledge of traditional cookery. When she had to cook a dish to express her feelings toward her deceased grandmother, she upgraded the okra dish of her grandmother by serving it in a tomato soup topped with parmesan, and grilled tuna. As Chef Roschfeld objected: "Tuna had nothing to do with your cuisine which is based on lamb, beef or chicken, or with your grandmother and your memories", she changed the tuna to chicken to the satisfaction of the chef who exclaimed: "Bless your hands. The dish tastes as if your grandmother prepared it."

What was, for Lama, a means of modernising traditional Palestinian dishes, was interpreted by Chef Roschfeld as an indication of her misunderstanding of the rules for upgrading dishes. He prevented her from using ingredients, which he considered as inappropriate to Palestinian dishes, but when she included items that he believed to be integral to Palestinian cuisine, he approved the dish that he labelled a Palestinian classic, even though it was not.

The second distinctive feature of Palestinian cookery that Lama introduced is cooking by intuition and feel. When assigned to cook under the guidance of Chef Gratowski, the owner of a successful restaurant in the Galilee who is inspired by Arab cookery, she chose to prepare a modern version of the *tabule*.[16] On this occasion, she protested against the irrelevance of Western measures to prepare Palestinian dishes:

Lama: I am serving tuna tartar over *tabule* but by using *maftul.*[17] We [Palestinians] don't add coriander to the *tabule*, but I will do because fish goes well with coriander.

Chef Gratowski: I suggest cutting each one of the herbs separately and keeping each one of them separately so you can control the amount you're using.

Lama: I don't want to do that. You have to trust me. I know what I am doing. I cook by intuition. I neither measure nor taste.

Gratowski: Why did you put so much lemon?

Lama: Because this is how I like it. You have to trust me.

Lama negotiates the principles of cooking with Chef Gratowski and of upgrading Palestinian dishes. She claims that her knowledge of Palestinian cookery allows her to be more confident in the use of traditional means of cooking, such as intuition and feeling, rather than being guided by a foreigner to her cuisine who wants to introduce western principles into Palestinian cooking.

Like many modern Palestinian women, Lama had no experience of preparing Palestinian classics. In the episode that centred on the preparation of dumplings, she prepared, for the first time, *shishbarak,* Palestinian dumplings filled with minced meat and slowly cooked in a yogurt sauce seasoned with mint. During the preparation, she said: "It is an Arab classic. I am trying to reproduce the movements of my mother and grandmother when they kneaded the dough, but I cannot reproduce the shape."

In her attempts to explain her difficulty in preparing *shishbarak*, Lama listed three characteristics necessary to prepare traditional Arab dishes: oral transmission of culinary knowledge from one generation to the next; a learning process that consists of trials and errors; and cooking by feeling. Her first attempt to make *shishbarak* failed, and the judges, with the aim of defining their taste, labelled them as 'Arab *kreplach*', an eastern European Jewish dumpling served in a chicken soup, with the texture of *kibbe* (balls of bulgur stuffed with ground meat and fried) or of *maamul*, a popular Arab cookie.

The third characteristic of contemporary domestic Palestinian cookery, abundance and generosity, was particularly visible when Lama prepared dishes that are served to guests. Laboriously prepared dishes, made of ingredients as expensive as they are of highly symbolical value, such as fillet of beef, were copiously served to the judges, even though the recipes did not require beef. When Lama dared to use fillet to make sausages, the chefs violently criticised her:

Chef Roschfeld: Preparing a sausage with fillet pisses me off. You are spoiled, and you use fillet because you like it. You think only about yourself, and not about the people for whom you cook. To prepare a dish that reflects modesty and frugality, by using fillet of beef is maddening.

Chef Shani: It shows how incapable she is to learn what she is supposed to learn.

Sausages are rarely consumed by Palestinians who are generally suspicious of frozen and industrialized meat products. Consequently, sausages are not associated with frugality or moderate financial means, but with modernity and affluence. A similar misinterpretation of her dishes occurred a few episodes later when she had to prepare a dish for Ms Anski, an ex-model who has opened the first farmers' market in Tel Aviv, and is known for her love of seasonal vegetables. Observing the rule of Palestinian hospitality that requires feeding the guest with expensive foods, she served fillet of beef accompanied by mushrooms cooked in a sauce composed of cream and peanut butter. This dish caused discontent:

Ms Anski: You have to know by now that I love spicy food and vegetables handled with care. Your dish makes me uncomfortable. You have not prepared it for me but for yourself. We asked you, several times, not to use fillet. But you won't listen to us.

Lama's attempts to show her respect for Anski by using Palestinian rules of hospitality were interpreted as an intentional manifestation of disrespect. Anski's argument, however, demonstrated how she and the chefs were poorly informed about Palestinian cookery and ethics, forcing Lama to have the same conception of hospitality and cooking as Jews have. The impression that Lama cooked according to principles with which she was not familiar disadvantaged her, even when her commission required the use of a Palestinian staple such as *pita* bread. While *pita* is consumed by Israelis in the same way that bread is used to make sandwiches, Palestinians use *pita* as a food-shovel to pick up the food from the plate.

Lama: It [to prepare *pita*] was supposed to be easy for me, but I couldn't think properly. Therefore, I prepared something I like to eat, a *pita* stuffed with meatballs made of fillet.

Ms Anski: It is the ugliest of all the dishes.

Chef Shani: The salad is terrible, the meatballs are dry. It is not edible.

Chef Roschfeld: This is what happens when you use fillet to prepare meatballs. We should not even bother discussing such a terrible dish.

The judges' comments recognised the function of *pita* bread in Israeli cookery, but ignored its role in Arab cuisine. The chefs disregarded Lama's difficulty in using a staple in a manner seldom used to her native cuisine. Moreover, Lama's choice of expensive fillet meat was also little appreciated, and revealed how limited was her knowledge of food items and of the role they fulfil in the meal.

When Lama made use of the basic principles of traditional Palestinian cookery, she was able to produce upscale dishes that were not an integral part of Palestinian cuisine. During the semi-finals, she prepared a dish based on the principle of cooking in layers, by using grape leaves to pad a fish covered with a cloth and cooked with olive oil, wine, lemon, tangerine juice and herbs. She explained: "I will use grape leaves in the way we cook stuffed vegetables. This is not a big deal if they are burnt as the fish will keep the aroma from the herbs."

Before laying the plates, she deboned the fish and placed little pieces of flesh on the top of a crusty potato puree, making the fish look like traditional festive Palestinian dishes such as the *mansaf*, rice topped with lamb meat and fried with onions and pine nuts.

> Chef Roschfeld: It is very aesthetic. The taste is superb.
>
> Chef Shani: It's very delicate and the tarragon gives it a fresh taste.
>
> Chef Cohen: It's the kind of dish that every chef would be proud to prepare.

However, as modern, daring and detached from traditional conventions as Lama tried to appear, she could not use her participation in MCI to demonstrate to the public the changes that Palestinian society and its cuisine were undergoing. She was cast as a representative of a traditional group, incapable of internalising the principles of the Israeli culinary scene, and lacking the skills and experience that make great cooks. In the last episode, when the finalists' families were present in the studio, Chef Cohen's farewell to Lama was:

> You're a fighter. You live neither in the Arab nor in the Jewish world, and both parties do not make things easy for you. You should be very proud of your daughter, Mr Shhade. May I give her a hug? I know that your culture requires I ask your permission.

Chef Cohen complimented Lama for daring to lead a life similar to that of Jewish women of her age, and called on her father to express his support of her unconventional choice. At the same time, however, he reinforced her belonging to a traditional group which sees women as subjected to paternal control. This interplay between modernity and tradition, as perceived by the judges, was presented as an integral part of the experience of Palestinian cooks.

Conclusion: MCI as a mirror of the Palestinian position in Israeli society

The analysis of the verbal exchanges between the Palestinian contestants and the chefs throws light on how the former are constrained to conform to the image of the traditional Arab, as perceived by the Israelis. Although the four contestants, Musa, Salma, Nof and Lama, presented the heterogeneous social make-up of Palestinian society in Israel, all of them had to negotiate their entitlement to different casting and to find alternatives to the hegemonic narrative of Palestinians, in order to fit into the requirement of the production and to maintain their chances, limited as they were, of staying involved in the public culinary scene. The participation of Palestinian contestants in MCI, and their ability to succeed in the show, does not imply that the culinary field is reversing or may challenge power relations in Israeli society. On the contrary, MCI is a clear example of how Palestinian contestants are manipulated and channelled, via the culinary field, into the role of the "Other" and even the 'exotic' who internalises the hegemonic discourse in order to increase the chances of benefiting from improved consideration in Israeli society.

This cooking programme is a reflection of the difficulties Palestinian citizens of Israel face in participating in, and being recognised by, Israeli society, as well as in having the heterogeneity of their community in terms of religious adherence, intellectual development and aspiration acknowledged. Their distinctive culinary features are not only ignored or not legitimated, but are also appropriated by their host society as belonging to its patrimony.

Notes

1 These dishes are those prepared by women who lack the financial means to feed their family with meat, fish or other expensive ingredients.
2 *Humusiot* are places that serve freshly made hummus only, and are frequented for a late breakfast or early lunch.
3 *Knafeh* is a sweet dish, made of dry thin noodles called *kada'if* and Arab cheese, which is baked and served hot.
4 *Baklava* is a pastry made of filo dough filled with nuts and seasoned with honey.
5 *Malabi* is a dessert made of milk or cream and sugar thickened with gelatin or cornstarch.
6 *Qataif* are thin dried noodles that are used for preparing deserts.
7 *Kusa Mahkshi* is squash stuffed with rice and a little meat.
8 *Ftier* is a thin *pita* bread stuffed with *za'atar*, a mixture of dried herbs, mostly sage leaves and sesame seeds, and cheese.
9 *Jiaozi* is a Chinese dumpling commonly eaten across Eastern, Central, Southern and Western Asia.
10 Nof's comment has to be read as: "I have decided to change the negative perceptions people have of Arabs."
11 *Kaek El Id* are cookies stuffed with dates.
12 *Bulgur* is dried cracked wheat.
13 Palestinians use the term 'fiancé' with reference to the person they are dating regardless of whether or not they are engaged.
14 *Ras-el-hanut* is a spice mix from North Africa which has been adopted by modern Palestinian women. It plays a role in North African cuisine similar to that played by *garam masala* in Indian cooking.
15 *Labane* is a soft cheese made of goats' milk, shaped into small balls, covered by olive oil and stored in jars.

16 *Tabule* is a salad made of fine *bulgur*, a lot of parsley and a few mint leaves, seasoned with olive oil and lemon.

17 *Maftul* are Palestinian couscous flakes.

References

Amal, J. (2007). "Nationalizing states and the constitution of "hollow citizenship": Israel and its Palestinian Citizens", *Ethnopolitics,* Vol. 6(4): 471–493.

Amal, J., Elias N. and Soker, O. (2011). "Cultural encoding and fake equality in popular reality shows: lessons from Israel", *Journal of Ethnic and Migration Studies,* 37(9): 1349–1366.

Andrejevic, M. and Colby, D. (2006). "Racism and reality TV: the case of MTV's road rules", in S. David and J. Escoffrey (eds.), *How Real Is Reality TV? Essays on Representation and Truth*, pp. 195–211. NC: McFarland & Company.

Appadurai, A. (1988). "How to make national cuisine", *Contemporary Studies in Society and History,* Vol. 30: 3–24.

Bauman, Z. (2002). *Society Siege,* Cambridge: UK. Polity Press.

Browne, R.D. (1996). *Electronic Media and Indigenous Peoples: A Voice of Our Own?*, Ames: Iowa State University Press.

Caspi, D. and Elias, N. (2011). "Don't patronize me: media by and for minorities", *Ethnic and Racial Studies,* Vol. 34(1): 62–82.

Collins, K. (2012). "A kitchen of one's own", *Camera Obscura,* Vol. 27(2): 1–23.

Cottle, S. (2000). *Ethnic Minorities and the Media: Changing Cultural Boundaries,* Philadelphia: Open University Press.

Downing, J. and Husband, C. (2005). *Representing 'Race', Racisms, Ethnicities and Media,* London: Sage Publications.

Elias, N., Amal, J. and Soker, O. (2009). "Illusive pluralism and hegemonic identity in popular reality shows in Israel", *Television & New Media*, Vol. 10(5): 375–391.

Ferrero, S. (2002). "Comida sin par. Consumption of Mexican food in Los Angeles", in W. Belasco (ed.), *Food Nations: Selling Taste in Consumer Societies,* pp. 175–193. New York: Routledge.

Gallagher, M. (2004). "What's so funny about iron chef?", *Journal of Popular Film and Television,* Vol. 31(4): 176–184.

Goddard, E. (2003). "Real life: the social geometry of reality shows", in M.J. Smith and A.F. Woods (eds.), *Survivor Lessons: Essays on Communication and Reality Television,* pp. 73–96. United States: Jefferson NC. McFarland and Company.

Gross, L. (1998). "Minorities, majorities and the media", in T. Liebes and J.Curra (eds), *Media, Ritual and Identity*, pp. 87–102. London, Routledge.

Gvion, L. (2006). "Cuisines of poverty as means of empowerment: Arab food in Israel", *Agriculture and Human Values*, Vol. 23(3): 299–312.

Gvion, L. (2009). "Narrating modernity and tradition: the case of Palestinian food in Israel", *Identities,* 16(4):391–413.

Gvion, L. (2011). "Cooking, food and masculinity: Palestinian men in Israeli society", *Men and Masculinities*, Vol. 14(4): 408–429.

Gvion, L. (2012). *Beyond Hummus and Falafel: Social and Cultural Aspects of Palestinian Food in Israel*", Berkeley: University of California Press.

Gvion, L. (2014). "Tradition and resistance. The case of Palestinian restaurants in Israel", *Journal of Intercultural Studies*, Vol. 35(4): 366–384.

Gvion, L. (2015). "Two narratives of Jewish food. 'Jewish' vs. 'ethnic'", in A. Helman (ed), *Jews and Their Foodways*, pp. 126-141. Oxford: Oxford University Press.

Hirsch, D. (2011). "Hummus is best when it is fresh and made by Arabs", *American Ethnologist*, Vol. 38(4): 617–630.

Hollows, J. (2003). "Oliver's twist. Leisure, labor and domestic masculinity in the Naked Chef", *International Journal of Cultural Studies*, Vol. 6(2): 229–248.

Hollows, J. (2002). "The bachelor dinner. Masculinity, class and cooking in Playboy, 1953–1961", *Continuum: Journal of Media and Cultural Studies*, Vol. 16(2): 143–155.

Holmes, S. and Jermyn, D. (2004). *Understanding Reality Television*, London: Routledge.

hooks, b. (1992). "Eating the other: desire and resistance", in bell hooks (ed.), *Black Looks: Race and Representation*, pp. 21–39. Boston: South End Press.

Jabarin, H. (2001). "Israeliness" looking into the future of Palestinians", *Law and Governance*, Vol 6: 53–86. (in Hebrew).

Johnston, J., Rondey, A. and Chong, P. (2014). "Making change in the kitchen? A study of celebrity cookbooks, culinary personas, and inequality", *Poetics*, Vol. 47: 1–22.

Kirby, L.A. (2013). "Cowboys of the high seas. Representations of working-class masculinity on deadliest catch", *The Journal of Popular Culture*, Vol. 46(1): 109–118.

Mintz, S. (1996). *Tasting Food, Tasting Freedom*, Boston: Beacon Press.

Newcomb, H. (2007). *Television. The Critical View*, New York: Oxford University Press.

Orbe, M.P. (2008). "Representations of race in reality TV: watch and discuss", *Critical Studies in Media Communication*, Vol. 25(4): 345–52.

Pozner, J. (2010). *Reality Bites Back*, California, Berkley: Seal Press.

Rabinowitz, D. and Abu-Baker, K. (2002). *The Stand Tall Generation: the Palestinian Citizens of Israel Today*, Jerusalem: Keter (in Hebrew).

Ranta, R. (2014). "Consuming Palestine: Palestine and Palestinians in Israeli food culture", *Ethnicities*, Vol. 14(3): 412–435.

Scholes, L. (2011). "A slave to the stove? The TV celebrity chef abandons the kitchen", *Critical Quarterly*, Vol. 53(3): 44–59.

Smith, G. (2012). "Barthes on Jamie: myth and the TV revolutionary", *Journal of Media Practice*, Vol. 13(1): 3–17.

Smith, G. and Wilson, P. (2004). "Country cookin' and cross-dressin'", *Television and New Media*, Vol. 5: 175–195.

Smith, M.J. and Wood, A.F. (eds.) (2003). *Survivor Lessons: Essays on Communication and Reality Television*, Jefferson, NC: McFarland.

Stein, R. (1998). "National itineraries, itinerant nations", *Social Text*, Vol. 16(3): 91–124.

8 The never-ending reinvention of 'traditional food'

Food practices and identity (re)construction among Bolivian returnees from Argentina[1]

Charles-Édouard de Suremain

Introduction

What migrants bring to light about their global situation – social, familial, economic or cultural – in the country of immigration is not always the same as how they actually live on a day-to-day basis. Beyond images, words and the more or less standardised discourses glorifying the founding experience of migration that migrants willingly stress themselves, there is often a tremendous discrepancy between practice and daily life.[2] Such a discrepancy, which exemplifies a classic methodological problem in anthropology – the distinction between what is told and what is done or felt – is by now relatively well documented as regards migrant populations.[3] On the other hand, the social situation of returnees in the homeland is still of minor interest for anthropologists as compared with that of refugees,[4] though of wider interest for the social sciences. This relative deficiency, varying in different regions of the world, is all the more regrettable in that ethnographical studies on returnees may contribute to the understanding of complex situations, in which the very processes of identity construction are at stake, through social stratification which is uplifting or degrading according to the state of the migrants or returnees. In this respect, the study of the food practices of returnees allows for questioning the interaction of migration with identity and with 'traditional food', notably, to what extent the social construction of migration, real or imaginary, is directly experienced through diet. Perception of migration, as success or failure, stems from the confrontation between what is eaten at home (here) and in the host country (there.) Food may provide a privileged access to a complete grasp of migrant identities 'on the move' or being constructed. In any case, a better understanding of the link between migration, food and identity allows for more accurate comprehension of the local significance given to 'traditional food', poverty and wealth and, more generally, to well- and ill-being.

In this article, I will provide some responses to these questions from the analysis of what the members of a Bolivian family, including children, who have lived in Argentina do eat, do not eat, wish to eat and wish not to eat after returning to Bolivia. I will show how food practices from here (Bolivia) and from there (Argentina) highlight the stigma of poverty and wealth, lack and abundance of resources, of 'bad' and 'good' health or positive and negative body images. The way an 'elsewhere food' enlightens – or informs – a 'here food' or 'there food' provides another way to explore more generally the interaction issue between social stratifications, identities and tradition which are at stake in the migration situation.

Data presented in this text were collected in Bolivia in 2003 during an interdisciplinary participative action-research financed by the European Community which investigated local perceptions on growth and development of children under five in Bolivia and Peru (1998–2003). As the programme aimed to improve relations between patients and professionals, I conducted ethnographic fieldwork in primary health care centres. I met the Quintero family, on which this present chapter is based, while I was observing interactions between caregivers of children in the waiting-room. I was immediately struck by how their particular situation would be meaningful and comparable to many other returnee situations. I did not conduct fieldwork in Argentina, but migrants often referred to the foods they consumed in that country. The method of the investigation is thus not, properly speaking, comparative, but the comparison of food consumption invoked by migrants gives us a means of understanding how they construct their discourses on practices in a country where they have lived but no longer live.

The Quintero family is composed of the householder, Julio, his wife Eulalia and their two young children, Justiño and Cristina. The family lives in Barrio Magisterio, one of the sub-quarters of Chávez Rancho, a peri-urban area of Cochabamba, the third city of Bolivia, which is located at an altitude of 2500 metres in the middle of the inter-Andean valley. Four kilometres distant from the downtown, Chávez Rancho has more than 40,000 inhabitants. It is divided into 31 districts (Organización Territorial de Base) and many informal sub-quarters are recognised locally. My choice of the Quintero family was determined by the fact that its situation and discourses are largely shared by family migrants in Bolivia, so that the data presented in the article may be common to this group.

During my twelve one-week to 10-day stays in Chávez Rancho, I coupled direct observation of food practices with the reconstruction of what I have called "intergenerational food life stories". In participative action-research, social and spatial contexts of the narrative and its historical background are the most important methodological premises to take into account. The objective has been to reconstruct, through successive interviews, the life of the Quintero family, by centring on some key life events (birth, marriage, migration, job, death, etc.). However, unlike standard life stories, interviews have been carried out with all the persons, 16 in total, who claim to belong or to be related to the Quinteros, sharing their daily life and having privileged relationships with them (Julio, Eulalia, their two children, their four parents and eight grandparents). Furthermore, I have focused the interviews with family members of different sexes, ages and, above all, of distinct generations, on food practices in order to understand the meaning of 'traditional food' in a migrant context. I have thus collected multiple types of information on supply, transformation, preparation, consumption, commensality, conservation, waste treatment and food's symbolic status; part of this information is presented here.

Each interview was conducted either at home or in a discrete place downtown (some food stores at the market place, some remote *chichería*), and lasted between one and two hours. Some of them (especially with the children) were recorded, but they have all been transcribed. The most meaningful data were collected through 'classic' ethnographic participant observation, by spending time with people, listening to their ordinary conversations, accompanying them in their daily duties and destinations (market, health centre, neighbours, etc.), sharing their feelings, experiences, thoughts and daily meals.

Relocalizados, indiecitos, damnificados: labelling the returnees

Like numerous young Bolivians, Julio (22 years), Eulalia (19 years) and their son Justiño (2 years) crossed the frontier between Bolivia and Argentina in 1994 in the hope of improving their life.[5] They stayed in Salta,[6] a town in the north-western part of the country, for nine years. Justiño started his schooling in Argentina; he was aged 11 when he went back to Bolivia at the end of 2002. Meanwhile, Julio and Eulalia uneasily moved from job to job in various sectors: construction work, public work, agriculture and horticulture for Julio, and maid or waitress work for Eulalia. Their daughter, Cristina, was born in 1999.

As for thousands of Bolivians, Julio's migration to Argentina was not definitive. His aim in migrating was to prove to himself that he could care for his wife and young son financially. He also wished to help his parents and grandparents financially, and his parents- and grandparents-in law. In Julio's mind, the money sent to his relatives (*remesas* or saving) that came from his migration had to prove his emancipation. He wished to succeed his father as the money provider, which would enable him to occupy the central position amongst the kindred. Unfortunately, the *remesas* have not allowed Julio to improve his economic means nor to acquire the dreamed of social status in the long term.

Before migrating to Argentina, the young couple lived with Julio's parents, according to an arrangement, quite common in popular urban settings, which is related to the patrilocality system adopted by peasants in Bolivia. In exchange for the use of the kitchen, patio, latrines and one room, Julio and Eulalia had to take responsibility for water and electricity expenses, house maintenance and, above all, food expenditure. The standard of living of Julio's parents was quite modest. His father, like many older inhabitants of Chávez Rancho, was a pit worker, unemployed during 1970s–1980s. In this region, the entire mining activity suddenly stopped, and the workers received from the government, as sole compensation, access to cheap housing (Gill 1997). The nickname given to these people, *relocalizados*, derives from a term signifying literally 'relocated' or 'replaced', but which refers implicitly and in a figurative manner to those 'who do not feel to be in their place'.

The socio-economic profile of Eulalia's parents is similar to that of Julio's: they are unemployed workers in mining activity. The eight grandparents of the Quintero couple, however, are poor Quechua peasants. They are '*indios*' or '*indígenas*' (indigenous) as they called themselves. The city-dwellers contemptuously nickname them '*indiecitos*' (little Indians). This pejorative appellation, depreciative and stigmatising, is recurrent for all indigenous Latin Americans, notably those residing in mountain regions. Ruined by the conjunction of recurrent droughts, land erosion and widespread dividing of lands due to inheritance, this generation of peasants ended up joining the small, basic hamlets in the surroundings of mining camps, and then integrated themselves there definitively with their children in the 1960s (Absi 2003; Nash 1979).

In 2003 when I met the Quintero family, both Julio and his wife were having great difficulty in finding jobs in Cochabamba, even occasional ones; their children had been integrated into the public school. Not only by neighbours and local residents, but also by their other relatives, Julio, Eulalia, Justiño and Cristina are called '*damnificados*' (disaster victims). This generic term usually identifies the victims of natural disasters such as earthquakes, rockfalls, and floods etc. which are frequent in the country, and in the region of Cochabamba in particular. It refers to those who have lost their houses and are sometimes precariously and temporarily re-housed thanks to public or private help (NGOs, Ministries, the Catholic Church, international institutions). The common use of *damnificados*, notably by the media, is a categorisation or a form of labelling which is more or less accepted and interiorised by the Quinteros.

Relocalizados, damnificados, indiecitos… Everything goes on as though these three substantives enable us clearly to identify three consecutive generations of people whose social status may be perceived as 'uncertain' in the long term. It is as if, inescapably, a particular family history used to be reproduced through generations: a family story for which the thread would be the uncertain fate of persons perpetually ranked, unranked or re-ranked against the background of social marginalisation, according to Pierre Bourdieu (1978). Ethnicity, in this context, is defined as a 'particular form of social interaction', permanently recomposed and reworked by historical events (Barth 1969).[7]

What is eaten 'here' and 'there'

It is worth understanding how the social construction of the origin, either real or imaginary, of protagonists sheds light on a few of our initial questions: what is eaten, not eaten, what foods are wished for and not wished for by the returnees, namely the Quintero family members? What the Quinteros eat daily since their return to Bolivia may be summed up in a few words: it is food that they ate before migrating to Argentina; food that they expected never to eat again. And what the Quinteros would like to eat now can also be summed up briefly: it is food that they used to eat in Argentina that they can no longer eat in Bolivia – namely the daily consumption of bread, meat and sodas. These three items, so-called 'traditional Argentine food' by Julio and Eulalia, constitute a strong identity issue for the Quinteros' family members.

In the Andes, wheat arrived along with colonisation and evangelisation in the sixteenth century. In the high plateau and valleys, agricultural systems were based on several cereals (maize, quinoa, amaranth), as well as on potatoes and beans, cultivated on small, scattered plots forming what J.V. Murra (1975) called the 'Andean archipelago'. Resources were dispersed in the mountains, a risky milieu. In anticipation of climatic accidents, households were able to stock and to exchange products (fish, game) with other areas such as the piedmont and the lowlands, for ensuring food availability in the long term. Thanks to this sophisticated socio-economic organisation system, during the pre-Colonial period, food was available and quite diversified.

In Bolivian villages, traditional food consumed by poor peasants has not changed very much since colonisation. Above 3000 metres, scarcity of combustible material makes it a real challenge to cook different dishes separately or consecutively. Meals are mostly constituted of one dish. Stocks (*caldos*) and soups (*sopas*) are numerous and comprise *chairo paceño*, the most popular soup composed of beef, young lamb, carrots, broad beans, peas, corn, potatoes, etc., according to region; *chankao*, a salty soup of small potatoes sometimes with a bone for fiesta days; *sopa de mani* made up of peanuts; *caldo de riñon*, a stock of lamb, pork or beef kidneys, and the less elaborate *sopa de fideos*, noodle soup. Cereals (corn, wheat, quinoa, sweet manioc), peas, broad beans and tubers (potatoes) are boiled or cooked in gruel. The pre-colonial *chuño* (dehydrated potatoes) continues to be consumed almost everywhere. Although soups and stocks integrate meats, this produce intake is very variable according to regions. While in the Andes, lamb or llama, after having been sacrificed, is grilled without salt on fiesta days, in the cities, these meats are not reserved exclusively to celebrations. In the countryside, it is not easy for the poorer people to buy *chicharrón*, ready-to-eat grilled pork, so they prepare *saisi*, a dish of beef with vegetables or *picante de pollo*, chopped chicken with vegetables. When such dishes are eaten, the remainder is smoked (*charque*), and then put into soups. *Silpanchos* (a flat and thin fried piece of chicken) and *tamales* (vegetable turnovers) are more usually consumed in the markets or in the streets. Spicy sauces (*llajwa, ají*)[8] are generously served separately with every dish. There is, in fact, no 'real meal' (*comida de verdad*) if at least one of these solid and liquid items is not present. The availability of these items depends on the region and the season, but the fundamental schema of one dish to constitute the 'real meal' remains the same.

Is bread always the 'food of the poor'?

Wheat is produced in Bolivia, but the local varieties are not suitable for making bread. Furthermore, mills and ovens are rare in the country due to scarcity of fuel. For the great majority of peasants, bread means 'food for rich people'. It is available mostly in big cities, and generally bought during journeys and migrations to cities for seasonal work or for visits to parents, for weddings, funerals and important religious ceremonies. It is such a highly valued food that city dwellers offer bread to their relatives living in the country during their visits. Bread may also be a birth present for the parents.

The production and marketing of bread are developed only in urban zones. Available in markets, in small district groceries and supermarkets, it is made in semi-industrialised bakeries. Although bread is present on the tables of the ordinary people in urban areas as well as in mining camps, it is not consumed casually at any time of day, and its quantity is rationed. At home, it is served at breakfast, with noon meals, and at supper with coffee or soup as a starter or as a meal in itself, according to the standard of living. Street food vendors sell bread as a half-baguette called *maraqueta* or as a small round loaf called *pan de batalla*.[9] Bread is also served in the afternoon at 'tea-time' (*la hora del té*) to accompany coffee, and tends, for the poorest, to replace dinner. Eating bread at tea-time is so important for Bolivians that those who do not have enough money to buy any, will take tea or coffee '*puro*' (pure), 'without bread'. In their minds, 'pure' means 'without bread': thus, it is not that tea-time in itself is more important, as a moment, than the consumption of bread. It is rather the contrary. Sometimes, when families are short of money, they replace bread by *pito* or wheat flour grilled in the pan.

In the Quintero family, the children have the privilege of being the main consumers of daily bread that they eat, first dipping it into a glass of soda, at the so-called tea-time. This regular and particular consumption apart, adults rarely take bread during ordinary meals. Among adults, Julio is the only one who eats bread quite frequently, particularly when his city wanderings lead him to eat, at tea-time, at little street stalls. Like many poor people, the only meal he can afford takes place at tea-time. It is for him a substitute for lunch (*comida*) and supper (*cena*). Tea-time is also a way to eat and to avoid his relatives' possible criticisms when he is unable to provide his wife with the money to purchase food.

The economic constraints of the poor in rural as well as in urban Bolivia mean they are not always able to buy bread. This fact is striking and strongly opposed to the bread status in the neighbouring countries of Bolivia such as Brazil, Chile or nearby Argentina, where it is considered the 'food of the poor' (Absi and Suremain 2010; Katz and Bak-Geller 2010). In Argentina, daily consumption of bread is common for rich as well as poor, children as well as adults. Bread is relatively cheap and affordable. It is never absent from tables or vendors stalls nor at home. It is part of every meal and is never rationed. Such a difference in the food standard of living between Argentina and Bolivia has constituted an important source of frustration for Quintero family members since their return.

Is meat really an ordinary food here and there?

Apart from the market-oriented lowlands of Bolivia (Amazonian department of Beni and Santa Cruz), cattle breeding in the highlands and in the valleys is mostly for agricultural work (bullock, donkeys and horses), wool production (sheep and camelids, i.e. llamas and *vicuna* or *alpacas*), commerce (pigs, goats, sheep, etc.) or for sacrifice in divination and healing rituals (llamas, guinea pigs), rather than for consumption. When I conducted this study in 2003, there was only one slaughterhouse for the whole city of La Paz. Regarding the local standard of living (minimum wage of 75 US dollars), meat is much too expensive (1.5 to 6 US dollars per kg). According to the evaluation of the Bolivian Ministry of Agriculture, the consumption of meat per head yearly was only 20 kg in 2005, placing Bolivia far away behind Argentina (around 50 kg per head), and especially Brazil (90 kg per head) listed among the highest meat-consuming countries in Latin America.

In poor urban and rural areas in Bolivia, people make a clear distinction between chicken (*silpancho*), entrails (heart, guts, liver, kidneys, etc.) and '*carne de verdad*' or 'real meat' which is flesh of cattle, horse, llama, pig, sheep etc. Except for *charque*, smoked and salted meat of the llama, and *aycha kanka*, dried and grilled meat, 'real meat' is not cooked and consumed as a specific dish – except when animals are sacrificed during fiesta days. Occasionally, pieces of meat and bones are stewed or boiled in soups. Even in the streets, meat is always consumed in extremely small quantities by all socio-economic strata of the population. In the *plato callejero*, the name of the 'plate' which is sold by vendors, the quantity of meat is limited to a small piece which is eaten in one or two mouthfuls.

The high value attached to meat means that every part of it is used. Bone, fat and rind are retrieved for preparing dishes such as soups. These soups may be prepared at home for medicinal purpose. They are supposed to cure many common health disorders (flu, cough, stomach pain). Prepared by *curanderos* (traditional healers), they have preventive virtues, protecting the body from recurrent illnesses or pains. The recurrence of particular health problems, such as *mal viento* (bad wind) or *susto* (unexpected fright), is considered a sign of severe disorder in the social sphere. This disorder may lead the individual and his/her family to infinite 'misfortune' (*daño*). Many preparations exist and are kept more or less secret by some specialists (Girault 1984).

Considered as a 'celebration meal' (end of pre-marital period or *sirvinakuy*, wedding, a child's first hair cut or *rutuchikuy*, etc.), meat consumption by the poorest is always a special or exceptional event. It involves considerable financial effort from every one of the kindred. During the celebrations, most of the dishes are made up of chicken or pig, but not beef which is far too expensive. Usually, the occasion is explicitly announced, highly praised and commented upon. This is the case during the *k'oa*, a festival named from an Aymara term which designates both a useful resinous plant and a form of 'collective meal'. *K'oa* takes place when a special event concerning a particular social group occurs, such as a birth, completion of a building or the end of some negotiation. For a *k'oa*, relatives, neighbours, friends or members of an association or a syndicate get together to purchase and to cook the food. The meal prepared and collectively eaten is called *aphtapi*. It is composed of Andean ingredients rarely consumed daily; meat, such as beef, is one of these foodstuffs as it is bought collectively. Today, *k'oa* and *aphtapi* have been largely re-appropriated by *Mestizos* and Whites, for celebrating certain events, notably their socio-political mass mobilisations.

Chicken, beef and pig, mixed with cheese and vegetables, are also used to fill the wheat turnovers (*empanadas* or *salteñas*), the light morning meal of the urban middle class and workers (students, employees, building workers, etc.). At dawn, middle class people consume entrails which are cooked in brochettes (*anticuchos*); they usually cover them with the spicy *llajwa* sauce. But these snacks are out of reach of lower status people such as the Quinteros. When they receive wages after occasional work, quite often in construction, they prefer to purchase chicken or 'real meat' at the butcher.

Due to their harsh and precarious socio-economic situation, the Quinteros eat 'real meat' only occasionally. It is impossible for them to spend so much while they have so much difficulty in affording daily food items. When they eat meat, it is often in the form of *charque* in stews and soups. In the poorest families, such as those who are sometimes in the Quinteros' situation, the oldest are deprived of meat and this situation is more or less accepted because of the property of meat which is considered as 'warming' according to the local humoural conceptions.[10] Eating meat, as old people say, would lead to numerous health problems and changes in character and behaviour: they could become too expressive and even aggressive; they would gain 'bad fat' (*mala grasa*) which would be a sign of a way of life inappropriate to their situation. In other words, not to eat meat is the distinctive food pattern of the 'oldest', and its abstinence perfects the body of the aged person. Therefore, the 'real meat' is preferentially given to the young people and pregnant women, to those who 'need blood to live'.

In highland Bolivia, the parallel between meat and blood-irrigation circulation of fluids is important and explicit. It is said that meat helps to maintain the organism's 'good functioning' and 'good growth' (Canessa 1999; Suremain *et al.* 2003). For the Quinteros and many Bolivians, Argentina is the country where people are supposed to eat more meat, and consequently, the country where people are rich and healthy, even when old. People know that the access to work and regular wages is a condition for affording meat, and unemployment problems, accentuating the high value attributed to meat for well-being and wealth, make the situation of the poorest unbearable.

Are soft drinks so abundant everywhere?

Regularly, the media recalls that Bolivia figures, among the countries with the lowest average consumption of milk in the world, estimated at about 40 litres per person per year,[11] due to the price of the milk, and its unavailability inherent to bad storage conditions, and amylase deficiencies in the population to digest it. The small milk intake is proportionally inverted by the huge volumes of soft drinks (*gaseosas*) drunk per inhabitant. Apart from soft drinks, an average of 50 litres of beer per head is consumed yearly, and *chicha*, a traditional drink of fermented corn, is also consumed in large amounts either at home or in *chichería* (see Katz and Lazos in this book).

In Cochabamba, opportunities to drink *gaseosas* are numerous for everybody. People consume soft drinks with friends, when they get their wages, and during any celebration. Soft drinks are numerous and they are present everywhere, in rural and in urban areas, on street stalls which are subsidised to advertise them, as well as in high-class restaurants. The choice of a particular *gaseosa* is dependent on economic and social status. The Quinteros put forward different reasons to justify their abundant consumption of soft drinks. As expressed by Eulalia, the motivation is hygienic: "water is not potable", medical: "*gaseosas* eliminates parasites" and nutritional "soft drinks fill up our stomach, they cut hunger, and they allow us to avoid tiredness… for cheap". For the poorest people and mostly the oldest and teenagers, soft drinks may occasionally replace a meal (*comida* at noon or *cena* at dawn). 'Light' *gaseosas*, i.e. products low in sugar, are also available on the market, but they are consumed only by the rich because of their high cost and their inability to bring satiety.

Drinking soft drinks depends on specific group affiliation, especially for the young, such as a specific football team sponsored by the trademark, and also on prohibition, enthusiastically promoted by the new sectarian Protestant churches which strictly prohibit alcoholic drink. In the case of conversions, which are numerous in the Andes, a new kind of conviviality is emerging slowly with more or less success and respect according to the individual (Magny 2008). Lastly, in exceptional cases, the boycott of a soft drink trademark by specific social groups, Coca-Cola notably, symbolises radical ideological choice. This movement occurred between 2001 and 2003 to oppose the US invasion of Afghanistan, after the September 11th attacks, a period locally called the 'third world war' (Suremain 2008). Therefore, the label consumed varies according to social categories and identity groups.

In Bolivia as well as in Argentina, alcohol is part of the fiesta and of the daily traditional food system. But natural soft drinks (fruit juices) and manufactured drinks can definitely be considered as traditional too, both in the countryside and in the cities. In the Bolivian highland, the *gaseosas* also occupy a particular place in domestic, public, collective and individual rituals. As reported of many Mexican rituals (Nash 2007), fizzy (gaseous) drinks are supposed to help people to burp, i.e. to evacuate 'bad energies' and 'bad feelings' from the body.

On the Quinteros' table, bread and meat are rarely present, but Eulalia emphasises that "there are always two-litre bottles of soft drink". She says that the preference of her children is for Coca-Cola while hers and that of her husband are for acidulated soft drinks which are also cheaper. In everyday life, a sort of silent negotiation occurs between her and her children, as she is in charge of shopping for food at the market. She states that she 'tries to satisfy everybody', at least, as regards this particular beverage. Eulalia laments that, in Argentina, she did not have to be so careful regarding soft drink brands, and she had sufficient means to achieve the socially valuable consumption of Coca-Cola.

Back to 'traditional Bolivian food'

The social and symbolic value given to certain 'traditional foods' by the Quintero family members, in the Bolivian context, throws light upon other economic, social and symbolic dimensions. These dimensions regularly stand out in discourses and practices and in the different food life stories collected.

In a life span, 'food memory' implies time levelling. If food memory is so pregnant, it is because it echoes various events (smells, colours, flavours) learned in early life and deeply interiorised by individuals. Thus, individuals, even children, remember from the past only what makes sense in the present; they reinterpret the past in the light of the present, which is real, imaginary or simply reconstructed. Evoking food of the present means evoking food of the past, but the only thing that really matters to people is to speak through food about what they are, what they were or what they would like to be.

Here and there: poverty and wealth, abundance and lack

In the Bolivian context, the symbolic importance given to bread, meat and soft drinks highlights, and mirrors, the ideal food model of Argentina as perceived by returnees. The return, even if temporary and simply a step before a new departure, reveals the spectrum of suffering and poverty among migrants. What happens in Bolivia is differently expressed in Argentina. In that country, bread and meat are archetypal foods, including for the poorest in urban areas – and despite the crisis (Aguirre 2004; Álvarez 2003), and despite the strong and long term alimentary crisis which affects not only the whole continent but the whole world for at least a decade. In Bolivia, where bread and meat are not even daily foods, their presence or absence, their quality or their mode of consumption reflects, constructs or reinforces social and local stratifications.

Like a great number of Argentineans from the urban and ordinary categories of population, the Quinteros never did eat meat every day during their stay in Argentina, but rather consumed rice, pasta, bread,[12] pizzas, with soft drinks to 'fill up' their stomachs (Aguirre 2004; Álvarez and Pinotti 2000). But the weekly consumption of meat in *asado* (grilled meat in open areas) has affected the Quinteros in the long-term, notably Julio. In fact, copying his Argentine neighbours he, as a male, used to prepare, keep an eye on and serve the Sunday *asado*. In this context, he was in a position to gain the prestige of being able to offer an abundant meal to his family, even to his guests. According to Álvarez (2003: 15–16):

> (…) grilled beef seems to occupy the national meal status: obviously, daily, women prepare diverse spicy and elaborate meals six nights in a row; the Sunday or free days, grilled beef [*asado*] is the only and unique meal typically cooked by a man. And this particular meal is supposed to represent the whole Argentinian national plate, in Argentina or outside'.[13]

Julio does not today regret his lack of integration into the Argentinian nation due to his migrant status, and his 'Indian type' low status. He was not, in fact, looking for such integration. He regrets rather his financial position at this time. Nowadays, in Bolivia, his income does not allow him to offer such a highly valued food to his family. Because of this, in terms of prestige and social capital, Julio is a 'loser': in Bolivia, he is no longer the householder who is capable of affording what one might be called an 'ordinary nourishing ritual'. His wife and children suffer from Julio's status decline. Eulalia regrets 'the good old days' and Justiño evokes with nostalgia "the time when Dad was taking care of everything, everything in the kitchen…".

Children lack meat, ideal adult food, far more than they do soft drinks and Argentinian candies (*golisinas*). Nevertheless, although the Quintero children are used to drinking as many soft drinks 'here' as 'there', the brands they consumed in Argentina are not available in Bolivia.

According to Bolivian social stratification and his new status, Julio is depreciated in his function of supplier of meat. For him, what is at stake is the symbolic value attributed to meat locally consumed compared to that of meat consumed in Argentina (beef, lamb or mutton). In Cochabamba, even though perceptions of llama meat are changing progressively and positively (the so-called 'fat and cholesterol free meat' cooked as an 'occidental beefsteak') among wealthy classes, this is not really the case in rural or popular urban areas. In Bolivian perception, notably in that of the oldest' one, the llama, and particularly the *charque,* is associated with the Indian-peasant world and agricultural work: "It is our own meat" (*es carne nuestra*) says Julio's father. *Charque* is consumed dried in soups and stews, but it is out of the question, at least as long as the elders are alive, to prepare llama meat in Argentinean *asado* way. In Bolivia, Julio can buy, from time to time, llama reduced in price or, very exceptionally, some pieces of chicken or pork, but in a quantity which is far from satisfying the claims of social recognition that he had in Argentina, and for which he is feeling a powerful nostalgia.

Good health, bad health and body image

Local perceptions of good and bad health, both related to body image, express the social stigma that the returnees seem to be burdened with. Especially the youngest, Justiño and Cristina, both feel that they are "somehow different; not the same, anyway" as expressed by Cristina, or "I just feel weak and ugly" as Justiño states. As far as their parents, Julio and Eulalia, are concerned, it is as if the 'Bolivian food tradition' were largely responsible for this situation. These particular perceptions confirm some of the most important trends in public health and the preoccupations of Latin America.

Bolivia is far from experiencing the same epidemiological situation and nutritional transition as Argentina, Mexico or Brazil, but it moves on progressively (Caballero and Popkin 2002). Nowadays, the prevalence of overweight children under five in Bolivia, evaluated by WHO in 2004 at 9.2 per cent,[14] is a little lower than that in Argentina estimated at 9.9 per cent in 2005 (Aguirre 2004). However, the prevalence of overweight children does not concern those belonging to the same social categories in the two countries: in Argentina, overweight (and obese) children are from poor backgrounds, while in Bolivia, it is rather a sign of wealth, *a fortiori* in poor rural areas where the phenomena is growing due to migrations.

In the eyes of the neighbours and relatives of the Quinteros, the criteria are not the same: to be 'tall' often means to be 'overweight'. Justiño and Cristina are thus regarded as different from other children: "they are taller" assert their grandparents proudly. It is precisely the quality of food consumed in Argentina that is supposed to have improved their body size, seen as more imposing than that of their peers who are growing up in Bolivia with 'traditional Bolivian food'.

Meat consumption during their stay in Argentina provides a reason as to why Justiño and Cristina were different from the others in growth and development. In a film I made with Nicolas Montibert on swaddling in Bolivia, a mother declares of her child (less than 10 years old) who was born and raised in Argentina that "he is made of another flesh… of Argentine meat" (Suremain 2007).

Regarding their physical appearance, Justiño and Cristina, aged 12 and five respectively during the investigation, assert that since they are living in Bolivia, they have lost 'weight', '*carne*' (meat, also flesh). Justiño, in particular, tries to keep his corpulence, something that, in his estimation, made him 'special' (*especial*) in comparison to his classmates when he arrived from Argentina. Here, his supposed overweight (in fact, he is relatively tall) is a sign of wealth and well-being while it was a common feature for migrants in Argentina. There, overweight people were simply assimilated to the mass of the 'poor' or ordinary people.

For their parents, Justiño and Cristina are now 'weaker' than they were in Argentina. It is obvious that the daily food consumed here does not permit their children to develop optimally or to grow normally. In fact, they borrow arguments from both biomedicine and from the humoural conception to express a powerful fear: that the physical stigma of the very difficult conditions under which they lived when they were children may appear again. In as much as this stigma could mark their body, they sense they will always have difficulties that must be hidden from the eyes of others.

Conclusion

The prevalence and social value given to foods is a privileged approach to comprehending social status and identity 'in the move' attributed to the returnees. At the level of discourse, food 'here' and food 'there' are opposites and exclude each other, in an unending rhetoric.

In the popular urban areas, the Argentinian poor do not eat like the Bolivian poor: they eat 'there' like the rich eat 'here'. This, at least, is the returnees' perception. Food or lack of food reminds the returnees every day of their condition as poor people in their homeland. This situation presents a configuration drastically different from that described by Françoise Lestage (2008) where she shows how the food circulation between Mexico and United States is a powerful vector for social and identity reproduction between migrants who move and those who stay. In this present context, there is no borrowing or adaptation at all, neither in food practices, in supplies nor in modes of preparation; there is no circulation of ideas and practices, nor creation of a new single and mixed form of identity through and thanks to food. On the other hand, Argentinian food, in the Quinteros' perceptions, remains the idealised food model and Bolivian food is, consequently, a counter-model not expected or valued by returnees.

Food opposition between the two countries crosses structures and reinforces construction of the local identity. It works even to stigmatise the body as the rich of 'there' are supposed to be taller and thinner than the rich of 'here', considered as small and fat. In other words, for returnees in Bolivia, protecting fatness signifies extending their temporary position as rich, knowing that such a position in the Argentinian context is only illusory. As Françoise Héritier correctly says (1985: 61): "The Other is the one who does not eat like oneself". Such perceptions remind returnees of 'who they are', 'what they are', and especially 'what they are not', according to the time and the spatial and social context.

If the paradox of returnees' identity is at stake daily, its intensity is lessened during festive meals. On these occasions, returnees get together in order to re-create some kind of local Argentine atmosphere. In the Bolivian urban milieu, ordinary people consume in celebrations meat, bread and soft drinks, i.e. food that is not really ordinary for them. Nevertheless, these dishes have a bitter taste: they give the illusory delight of the wealth that the returnees thought they possessed on the other side of the boundary. The feast which has nothing in common with the Argentinian *asados*, is never 'complete'. As Eulalia complains: "there is always something [food] lacking. (…). It is a kind of meat (*la clase de carne*) that we eat, this bread which lacks savour (*no tiene sabor*)… Here, people only drink beer [and not more prestigious soft drinks]". This is precisely the 'something lacking' which involves for returnees the feeling of status loss; it is this 'something lacking' which is so present by its absence 'here' in Bolivia, a social and cultural universe where it has a form, a function and a significance opposite to the one it has 'there', in Argentina.

Notes

1 This text is the revisited and completed version of a shorter article published in 2011 in the online review *Anthropology of Food* (www.aof.revues.org).

2 On the methodological consequences of the gap between discourses and practices in food research, see F. Xavier Medina (2004).

3 See W. Tomas and Florian Znaniecki (1996), N.G. Schiller *et al.* (1995), Françoise Lestage (2008) and, more recently, the last volume of *Hommes & Migrations* (2010). As referring to migrants' food in France, see Élodie Razy (2006).

4 On 'voluntary' returnees, see Doreen Massey *et al.* (1991), Emmanuel Calvo (1997), and Diane E. King (2008). The issue of 'forced' migration is a very different question but it will not be discussed here.

5 See Geneviève Cortes (2000), Tanja Bastia (2007), Jorge Dandler and Carmen Medeiros (1988) on migrations inside Bolivia and abroad.

6 In 1990–2000s, Salta, a city located in the province of the same name, had nearly 470,000 inhabitants; 50,000, nearly 8 per cent of the population, were temporary or permanent Bolivian residents (Guevara 2004).

7 This particularity is essential in Latin America: to quote Judith Friedlander's words (1977), one is always 'the Indian of the others'. On socio-ethnic categories and denomination issues in Bolivia, see Jean-Pierre Lavaud and Isabelle Daillant (2007).

8 *Llajwa* is a commonly used spicy sauce composed of red-fleshed tomato, chopped red pepper (*locoto*) and *quirquiña*, an aromatic herb. *Ají*, a variety of red pepper, is a generic term for any kind of spicy sauce with pepper.

9 Each costs almost 15 cents.

10 Literature on humoural concepts in Latin America is abundant, but it deals especially with representations of the disease and its fundamental principles. See George M. Foster (1987). For a study of the humoural system related to food, see Charles-Édouard de Suremain *et al.* (2002).

11 See the report: http://www.fao.org/docrep/012/i1522e/i1522e02.pdf (retrieved on 7 September 2011).

12 On the scale of Latin America only Chile, and especially, Uruguay and Argentina, are countries where bread is consumed daily (Katz and Bak-Geller 2010).

13 '*(...) el asado de carne vacuna aparece acaparando el status de comida nacional: si durante seis noches a la semana las mujeres son las que llevan a la mesa las cenas frecuentemente integradas por un conjunto diverso de ingredientes, condimentos y procesos de elaboración, el asado de los domingos al mediodía o de los feriados es la sola y única comida típicamente preparada por un hombre. Y ésta es la que parece representar a la Nación Argentina, tanto en su propio territorio como en el exterior*'.

14 www.who.int/nutrition/databases/infantfeeding/countries/bol.pdf (retrieved on 7 September 2011).

References

Absi, P. (2003). *Les ministres du Diable. Le travail et ses représentations dans les mines de Potosí, Bolivie*, Paris: L'Harmattan.

Absi, P. and Suremain, C. É. de (2010). "Andes boliviennes (Traditions du pain dans les)", in J.P. de Tonnac and S.L. Kaplan (eds.), *Dictionnaire universel du pain*, pp. 52–55. Paris: Robert Laffont.

Aguirre, P. (2004). *Ricos flacos y gordos pobres. La alimentación en crisis*, Buenos Aires: Capital Intelectual.

Álvarez M. (ed.) (2003). "La cocina como patrimonio (in)tangible", in *Primeras Jornadas de Patrimonio Gastronómico La Cocina como Patrimonio (In)Tangible*, pp. 11–26. Buenos Aires: Comisión para la Preservación del Patrimonio Histórico Cultural de la Ciudad de Buenos Aires.

Álvarez, M. and Pinotti, L. (eds.) (2000). *A la mesa. Ritos y retos de la alimentación Argentina*, Buenos Aires: Grijalbo.

Barth, F. (ed.) (1969). *Ethnic Groups and Boundaries. The Social Organization of Cultural Difference*, Boston: Little, Brown and Company.

Bastia, T. (2007). "From mining to garment workshops: Bolivian migrants in Buenos Aires", *Journal of Ethnic and Migration Studies*, Vol. 33(4): 655–669.

Bourdieu, P. (1978). "Classement, déclassement, reclassement", *Actes de la Recherche en Sciences Sociales*, Vol. 24: 2–22.

Caballero, B. and Popkin, B.M. (eds.) (2002). *The Nutrition Transition: Diet and Disease in the Developing World*, London: Academic Press.

Calvo, E. (1997). "Toujours africains et déjà français: la socialisation des migrants à travers leur alimentation", *Politique Africaine*, Vol. 67: 48–55.

Canessa, A. (1999). "Making persons, marking differences. Procreation beliefs in Highland Bolivia", in P. Loizos and P. Heady (eds.), *Conceiving Persons. Ethnographies of Procreation, Fertility and Growth*, pp. 69–87. London-New Brunswick: The Athlone Press.

Cortes, G. (2000). *Partir pour rester. Survie et mutation de sociétés paysannes andines (Bolivie)*, Paris: IRD Éditions.

Dandler, J. and Medeiros, C. (1988). "Temporary migration from Cochabamba, Bolivia to Argentina: patterns and impact in sending areas", in P. Pessar (ed.), *When Borders Don't Divide: Labour Migration and Refugee Movements in the Americas*, pp. 8–41. New York: Centre for Migration Studies.

Foster, G.M. (1987). "On the origin of humoral medicine in Latin America", *Medical Anthropology Quarterly*, Vol. 1(4): 355–393.

Friedlander, J. (1979). *L'Indien des autres. La réalité de l'identité indienne dans le Mexique contemporain*, Paris: Payot.

Gill, L. (1997). "Relocating class: ex-miners and neoliberalism in Bolivia", *Critique of Anthropology*, Vol. 17(3): 293–312.

Girault, L. (1984). *Kallawaya, guérisseurs itinérants des Andes. Recherches sur les pratiques médicinales et magiques*, Paris: ORSTOM.

Guevara, J.P. (2004). "Migraciones bolivianas en el contexto de la globalización", *Alternativas Sur*, Vol. 3(1): 171–187.

Héritier, F. (1985). "La leçon des « primitifs", in Collectif (ed.), *L'Identité française*, pp. 56–65. Paris: Tierce.

Hommes & Migrations (2010). Cuisines et dépendances, Vol. 1283.

Katz, E. and Bak-Geller, S. (2010). "Amérique Latine (Traditions du pain en)", in J.P. de Tonnac and S.L. Kaplan (eds.), *Dictionnaire universel du pain*, pp. 41–46. Paris: Robert Laffont.

King, D.E. (2008). "Back from the "Outside": returnees and diasporic imagining in Iraqi Kurdistan", *International Journal on Multicultural Societies*, Vol. 10(2): 208–222.

Lavaud, J.-P. and Daillant, I. (eds.) (2007). *La catégorisation ethnique en Bolivie. Labellisation officielle et sentiment d'appartenance*, Paris: L'Harmattan.

Lestage, F. (2008). *Les Indiens mixtèques dans les Californies contemporaines, Migrations et identités collectives*, Paris: Presses Universitaires de France.

Magny, C. (2008). "Quand on ne peut plus boire d'alcool ni mâcher de feuilles de coca". *Anthropology of Food*, Modèles alimentaires et recompositions sociales en Amérique latine, S4. http://aof.revues.org/index2972.html (retrieved on 7 September 2011).

Massey, D., Douglas, S., Alarcon, R., Durand, J. and González, H. (1991). *Return to Aztlan: The Social Process of International Migration from Western Mexico*, Berkeley: University of California Press.

Medina, F.X. (2004). "Tell me what you eat and you will tell me who you are: methodological notes on the interaction between researcher and informant in the anthropology of food", in H. MacBeth and J. MacClancy (eds.), *Researching Food Habits. Methods and Problems*, pp. 55–62. Oxford: Berghahn Books.

Murra, J.V. (1975). *Formaciones económicas y políticas del mundo andino*, Lima: Instituto de Estudios Peruanos.

Nash, J. (1979). *We Eat the Mines and the Mines Eat Us: Dependency and Exploitation in Bolivian Tin Mines*, Columbia: Columbia University Press.

Nash, J. (2007). "Consuming interests: water, rum, and Coca-Cola from ritual propitiation to corporate expropriation in Highland Chiapas", *Cultural Anthropology*, Vol. *22*(4): 621–639.

Razy, É. (2006). "Les migrants ont-ils des manières particulières d'habiter ? L'exemple Soninké", *Hommes & Migrations*, Vol. 1264: 77–87.

Schiller, N.G., Basch, L. and Szanton- Blanc, C. (1995). "From immigrant to transmigrant: theorizing transnational migration", *Anthropological Quarterly*, Vol. 68(1): 48–63.

Suremain, C.-É. de (2007). "Au fil de la *faja*. Enrouler et dérouler la vie en Bolivie", in D. Bonnet and L. Pourchez (eds.), *Du soin au rite dans l'enfance*, pp. 85–102. Paris: Erès.

Suremain, C.-É. de (2008). "Shawarmas contre MacDo. Mondialisation et standardisation alimentaire à l'épreuve des contestations identitaires (Bolivie)", *Anthropology of Food*, Modèles alimentaires et recompositions sociales en Amérique latine, S4. http://aof.revues.org/sommaire2763.html (retrieved on 7 September 2011).

Suremain, C.-É. de, Guttierrez, B., Maria, E. and Lefèvre, P. (2002). "El buen uso de lo "cálido" y de lo "frío". La alimentación y sus beneficios perc*ibid*os para la salud de la madre y del niño en Bolivia", *Actas del IIIer Congreso Virtual de Antropología y Arqueología (Argentina)*.

Suremain, C.-É. de, Lefevre, P., Rubín de Celis, E. and Sejas E. (eds.) (2003). *Miradas cruzadas en el niño. Un enfoque interdisciplinario sobre la salud, el crecimiento y el desarrollo del niño en Bolivia y Perú*, La Paz: Plural-Institut de Recherche pour le Développement-Éditions de l'Institut Français d'Études Andines.

Tomas, W.T. and Znaniecki, F. (1996). *The Polish Peasant in Europe and America: A Classic Work in Immigration History*, Urbana: University of Illinois Press, 1st publication 1918.

9 What is a healthy diet?

Some ideas about the construction of healthy food in Germany since the nineteenth century

Detlef Briesen

This chapter deals with the history of how 'healthy' food has been evolved in Germany since the late eighteenth century. I must say at the outset that I cannot give more than an overview of this broad and complicated topic.

Firstly, from the historical perspective, there is no national 'German' food. Food consumption in the German speaking countries was, until the mid nineteenth century, influenced rather by regional cooking patterns (south-east, south-west, and north-east) which were mainly an outcome of differences in climate, prosperity and customs, and by the French tradition of 'cuisine bourgeoise'.

The general finding of cultural history is that nutritional standards in the German speaking countries have declined steadily since the fourteenth century. Numerous reports from the first two centuries of the early modern period tell of an abundant and sufficient diet for all social strata. Daily eating was based on large quantities of meat, poultry, sausage, cheeses, milk, beer and wine. With the crisis, ongoing since the late sixteenth century, which saw a sharp decline due to climate change and continuous warfare, nutritional standards for most Germans steadily decreased, reaching an all time low most likely around 1800. Severe crises, in particular between 1600 and 1850, led to two developments: an increase in social differentiation by food quality, with ostentation exhibited by the upper classes, following the Italian, and later, the French example, and by the spread of 'ersatz' food especially for the lower social strata. The daily diet of the pre-industrial pauper class consisted mainly of large quantities of carbohydrates, alcohol and ersatz coffee (based on chicory or grains), with considerable regional variation and deeply influenced by the different level of social polarisation in various 'German' regions. European ethnology had already by the 1960s carved out typical regional patterns of diet: in the poor German north and north-east, the large numbers of urban and rural paupers survived mainly on millet and grain 'soups' for breakfast, and potatoes, brandy, and ersatz coffee for the other meals of the day. The diet of the regional nobility which was beef-based sharply contrasted with this pattern. In other German regions, food was to a lesser degree an element of social differentiation: in the south-west, meals consisted of noodles, wine, cider and vegetables, but of less meat, and the diet was more socially inclusive. There, people already followed the French custom of eating bread for breakfast and cakes in the afternoon. The same was true for the south-east including Austria with its dumplings and beer and the traditional, even medieval, system of only two meals per day (Briesen 2010). The poverty and scarcity of food in the German speaking countries directly influenced the reform movements of the second half of the nineteenth century. In particular, the growth of agriculture and industrialisation changed the pattern of diet in the German speaking countries significantly after 1800, introducing commodities like pork or beer into the mass market, very soon to be interpreted as traditional 'German' diet.

Secondly, for approximately 60 to 80 years after 1850, the German speaking countries, in particular the German Empire of 1871, and the German speaking academic world which covered large parts of central, northern, eastern, and south-eastern Europe, became the centre of food reform of the industrialised world. The concept of industrialised food as well as life reform alternatives were mainly developed in the German speaking countries, making them the hotbed of the debate on healthy food, but also diversifying the food consumed by Germans. Thirdly, after 1945, (West) Germany was characterised by the same trends in food consumption as most of its neighbouring countries. But it is always good to have a closer look at the German example because the debate on healthy diet was, in particular between 1800 and 1950, fought with vigour, and even fanaticism. During that time, Germans contributed significantly to the Age of Extremes (Hobsbawm 1994).

Today, the debate on health policies in European countries, like Germany, focuses to a considerable degree on efforts to promote health by creating healthy lifestyles. Such attempts are designed to reduce the costs of healthcare significantly and, in particular, to provide a preventive orientation as a universal means to forestall human suffering, disease or even untimely demise. Seen from an historical perspective, these efforts have been neither new nor innovative: prevention by better or controlled behaviour and consumption had, in fact, always been a constant factor in the health history of humankind and, in particular, in the history of human diet. But what actually is a healthy diet or even disease prevention through healthy diet? A closer look shows that a prevention-oriented approach has some particularities and that the entire concept is not so easy to identify. A healthy diet can be based on some specific limitations or on avoiding certain behaviour, such as smoking or taking drugs, or consuming alcohol, except moderately, and excessive intake of salt, fat and sugar. There is a broad consensus in science and amongst the public about what not to do to damage your health, at least in theory. But, as always in social and life sciences, the problem is the argument about what humans should consume to improve their health. Though there should be no doubt about progress in nutritional science over the last 200 years, the positive precepts for a better lifestyle are still often based on mere converse arguments from scientific findings on the negative results of consumption patterns, or even belief systems, or personal preferences of their apologists, in particular, in nutrition. Again and again in the history of healthy diet, experts took views which later proved to be wrong or even harmful.

One of the most striking particularities of the recent debate on healthy nutrition is that these ideas from the history of the discourse on food are still alive. Even the experts of antiquity have their say today. The entire chain of concepts from antiquity until the post-modern age forms different layers of recommendations and proscriptions about which food is healthy and which unsound. This chapter mainly attempts to identify these different efforts to define healthy food, and to understand the various ideas, ideologies, concepts, and their contemporary relevance (Briesen 2010).

Humoural pathology: regaining cosmic balance

An initial reply to the question of what the quintessence of a healthy diet is, is deeply embedded in the old European tradition. Until today, humoural pathology has played a crucial role in defining and propagating the idea of proper food, often combined with medical approaches such as the still prevalent herbalism of Hildegard von Bingen (circa 1098–1179). According to these ideas of a bland or light diet, personal health can be achieved if the human diet is composed according to the universal or cosmic principle of balance or harmony. This idea even formed the mainstream of European concepts of healthy food until the middle of the nineteenth century, usually being traced back to Greek and Roman thought, though most of the medical and nutritional knowledge of antiquity was lost after the fifth century. Therefore, the antique tradition is an outcome of a process of interpretation of a very selective corpus of texts by medieval medicine. But, as such, the tradition of humoural pathology mainly consists in a system of recommendations to prevent ailments and illness by appropriate behaviour, and first and foremost, by balanced diet – one reason of course was that traditional medicine was hardly ever able to cure (serious) disease. Prior to the emergence and success of academic medicine, the art of healing was basically limited to a system of prevention. As many contemporaries nowadays share a deeply critical attitude towards biomedicine, humoural pathology and its medications, prescriptions and concepts for a healthy lifestyle are relevant even today.

Hence, in the foremost method of putting together a healthy diet in the German context, the great tradition of Hippocrates of Kos (circa 460–370) still plays an important role. His ideas – or rather the ideas of a group of Greek physicians publishing under his name – are characterised by a significant equalisation of cosmology and human health. The fundamental volume, *De Diaeta*, explains ailments and diseases as an outcome of disruption of a natural state of equilibrium caused by immoderate and intemperate behaviours (Potter and Gundert 1998; Gundert 2000; Mazzini 2000). To counterbalance the harmful consequences of both behaviours, the disciples of Hippocrates developed rules and standards for a healthy lifestyle, including daily routine and an optimal balanced diet. Humoural pathology became constitutive in the sense that it transferred the ideas of ancient physics into a medical theory: the four elements, earth, water, air and fire were put on the same level with the four human temperaments or types of personality (melancholic, phlegmatic, sanguine and choleric), and the four body fluids (black bile, phlegm, blood and yellow bile).

According to Hippocrates and his disciples, many ailments and diseases can be avoided by promoting the optimal flow of body fluids through adequate food which corresponds with the general needs of a particular personality. The temperaments are of utmost importance, but other factors should not be ignored, including profession, age and weather. The optimal Hippocratic diet is based on bread and meat, fish, fruits, vegetables and milk, only consumed moderately.

Compared to the original Hippocratic ideas, Galen of Pergamum (circa 129–199) simply gave more detailed information regarding a healthy diet. He generally recommended eating bread and pork and refraining from eating vegetables and fruits except for grapes, which may explain why grapes are brought to hospitalised patients as a present even today. Many of Galen's ideas can still be found in the cookbooks of the nineteenth and twentieth centuries: pears are cooked in red wine for detoxification, hare's meat is always chopped up in small pieces to destroy the aphrodisiac effects of that most sinful animal, green salad is a 'cold' food to be heated up with hot vinegar to make it digestible. Evident once again are the links between cosmic, physical and medical principles. The concept of achieving a healthy diet by following general principles had been promoted since Hippocrates and Galen. Disease and health were understood respectively as the wrong or right balance of the flow of body fluids, and again and again, the concept has been repeated until today, in the writings of German thinkers such as Immanuel Kant, Rudolf Steiner, Alfred Adler, Erich Adickes, Eduard Spranger, Ernst Kretschmer and Erich Fromm, and others in Europe such as Paul Carton in France.

Healthy *mischkost*: diet as the perfect blend of nutrients

A second and still dominant concept of healthy diet focuses on the idea of a pleasant, mixed, varied or balanced food intake (*gesunde mischkost*). The concept is a direct outcome of modern science, modern chemistry and a nutritional science, in particular, that emerged after 1840, deeply influenced by the German chemist Justus von Liebig (1803–1873). '*Gesunde mischkost*' (varied diet) spread especially in the German speaking world after 1950, promoted by scientists like Werner Kollath (1892–1970) (Kollath 1942) and Ernst Kofrányi (1908–1989) (Kofrányi and Wirths 1994). Varied diet set the standards in nutritional science, dietetics and medicine for several decades after the Second World War, and was energetically propagated by the very influential Deutsche Gesellschaft für Ernährung (DGE) (GDE. German Nutrition Society).[1] It was nearly issued by the government, but the state and experts in post-war West Germany avoided any direct interference into the lifestyles of German citizens after the experience of the Nazis and their ideas of vegetarianism, temperance and smoking-bans, to which I will come back in the following sections.

Varied diet results from the falsification of the concept of humoural pathology, a long process which started with the new understanding of the functioning of the internal organs by alchemists and iatrochemists. The first modern chemists, such as Antoine-Laurent Lavoisier (1743–1794) and Claude Bernard (1813–1878), discovered that digestion was not an internal cooking process, but a chemical process: metabolism produces energy by digesting nutrients such as fat, carbohydrates and proteins, and decomposes food to integrate its micronutrients into the human body. The particular achievement of Justus Liebig was to elaborate a new consistent dietetics from the rather fragmented contemporary knowledge. For him, two types of nutrients exist: first, proteins which provide the human body with energy for muscle and brain functioning. The second type, fat and carbohydrates, only delivers quantities of energy to the body.

The priority that Liebig gave to proteins had two consequences: on the one hand, academic dietetics overestimated until very recently, the necessary amount of daily amino-acid intake, and sometimes even supported ideas such as a diet completely based on meat, or the so called low glycemic diet, which propagates a low glycemic index as a precondition for slimming.[2] On the other hand, the studies of Liebig and his students demonstrated that the protein intake of the contemporary underclasses of Europe was simply not sufficient. Since then, eating meat has meant physical and mental fitness, and it has become an issue of social justice: sufficient and adequate food for everyone. Liebig himself – by his innovations like Liebig's Extract of Meat – and his disciples, like Jacob Moleschott (1822–1893), set healthy nutrition on the agenda of social reform. Already in 1858, Moleschott's book (Moleschott 1858) on dietetics was published in its third edition. It put strong emphasis on a varied diet consisting of meat, fruits and vegetables, and the particular blend was also to be designed to fit personal preferences, seasonal products and income. For the first time, a system of nutrition was proposed to a broader public which was not to be based primarily on regional traditions or high-class cooking habits, but on the particularities of human physiologies, personal needs and preferences. Within Moleschott's system of varied or balanced food, more expensive products could be replaced by cheaper ones (beef by lentils, for example). This has been the basic concept of all food pyramids which advise customers how to compose their daily diet until today.

There has been a long and lasting debate on varied diet since its advent around 1850. One result was that the daily recommendations for protein intake steadily decreased. Today, meat is no longer the necessary precondition for a healthy diet as it was some 150 years ago. Research also demonstrated that the human diet must consist of more than only protein, fat and carbohydrate. After 1911, vitamins, minerals and phytochemicals were discovered, and their relevance for the human body understood. Therefore, the idea of a varied diet has experienced significant changes over the past 150 years. Nevertheless, today the concept is still the basis of a scientifically constructed diet in Germany.

Lebensreform: healthy food follows nature

Lebensreform (life reform) claims that a healthy diet must follows nature's imperatives. The idea of natural food had two heydays in the German speaking world: the natural food of *Lebensreform* (approximately from 1890 until 1940) and organic or eco-food (in the Federal Republic since the early 1970s). Natural food is not synonymous with the dietetic concepts of humoural pathology nor is organic food an immediate outcome of *Lebensreform*.

Lebensreform and its nutritional ideas were directly influenced by vitalism, a doctrine which advocated the idea that living organisms are fundamentally different from non-living entities. The idea of a vital spark, a vital energy, or in its French original an '*élan vital*' emerged in the late eighteenth century as a result of the crisis of humoural pathology, alchemy, iatrochemistry, and mechanism. Vitalism claimed to have a solution for the traditional dichotomy of body and soul in occidental thought, and was propagated strongly by the cultural criticism of the late Enlightenment, in particular by the '*principe vital*' of Jean-Jacques Rousseau (1712–1778). The crucial question of vitalism has always been that it argues that elemental or natural forces are linked in a non-intelligible way with different aspects of (human) vital energy. Natural forces like water, wind, air or sunshine have a direct impact on the vital spark, on the body and soul of an individual. Therefore, the concept of vitalism combines philosophy, physics, chemistry, medicine and dietetics simultaneously. Healing by restoring the impact of nature's forces on human diet is thus fundamental for vitalism in general, and its ideas of healthy food in particular. As dietetics, *Lebensreform* generally advocated a grain-based diet, because grain optimises the intake of natural elements from water, wind, air and sunshine. This construction of healthy food has been very popular in Germany until today; and pioneers of the *Lebensreform* like Wilhelm Hufeland (1762–1836),[3] Johann Schroth (1798–1856) and Sylvester Graham (1794–1851) still have their disciples.

Lebensreform became a sort of social reform movement widespread in German speaking countries especially after 1880. While analysing its main ideas, one has to stress that it was far from advocating regressive, or even reactionary food concepts. Firstly, traditional European food systems had often stressed the value of meat consumption; on the contrary, many reformers since 1880 advocated vegetarianism or even veganism. An even more decisive change came, secondly, with the concept of raw food (unprocessed foodstuff); from antiquity until the early twentieth century, European dietetics had always promoted the cooking of food to improve its digestibility. Now reformers like Emil Drebber (1873–1943) and Max-Oskar Bircher-Benner (1867–1939) advised eating as much unprocessed food as possible to improve the intake of precious micronutrients and the consumption of large quantities of raw vegetable fibres.

Lebensreform was also a response to the problems of a modern society and its food processing industry. Around 1900, in West European and North American countries, food was available with wider choices and in greater quantities than ever before. The downside of these improvements was very often low quality of meat, vegetables, fruits, and grains. In Germany, for example, the consumption of white sugar increased tenfold between 1850 and 1900. It was an outstanding achievement of *Lebensreform* to interpret quantitative affluence in the consumption of high energy refined grains, sugar, salt, meat etc. as lack of quality and source of malnutrition and lifestyle diseases. One main difference between the vitalism of the late eighteenth century and the *Lebensreform* after 1880 was that the latter finally had to demonstrate its claims scientifically. In that context, many reformers acted dubiously, drawing wrong conclusions from experiments, or developing wrong interpretations for working therapies and theories.

The Swiss Max-Oskar Bircher-Benner (1867–1939) set an outstanding example of an excellent reform concept which, by theoretical legitimation, was pure nonsense. Bircher-Benner was no doubt the most influential nutritional reformer of the first half of the twentieth century. His dietetics was mainly based on the idea of increased consumption of fruits, berries, nuts, legumes and cereals. His nutritional reform concept proved to be useful, uncomplicated and healthy, but his explanation of the curative effect of his diet was a rather dubious one. He claimed that fruits, berries, nuts, legumes and cereals provide the human body with a sufficient amount of photons (*lichtquanten*, light quantum) – the real source of vital energy! (Bircher-Benner 1944)

The physician Mikkel Hindhede (1862–1934) went even further and took the events in his home country, Denmark, during the First World War, as a gigantic experiment. Even in a country not directly involved in the fighting, the war led to a severe supply crisis. Hence, the Danish government introduced a system of rationing for commodities like meat and alcohol. As a result, mortality and morbidity decreased in Denmark. Hinhede's explanation was that meat and alcohol consumption weakens vital energy; from this wartime experience, he drew the conclusion that the vital spark, not only of an individual, but of an entire nation, could be restored by lacto-vegetarianism, sun and air baths, and therapies to increase resistance by physical exercise and mental training. As Hindhede, like most Scandinavian scientists of his time published in German, his ideas were received in Germany with great interest. The construction of lacto-vegetarian eating as a tool to harden the individual and the society for the struggle of life brought him much support from the right wing of the political spectrum in Germany, and later deeply influenced the ideas of the Nazi movement on healthy 'German' vegetarian food (Hindhede 1922).

No wonder that, on the one hand, after 1933, many life reformers in Germany sided with National Socialism, and that, on the other hand, many important National Socialists like Heinrich Himmler or even Adolf Hitler himself, strongly supported the *Lebensreform* including vegetarianism, temperance and no smoking rules. But the intensive efforts of some portions of the Nazi movement to enforce a healthy, vegetarian German food were hardly ever strictly carried out or successful. The hardships of wartime for most Germans had rather the opposite effect: as long as cigarettes and liquor were available, their consumption during the Second World War increased significantly, and a good cut of meat became, in particular after the war, the most desirable of pipe dreams.

The ties between the *Lebensreform* and the Nazi movement, and a general refraining from the idea of direct interference into human lifestyles, made diet reform objectionable in West Germany after the Second World War. Diet reform, vegetarianism or even the idea of a German food after 1945, had a rancid flavour for several decades, and its products and concepts were limited to a niche market for these reasons. Eco-food therefore was a re-discovery of an important tradition of the German speaking world, and it was reintroduced in the early 1970s as an imported concept from the US – as we will see later in the section on negative nutrition.

International nutrition: sciences, industry and government

Another important way to define healthy food is 'international nutrition'. It is closely related to the idea of varied food, but is on a larger scale if we consider the links between scientific dietetics, the food industry and governmental regulation of markets and products. The powerful triangle of science, industry and government, asserts that it provides the population with safe and high quality foodstuffs, highly standardised by production, packing, taste, hygiene etc. International nutrition came into being between 1870 and 1940 in the US, as part of a significant economic and cultural change and related to an enormous increase in food production in the 'land of plenty', and was later promoted by the political dominance of America (Levenstein 1988, 1993).

Whereas traditional cooking and good taste was defined in Europe, mainly in France, Germany became the centre of the debate on 'modern' food in Europe in the nineteenth century, in the world of industry as in life reform. After 1900, the centre of the food industry and nutritional research slowly shifted to the US. While researchers like Russell H. Chittenden (1856–1943) or Elmer McCollum (1879–1967) were equipped with resources (labs, staff, budgets), German scientists after the turn of the century could only dream of such things. The outcome of a specific combination of affluence, big science and big business was that world-class research on nutritional science was focused more and more in North America, as is evident in the history of vitamin research after 1920, and of lifestyle diseases after 1950. Many actors in the US strongly supported research on human food, including universities, state and federal governments and, first and foremost, the Department of Agriculture in Washington under its head, Harvey Washington Wiley (1844–1930). Wiley was at the same time the leading personality in the American pure food movement which uncovered countless food scandals in the US, and had inaugurated in 1906 the Federal Food and Drug Administration (FDA). The FDA started as an inspection authority to fight fraud, forgery and lack of hygiene in food production and transport, all of which required empirical studies. These led to a change in the activities of the FDA after the Second World War; since then, it has defined the recommended daily allowances (RDAs) that, until today, have set the worldwide standards for food security from the perspective of science, big business, and government.

No wonder that FDA's food research became directly linked with associations of producers (like the dairy industry) and big food companies like General Foods, Standard Brands and General Mills! Research on nutrition and the abundance of foodstuff led to significant innovations in the American food market: processed foodstuffs, such as breakfast cereals, canned fruits, meat, vegetables, pickles and condiments, ready-made meals, frozen food, vitamin pills, fortified flour, salt, milk, curd etc. American affluence also promoted the mass commercialisation of sales and marketing and, interestingly, was combined with another concept originally developed in Germany – the idea of a varied or mixed diet.

The concept of *gesunde mischkost* (varied diet) was brought to the US by Ellen S. Richards (1842–1911)[4] and Mary Hinman Abel (1850–1938) where it was called 'new nutrition'. As in Europe, it was mainly designed as a contribution to social reform, and taught in home economics courses. By eating better and more cheaply, the American middle and underclass was to be enabled to save assets for higher quality housing, clothing and education. But due to the higher levels of prosperity and affluence in America compared to Europe, the concept of new nutrition was slowly transformed from predominantly social to health reform. The dominance of health gained more momentum with additional scientific discoveries after the Second World War, and paved the way for 'newer nutrition' or the international nutritional style. The latter is, until today, heavily based on industrial food production, the commercialisation of nutritional food, advertising and the general notion that consumers can combine various types of processed food to consume RDAs which are sanctioned by governmental institutions. The concept of international or newer nutrition asserts that it provides consumers with safe and hygienic food and all nutrients required for health, physical and mental fitness. It was widely introduced in European countries like West Germany after the Second World War, and deeply transformed the systems of regional food and scarcity which were prevalent until then. With the construction of its RDAs and food pyramids, the concept of international nutrition established a new, rather ambivalent style of consumption with benefits and downsides. On the one hand, it introduced larger quantities of dairy products, fruits, fish, vegetables and lighter meals into the pattern of consumption in Germany; but on the other hand, it promoted especially highly processed products which contain by far too much sugar, fat, salt and substances of dubious origin.

Negative nutrition: food is healthy if not proved harmful

Since the end of the 1950s, we can observe another notion of healthy food. It is not characterised by specific recommendations as to what people should eat in moderation, or even as much as possible, as dietetics so far had stressed. The new doctrine is based rather on the opposite idea – to be in general sceptical about what to eat, and in particular, about any advice derived from science, administrations and commercials, and to distrust every definition of healthy food propagated by big food companies. Due to its sceptical or critical basic orientation, the notion was called 'negative nutrition' by Warren J. Belasco (1989). In its multiple variations, negative nutrition is today the basis of consumerism, and is linked with critical research on food, and with consumer protection, environmentalism and organic food. The entire movement has benefited from scientific evidence on harmful food and consumption, and from food scandals in particular.

Negative nutrition, first, obtained acceptance due to the results of critical nutritional research, especially with the discoveries of the Framingham Study. The latter was started in 1950 as an attempt to understand the enormous contemporary increase in cardio-vascular disease. The innovation of the Framingham Study was that it initially suspected human lifestyles to be the main cause of heart attacks and strokes. The study surveyed a cohort of 6,507 individuals from the small town of Framingham in Massachusetts, US, to evaluate the prevalence of six risk factors related to cardio-vascular disorders: high blood pressure, smoking, insufficient exercise, elevated blood lipids, obesity and diabetes. The research did not only demonstrate that the latter risk factors – elevated blood lipids, obesity and diabetes – depended on food habits, but also, that the existing food recommendations with their high amounts of animal fat and amino-acids contributed significantly to the development of cardio-vascular health problems. And when the first studies on cholesterol were published in 1961, the American consumers were panicked by the idea that their officially recommended diet was not only unsound, but deadly. Most of the foodstuff experts had so far praised as being healthy – milk, butter and beef – contained a killer substance: cholesterol, which caused strokes and heart attacks. Cholesterol and its allegedly terrible side-effects produced the first modern food panic which swept rapidly from the US over Western Europe.

The idea of cholesterol did not only re-introduce distrust and even fear into western post-war societies and their notions about healthy food, it also sped up the search for alternatives. An obvious solution was the consumption of reputedly beneficial margarine and other cholesterol-free products which were strongly advocated by food companies. Another outcome of the cholesterol panic was an intensive search for alternatives. For the first time, it became evident that the concept of international nutrition was based merely on north-western European cooking traditions, French with British and German variations. But were not Mediterranean, Japanese or Chinese food habits by far healthier? Hence the cholesterol panic entailed a long lasting debate on healthy eating, but it took more than 20 years before the respective RDAs were modified in North America and Western Europe. From the late 1970s, Americans, Germans etc. were officially encouraged by their national food administrations to consume less animal fat and protein and more fish, fruits, vegetables, and cereals and to use olive oil, the emblematic oil of the 'healthy' Cretan diet, as idealised today.

Negative nutrition became increasingly popular due to the impact of several environmental and nutritional scandals from the late 1950s. In 1958, the carcinogenic effects of some chemical nutritional additives were discovered, and use of additives, pesticides and herbicides became dubious after the trailblazing research by Rachel Carson (1907–1964) on their disastrous impact on wildlife and human health (Carson 1962). More environmental and unsafe food scandals followed her highly popular book *Silent Spring*: mercury in freshwater fish, arsenic in chicken meat, hormones in beef, salmonella in canned soup, beef from 4D-cows (dead, dying, diseased, disabled), botulinium bacillus in pizza, rat hairs in hotdogs and DDT in human breast milk. These scandals deeply impressed the public in the US and caused strong reactions in Western Europe. They peaked in the US in 1979 with the accident at the Three Mile Island Nuclear Generating Station, in Harrisburg, Pennsylvania, and with the atomic disaster in Chernobyl in Ukraine in 1986. In West Germany, as in other European countries, mushrooms, berries and even breast milk were considered harmful substances. Hence, negative nutrition also reached Germany and was popularized by specific European or German food and environmental scandals. Already in 1982, the Cologne Katalyse-Umweltgruppe, an NGO dealing with food and environmental scandals, summed up how dubious and harmful the products of the food industry had become: emulsifying agents in sausage, salmonella in poultry, lead, cadmium, pesticides and phosphates in marine and freshwater fish. By drinking milk someone ingested considerable doses of DDT, lindane, heavy metals like thallium and rodenticides (Katalyse-Umweltgruppe 1982).

Negative nutrition entailed a boom in organic or eco-food and vegetarianism, and further stimulated the emergence of critical consumerism. A good example is given by Foodwatch, an NGO founded by Thilo Bode, the long-term general manager of Greenpeace International, which advocates no positive concept of healthy food, but is rather based on a deep criticism of contemporary dietetics, foodstuff and all ideologies and claims of the constitutional value of any nutrition science. Foodwatch demands better controls of big food companies, and in particular, a sustainable, eco-friendly agriculture, and a responsible way of food consumption (Bode 2007).

Healthy food and lifestyle: eat what you believe in

Negative nutrition contributed distinctively to the further diversification of the construction of healthy food during recent decades, though all prevalent contemporary notions are more or less directly linked with all the other above mentioned concepts – cosmic balance, varied and processed industrial nutrition, organic food and, again, negative nutrition. The change over the past three or four decades is not caused by another new food concept, but rather entailed two important socio-cultural changes.

First, in Western countries and in Germany in particular, health-conscious behaviour and diet have recombined with social and educational status: the concepts of varied diet and international nutrition were egalitarian – the new interpretations of sane consumption are socially exclusive. Upper and middle class people have significantly modified their consumption style. Whereas the lower social strata, today often stigmatised by the term 'precariat' (a social class formed by people suffering from conditions of existence without predictability or security), still enjoy salty snacks, sweets, cigarettes and a good chunk of meat, and take in particular the latter as an indicator of delicious and prestigious food, the diet of the well-off has become more abstemious. Especially younger persons with higher education tend towards vegetarianism and to refraining from smoking, whereas the better educated and wealthier part of the over-40s have begun to take periodic medical check-ups very seriously, especially if they show non elevated blood lipids, and ideal body weight indices. Confronted with an enormous abundance of food, this ideal is only achieved through a lifelong struggle and permanent abstention from favourite food, sometimes facilitated or justified by post-modern notions of salubrious behaviour like slow food[5] or LOHAS (low impact on health and environment).

During the recent decades, the construction of a healthy diet has been part of a new social polarity between the less prosperous and less educated social strata on the one hand, and the 'superior' ones on the other. A good indicator of the recent social exclusion by salutary consumption is hip size. The notion of the slim, healthy, active, successful and beautiful has spread from the US to Western Europe and, in both cases, members of migrant communities, minorities and, in general, lower social strata, are easily identified not only by face, dress or language, but by their waist circumference and the size of their bellies. Historically, this is a fascinating development as in the European context, stately size and weight have been considered indicators of health and prosperity for a very long time (Kiple 2007).

Secondly, healthy food has not only become socially exclusive, it has also been integrated into lifestyle concepts. The latter form the core of social and cultural differentiation in post-modern societies today: in the German case, as *Sinus-Milieus* which attribute with determinism to societal groups classified according to social stratification (upper, middle, lower class) value orientation (tradition, modernisation/individualism, performance/hedonism). These milieus define general patterns of belief, behaviour and consumption, and therefore deeply influence typical food preferences. Hence, and as a general rule, lifestyle and lifestyle concepts are related to the above mentioned fundamental concepts of healthy food: cosmic balance, varied and processed industrial food, organic food and negative nutrition. According to this general pattern, consumers follow advice from dietetics related to their lifestyle concept and more or less differentiated into detailed regulations about what to eat and what not. I will give only some examples. The concept of organic food puts emphasis on the growth of products under natural and reasonable conditions. That of functional food means that it contains various additives to further promote the tasty effects of the respective foodstuff. Fine food is nothing but the tradition of French and Italian haute cuisine, sometimes enriched with German regional products such as regionally or locally typical breads, fish, vegetables or specialties. Ethnic cuisine refers to cooking patterns other than the European one, in particular from China, Japan and South-East Asia. The concept of wellness through foodstuff comes with the idea that, for example, the consumption of certain lactobacillaceae in yoghurt, or salt from the Himalayas, may not only increase the consumer's health but also improve mood and temper. Convenience food stands, based on the idea of an improved international nutrition, provide the consumer with fresh, hygienic, tasteful and easy to prepare ready-to-eat meals. And evidently all post-modern lifestyle foodstuff is incredibly healthy…

Conclusion

Historians must be humble: they explain societal developments after those developments have taken place, and they are far from able to give detailed advice as to which food is healthy and which harmful. Nevertheless, three aspects of the relation between historical developments and the construction of a healthy diet are made obvious here. First, in the German context (as in the context of any other country) since the late eighteenth century, the construction of healthy food depends on general reference systems and their historical progress: economics, technology, science, fashion and general notions, ideas and beliefs, both crazy and reasonable. Secondly, consumers follow these concepts often without detailed knowledge of their backgrounds and consequences, or at least they use these concepts to justify their daily consuming patterns. And thirdly, healthy nutrition does not simply exist; it is a human construction which is subject to historical change, including phenomena such as discoveries, discourses, fashion, availability etc. The particular problem with healthy food is that, even after more than 200 years of intensive research, we still know more about harmful foodstuffs than about the healthy ones. Concepts of healthy diets and their respective development are still mainly based on reverse arguments, and hence, our caution and discrimination are required.

Notes

1 See the excellent overview over the history of DGE by Jörg Melzer (2003).
2 The Dukan diet, developed by the French medical practitioner, Pierre Dukan, is the best illustration of a current protein-based diet. This regimen has recently gained great notoriety in the world for its rapid results in weight loss, but it is highly debated by dieticians because of its imbalance in micronutrients, an imbalance which can induce tiredness, weakness, cardiovascular diseases and athero-thrombosis, of its deficiency in fibres and its level of amino-acids, four times superior to the recommended dietary allowances, which can cause renal failures. Moreover, this diet has two important inconveniences: it is expensive due to its products rich in proteins (of natural origin or by fortification), and its discontinuity means a rapid weight gain.
3 See Christoph Wilhelm Hufeland (1797)
4 See Ellen S. Richards (1900).
5 Slow Food was founded in Italy by Carlo Petrini in 1986. The international movement, with more than 100,000 members worldwide, attempts to preserve traditional and regional cuisine by encouraging the production of regional or locally characteristic foodstuff.

References

Belasco, W.J. (1989). *Appetite for Change: How the Counter Culture Took on the Food Industry, 1966–1988*, New York: Cornell University Press.

Bircher-Benner, M.-O. (1944). *Kranke Menschen in diätetischer Heilbehandlung*, Zürich: Wendepunkt-Verlag.

Bode, T. (2007). *Abgespeist. Wie wir beim Essen betrogen werden und was wir dagegen tun können*, Frankfurt: Fischer Verlage.

Briesen, D. (2010). *Das gesunde Leben. Ernährung und Gesundheit seit dem 18*, Frankfurt : Jahrhundert.

Carson, R. (1962). *The Silent Spring*, Boston: Houghton Mifflin Co.

Gundert, B. (2000). "Soma and Psyche in Hippocratic Medicine", in J. P. Wright and P. Potter (eds.), *Psyche and Soma: Physicians and Metaphysicians on the Mind-Body Problem from Antiquity to Enlightenment*, pp. 13–35. Oxford: Clarendon Press.

Hindhede, M. (1922). *Die neue Ernährungslehre*, Dresden: E. Pahl.

Hobsbawm, E. (1994). *The Age of Extremes: The Short Twentieth Century, 1914–1991*, London: Michael Joseph.

Hufeland, C.W. (1797). *Die Kunst das menschliche Leben zu verlängern*, Jena: AkademischeBuchhandlung.

Katalyse-Umweltgruppe, K.V. (ed.) (1982). *Chemie in Lebensmitteln*, Köln: Zweitausendeins.

Kiple, K.F. (2007). *A Movable Feast. Ten Millenia of Food Globalization*, Cambridge: Cambridge University Press.

Kofrányi, E. and Wirths, W. (1994). *Einführung in die Ernährungslehre*, Frankfurt: Umschau Verlag.

Kollath, W. (1942). *Die Ordnung unserer Nahrung. Grundlagen einer dauerhaften Ernährungslehre*, Stuttgart.

Levenstein, H.A. (1988). *Revolution at the Table: The Transformation of the American Diet*, New York: University of California Press.

Levenstein, H.A. (1993). *Paradox of Plenty: A Social History of Eating in Modern America*, Oxford: Oxford University Press.

Mazzini, I. (2000). "Diet and medicine in the Ancient World", in J.L. Flandrin, and M. Montanari (eds), *Food: a culinary history from antiquity to the present*, pp. 141–152. New York: Penguin.

Melzer, J. (2003). *Vollwerternährung, Diätetik, Naturheilkunde, Nationalsozialismus, Sozialer Anspruch*, Stuttgart: Franz Steiner Verlag.

Moleschott, J. (1858). *Lehre der Nahrungsmittel,* Für das Volk. 3, Erlangen: F. Enke.

Potter, P. and Gundert, B. (1998). "Hippokrates aus Kos", in Der neue Pauly, *Enzyklopädie der Antike*, pp. 590–599. Stuttgart: Band 15.

Richards, E.H. (1900). *The Costs of Living as Modified by Sanitary Science*, New York: John Wiley.

10 Are traditional foods and eating patterns really good for health?

A socio-anthropological inquiry into French people with hypercholesterolaemia[1]

Tristan Fournier

Introduction

Food modernity and traditional foods

Western countries are coping with a paradoxical situation regarding food. While one might suppose that an abundance of food would have brought serenity to a great majority of people, the relationship with food remains characterised by anxiety which is linked with several issues. First, a medicalisation process (Lupton 1995), that results from both scientific advances and increase in individual responsibility (Crawford 1977), has emphasised the nutritional dimension of food. As a consequence, nutritional safeguards have increased, but the effects may be counter-productive as they induce "dietary cacophony" (Fischler 1993). Then, a second paradox in food modernity results from the first one: although food has never been as safe as it is today, at least from the sanitary point of view, people are afraid of what they eat (Apfelbaum 1998), and especially of its possible impact on health, body and identity. French sociologist Claude Fischler (1993) has underlined the symbolic risks of incorporating 'Unidentified Food Objects' (UFOs). Lastly, globalisation is supposed to involve the homogenisation process of food which may reduce identity markers (Ritzer 2004).

All these elements are possible factors in a traditional food revival. The way in which traditional foods can be defined constitutes one of the core questions of this book. For some authors, the 'traditionality' attributed to products refers mainly to a historical rootedness of consumption and/or to philosophical or religious beliefs. For others, a foodstuff can be qualified as traditional if it is produced in a specific territory and eaten by the members of a specific community. These definitions are close to that of the European Food Information Resource Consortium which emphasises the historical dimension of traditional foods ("prior to the Second World War") as well as the specific features related to ingredients, composition and type of production

(Weichselbaum *et al.* 2009). Not only are the consequences of this traditional food revival visible at the institutional level through the global promotion of food heritages (Food inventories in European countries; the French gastronomic meal at the UNESCO Intangible World Heritage, 2010; creation of quality labels in Europe; etc.), but also at the consumers' level as this traditionality may reassure them with regard to both their health and identity. This particular representation merits consideration and discussion.

Analysing traditional foods and eating patterns

The present paper aims to analyse the influences of traditional foods on health and offers the hypothesis that, contrary to general assumptions, such foods may also have some negative nutritional effects. To achieve such an aim, both foods and eating patterns must be questioned. The socio-anthropology of food has stressed that the type, quality and quantity of food have to be considered when analysing the relation between food and health, but are not sufficient to understand it as a whole. The consumption of a foodstuff depends as well on contextual, social and cultural factors. Numerous social scientists have demonstrated that the relationship between mankind and its food is greatly influenced by socio-cultural dimensions, as far as food production techniques (Poulain 2002a), choice of edible products (Fischler 1988), food habits (Mäkelä 2000) and even nutrition are concerned (Garine 1979). From the concept of "social space" that Georges Condominas (1980) had elaborated to theorise about the relation between a social group and its environment, Jean-Pierre Poulain (2002a) has created the concept of *espace social alimentaire* (food social space) to describe the organisation of a society as regards food and eating. Actually, human food is structured by two types of constraints: ecological ones which lead individuals to adapt to their biotope, and biological ones which mainly result from their omnivorous status. The food social space allows for identifying that, in parallel with these constraints, a kind of 'breathing space' exists where the social and cultural dimensions are very much involved. In practice, six dimensions have to be considered: edible products, food production, culinary aspect, food habits, temporality and social differentiation. This concept allows for understanding that societies which are characterised by the same constraints do not always share the same food production techniques, promote the same foods or adopt the same table manners. Thus, the food social space aims at identifying the eating pattern of a social group which consists in a set of skills and information accumulated from generation to generation, allowing for the selection of resources from the natural milieu, for their preparation in edible form, and then, in dishes, and finally for their consumption. Eating patterns, which are particular configurations of the food social space, represent too a system of symbols which takes part in the construction of social and cultural identities and allows for internal and external processes of differentiation (Poulain 2002a). Analysing the influences of traditional foods on health, therefore, calls for considering both foods and eating patterns.

Questioning food and health in France, 'the country of processed meat and cheese'

In France, the relationship that people have with food is characterised by the emphasis on taste, commensality and conviviality, eating synchronism and structure of meals (starter, main dish, cheese and dessert). These dimensions which structure the French eating pattern may be recognised as traditional and related to French gastronomy (Rozin *et al.* 1999; Poulain 2002b). Among traditional foods, many are made from animal fats, such as processed meat or cheese. The latter has a major role as its consumption constitutes a specific stage of the meal (between main dish and dessert), especially of dinner. French people are, along with Greeks, the biggest consumers of cheese in the world: in 2011, about 26.3 kg per head; for comparison, in Spain and USA, its consumption was, respectively, 9.6 kg and 15.1 kg per head while in China only 0.2 kg (CNIEL 2013).[2] Moreover, cheese is consumed by approximately 85% of French people, at least once a day. In this chapter, the traditional foods that I will present belong more to food categories (for example, 'cheese') than to specific foods of these categories (for example, 'Roquefort', a French cheese).

The traditionality assigned to certain foods may have some important effects on health, positive as well as negative, and it is thus relevant to address it. I will investigate the influences of traditional foods and eating patterns on health through French people affected by hypercholesterolaemia. Why hypercholesterolaemia? This dyslipidaemia constitutes a food-related problem (except in cases of family pathology) and, as soon as it is detected, the patient receives dietary recommendations.[3] According to national and international guidelines (AFSSAPS 2005; Grundy *et al.* 2004), dietetic prescriptions consist in reducing the consumption of foods that contain a high level of saturated fats, notably dairy products or processed meat, along with maintaining an adequate intake of mono- and poly-unsaturated fats (olive oil, fat fishes etc.). The situation of hypercholesterolaemia is all the more interesting to analyse in that this problem remains one of the most important modifiable cardiovascular risk factors. It is estimated to be responsible for 4.4 million premature deaths per annum worldwide (WHO 2002) and affects 20% of the French population (Ferrières *et al.* 2009). However, compliance with diet remains one of the main difficulties encountered by hypercholesterolaemic individuals (Kotseva *et al.* 2009): sooner or later, the dietetic advice is ignored. Some social determinants of the dietary compliance of French people with hypercholesterolaemia, already identified and published elsewhere (Fournier and Poulain 2008; Fournier *et al.* 2011), deal with age, sex, perceptions of hypercholesterolaemia and socio-cultural aspects of food. The socio-cultural features will be more precisely analysed here as food traditionality (both foods and eating patterns) may constitute a risk factor with regard to such a chronically food-related problem.

In the first part, I will present the methodology used for analysing the impact of food traditionality on compliance with the prescribed diet for French people affected by hypercholesterolaemia. Then, from the results, I will discuss two subjects: firstly, reasons for which people keep on eating various 'risky' foods, notably those regarded as traditional, even though they are proscribed, and secondly, influences of the French eating pattern on dietary compliance, particularly with regard to taste and commensality/conviviality. The object of this chapter is to show that traditional food does not automatically mean 'good health' and the traditionality attributed to foods and eating patterns together needs to be taken into account by health professionals if compliance with diet and food traditionality is to be improved.

The surveys: investigating food traditionality and health

Data presented in this paper are from a PhD thesis in sociology which has attempted to answer a question originating in the medical milieu: why do some hypercholesterolaemic individuals not comply with their doctor's dietetic advice although exposed to cardiovascular risks? Three methods were used to explore the question: in-depth interviews with 21 hypercholesterolaemic individuals; a focus group of eight individuals to enlarge the 'interviewer–interviewee' view; and a questionnaire designed according to comprehensive data and submitted to 802 individuals by phone. According to the French law regulating clinical research (Loi Huriet),[4] this survey did not require any particular ethical committee or data protection board approval.

Qualitative surveys: in-depth and focus group interviews

The qualitative survey was carried out so as to investigate the reasons for which hypercholesterolaemic French people are not compliant with the dietetic recommendations in the long term. In the review of the literature, four issues were identified as central and influential in building the guideline for both in-depth interviews and the focus group: 1) eating patterns of individuals; 2) individuals' relationships with the medical environment; 3) individuals' perceptions of cardiovascular risks and 4) 'disease' management by individuals. Socio-demographic characteristics were asked for at the end. In-depth interviews and the focus group interviews were recorded and then transcribed in full for analysis.

Selection and socio-demographical characteristics of the subjects have been described previously (Fournier and Poulain 2008). To sum up, people interviewed in-depth and individually were from 25 to 69 years old. One third lived alone, one third in couples and one third in families. Women were slightly over-represented. The members of the focus group were from 24 to 79 years old; half of them lived alone and the other half in couples. Men and women were equally represented.

Four main determinants of non-compliance with diet have been identified in this qualitative study which are: 1) the eating pattern of the individuals based on their socio-cultural identities, routines, food handling etc.; 2) the social contexts with its situational and interactional dimensions that characterise food intake; 3) the relations that the individuals have with the medical milieu (doctor–patient relationship, 'sick role') and 4) risk perceptions by individuals on hypercholesterolaemia ('optimistic biases').

Quantitative survey: cohort study

A quantitative survey was carried out as a second step, the perspective being to validate the qualitative results on a large and representative sample of this population and also to document the hypercholesterolaemic French population in terms of socio-economic and socio-demographic status, as such data does not exist in France. The questionnaire, made up of 58 closed and multiple-choice questions, was designed to be completed in around 25 minutes. Since socio-demographic characteristics are related to the private life of the interviewee, these were asked about at the end so that confidence in the interviewer was first established.

The questionnaire was put together from the four main issues of the interview guideline which were: 1) eating pattern (with questions on eating habits, level of involvement in food chores, nutrition knowledge, food choices, diet experiences); 2) identification of metabolic diseases and relationships with the medical environment (history and aetiology of the dyslipidemia, number and types of cardio-vascular risk factors, and form of 'health locus of control'); 3) perception of cardiovascular risks (perception of the frequency, the seriousness and the fear of the disorder, and social representations of hypercholesterolaemia) and 4) disease management (role of family environment, impact of medical milieu and media, frequency and reasons for dietary lapses, 'coping strategies'). A pre-test was conducted on 20 individuals excluded from the final sample in order to investigate whether the questions were both comprehensible and discriminatory.

The construction of the sample and the socio-demographic characteristics of this population have been published (Fournier *et al*. 2011). In brief, the average age was 60 years old (SD=14.2) and 50% of individuals were retired, living mainly in couples. 30% had only basic education levels, but 45% belonged or had belonged to the middle socio-professional category.

As my main objective was to analyse the influences of socio-cultural aspects of food and eating on dietary compliance, two variables had to be elaborated: one regarding 'eating pattern' and the other 'compliance with diet'. As for the eating pattern variable, a distinction has to be made between social and cultural levels. Indeed, 'real' food practices and representations of individuals and social groups may differ from the French eating pattern which, in line with the gastronomic heritage, tends to constitute the eating reference. Because of this association, an 'eating style' variable, identified by dint of the question: 'what does eating mainly represent for you?' was added to the questionnaire. Individuals had the choice of responding by 1) 'to be in the family or with friends', 2) 'an enjoyable activity', 3) 'a way of maintaining health and protecting myself against illness', 4) 'a way of expressing ethical, political and ecological convictions' and 5) 'a necessary function', and their responses were classified as 1) 'convivial', 2) 'hedonistic', 3) 'prudent', 4) 'political' and 5) 'functional' in the analysis. Then, as a self-reported dietary prescription is likely to be biased, a separate 'compliance with diet' variable was built, using four variables: 1) declaration of a lipid-lowering diet; 2) self-reported infringements of diet prescription; 3) difficulties in following dietary prescriptions and 4) response of individuals to exposure to cheese. This last variable is relevant because cheese is a traditional food in France and its consumption was identified in the qualitative surveys as being the most difficult to regulate by people affected by dyslipidemia. Using this factor in the compliance with diet variable meant that statistically, *n* (802) was reduced to 729, as nearly 9% of people declared that they never consumed cheese. Results, classified into 'compliance' and 'non-compliance' with diet, were then crossed with independent variables.

Statistical results presented in this article are given in percentages and means; the standardised residuals are indicated in the crosstabs. Bivariate analyses were performed by using SPSS Software (VS 14.0) and categorical data were analysed by the Chi-squared test with a statistical significance at $P \leq 0.05$.

How food 'traditionally ' influences dietary compliance?

The section devoted to discussing results of the three surveys (cohort, in-depth interview and focus-group) is divided into two parts in order that both traditional foods and eating patterns are considered. The first part deals with the consumption and representations of traditional foods by hypercholesterolaemic people and the second with the influence of the French eating pattern on the compliance with the prescribed diet.

Table 10.1 Methodology

Tool	*Sample*	*Recruitment*
In-depth interviews	21	• LDL-cholesterol[a] level upper to 1.6g/l of blood • No other CV[b] pathologies (diabetes, hypertension) • Varied socio-demographic criteria (age, sex, family situation, socio-professional categories)
Focus group	1 group of 8	• LDL-cholesterol[a] level upper to 1.6g/l of blood • No other CV[b] pathologies (diabetes, hypertension) • Varied socio-demographic criteria (age, sex, family situation, socio-professional categories)
Questionnaire	802	• Sample representative of the French population • Quotas applied for sex, region of residence, and size of urban area • Monitored by a physician for a cholesterol problem

a LDL-cholesterol: Low-Density Lipoprotein cholesterol, known as "bad" cholesterol
b CV: cardiovascular

Traditional food promotion and dislipidaemia: between knowledge and practice

Medical literature stresses that compliance with dietary prescription remains one of the main difficulties in coping with hypercholesterolaemia (Kotseva *et al.* 2009). In this section, I will analyse the role in this issue of traditional foods. Firstly, I will investigate the level of nutritional knowledge of the interviewees in order to ascertain if the consumption of foods proscribed by the doctor is due to lack of information. Secondly, I will document the positive representations of traditional foods that I will analyse with the help of anthropological concepts of 'magical thinking' and the 'principle of incorporation' which are useful for comprehending why people keep on eating risky foods. Lastly, I will emphasise cheese consumption which seems to be the most difficult for individuals to regulate.

Nutrition knowledge and dietary deviations

Since difficulties regarding compliance with the dietary prescription are documented in the medical literature, one may hypothesise that individuals do not know the basic dietetic recommendations. From the responses of interviewees to questions on nutritional knowledge, some differences between foods to be avoided and those to be favoured have emerged. According to the results of the cohort, vegetables (67%), fruits (54%), fish (41%) and green vegetables (26%) are mentioned as foods that may be eaten regularly if the cholesterol level is high (Table 10.2); they are consistent with nutritional recommendations of the national and international guidelines (AFSSAPS 2005; Grundy *et al.* 2004). Among the foods to be avoided, red meat (57%), processed meat (44%), butter (39%) and cheese (26%) are mentioned (Table 10.2); their consumption is restricted in case of hypercholesterolaemia because of their high level of LDL-cholesterol. Nevertheless, other food categories also rich in LDL-cholesterol, such as eggs or organ meats, are not mentioned by individuals. Therefore, in general, hypercholesterolaemic people have a reasonable knowledge of nutrition and the hypothesis of lack of knowledge cannot be validated. This dichotomy between knowledge and practice is entirely in line with other studies, leading to the conclusion that compliance with dietary prescription does not depend only on the learning of nutritional composition of food (Henson *et al.* 2010).

The comparison between foods to be avoided and those eaten during dietary lapses reveals some interesting features (Table 10.3). First, processed meat is worthy of being investigated because it is largely perceived as a food to be avoided (44%) while it is frequently consumed during dietary deviations (named by 39% of people). This phenomenon implies a gap between social norms and practices, which is a well-known limitation in food studies as shown by Poulain (2002b). The discussions in in-depth interviews and in the focus group also revealed that processed meat is often reported as food to be avoided, and its consumption may be accompanied by a kind of easily identifiable guilt. The discrepancy between knowledge and practice clearly shows that hypercholesterolaemic people distinguish between what they should, and should not, eat. It is pointed out

Table 10.2 Foods classified as to be avoided or favoured by hypercholesterolaemic French individuals (cohort survey - each food was enquired about individually)

	Number (%)
Foods to be favoured (n=802)	
Vegetables	534 (66.6)
Fruit	429 (53.5)
Fish	328 (40.9)
Green vegetables	206 (25.7)
Starchy foods (rice, pasta)	66 (8.2)
Water	44 (5.5)
Cereals, bread	31 (3.9)
Pulses	22 (2.7)
'Anti-cholesterol' products[1]	15 (1.9)
Hot drinks (tea, herbal tea)[2]	7 (0.9)
Other[3]	175 (21.8)
Didn't know	38 (4.7)
Foods to be avoided (n=802)	
Red meat	455 (56.7)
Processed meat	354 (44.1)
Butter	312 (38.9)
Cheese	211 (26.3)
Egg	150 (18.7)
Cakes	88 (11.0)
Dish with rich sauce	83 (10.3)
Alcohol (wines and other alcohols)	74 (9.2)
Snacks	13 (1.6)
Other[4]	201 (25.1)
Didn't know	7 (0.9)

Notes

1 Individuals who named 'anti-cholesterol products' talked about functional foods such as margarine that aims at lowering cholesterolemia.
2 In France, 'herbal tea' often refers to verbena or lime-blossom tea.
3 Especially 'chicken meat'.
4 Especially 'sugar', 'oils', 'French fries' and 'chocolate'.

in other studies (Peretti-Watel 2000) carried out in the field of risk and health, which highlighted the common perception, that 'risky individuals' are those with issues such as addiction, or homosexuality in the case of HIV-AIDS. This restrictive perception of risks may explain the non compliance with processed meat avoidance despite the fact that this large food category is made up of both lean (cooked ham) and very fat (potted meat or *pâté*) products. By comparison, other foods such as butter or red meat mentioned as foods to be avoided (39% and 57% respectively) are less often eaten during dietary lapses (18% and 24% respectively). The foods which tend to be more frequently eaten during dietary deviations are cheese (50%), processed meat (39%) and cakes (33%). Nevertheless, the risk perceived in the consumption of products is variable from one category to another: cheese, cakes and snacks are rarely classified as foods to be avoided (26%, 11% and 2% respectively) while they contain high levels of fat (except for skimmed cheese), and are commonly consumed (50%, 33% and 21% respectively). These discrepancies invite the examination of several hypotheses. Firstly, festive or occasional consumption, in the case of cakes for example, may lead people to consider certain categories of foods as not risky even if they sometimes eat them. Regarding snacks, they are not referred to in 'institutionalised' food practice in France, at least among the older persons interviewed.[5] Lastly, the fact that the representation of cheese vacillates between 'bad food' and 'good food' merits particular attention as I will show later.

Table 10.3 Foods eaten during dietary deviation compared with foods individuals believed should be avoided (cohort survey - each food was enquired about separately)

	Number (%)	
	Foods eaten during dietary deviations (n=670)	*Foods considered 'to be avoided' (n=802)*
Cheese	337 (50.3)	211 (26.3)
Processed meat	262 (39.1)	354 (44.1)
Cakes	221 (33.0)	88 (11.0)
Dish with rich sauce	188 (28.1)	83 (10.3)
Red meat	161 (24.0)	455 (56.7)
Alcohol (wines and other alcohols)	154 (23.0)	74 (9.2)
Snacks	140 (20.9)	13 (1.6)
Butter	118 (17.6)	312 (38.9)
Egg	118 (17.6)	150 (18.7)
Other	52 (7.8)	201 (25.1)
Didn't know	6 (0.9)	7 (0.9)

'Magical thinking' and the 'principle of incorporation': theories still very much alive

The concept of 'magical thinking', used for the first time in anthropology (Tylor 1871; Frazer 1995 [1890]), is useful in better understanding why the consumption of certain foods is so difficult to regulate. In food studies, this concept refers to a form of reasoning in which the representation of a foodstuff constitutes an important factor in the food choice process (Rozin 1976; Fischler 1994). The foodstuff is symbolically impregnated with values – perceived as positive or negative – which, incorporated by the eater, may influence his/her' nature, behaviour and identity.[6] The concept of magical thinking is close to the 'principle of incorporation' defined by Fischler (1988) which is that 'you are what you eat.' This works, not only at the nutritional level (the food's nutrients are becoming our own body), but also at the social level (eating a foodstuff which is much-valued in a social group makes us more thoroughly integrated into this group) and at the symbolic level (qualities of an eaten foodstuff are influencing our identity). Incorporating a particular foodstuff means incorporating its nutritional, social and symbolic properties. Together, magical thinking and the principle of incorporation constitute a very effective lever for food decision processes. They are also useful in analysing the social representations that hypercholesterolaemic individuals have about traditional foods and their nutritional impact. These concepts act at two levels which have to be distinguished one from the other.

On the one hand, in the case of hypercholesterolaemia, the great majority of foods which must be avoided comes from animals (unskimmed dairy products, red meat, processed meat, etc.) and comprises various traditional foods in France. These foods play an important role in the social and cultural identities of people who consume them (Vial 1993; Méchin 1997). I have previously shown that foods the consumption of which is particularly difficult to regulate are deeply rooted in the culture. People often exclaim: "Why stop consuming processed meat as a starter when my family has always done that?" Between identity and health, the relevant question is: what is the most profitable for the eater? Then, social representations of traditional foods must be linked to 'lay knowledge' about dietetics. For example, milk and dairy products enjoy a positive representation in terms of nutrition for French people because of their traditionality. This representation is strongly instrumentalised by food marketing that uses the concept of magical thinking and the principle of incorporation in its advertisement, focusing on the traditionality, purity and health of dairy products to enhance its sales. And thus, recommendations to reduce the consumption of dairy products may induce some cacophony (Fischler 1993). In addition, the representations of traditional foods are socially determined, notably in terms of gender (Counihan and Kaplan 1998). For example, red meat constitutes an important food for men as it symbolises strength. In several interviews and in the focus group discussions, some men stated that "red meat gives muscles". Recommending reduction of red meat intake could, indeed, have different meanings and consequences for men and for women. To a great extent, representations of medical diets are deeply gendered (Gough

2007). In terms of social classes, some differences have already been identified (Bourdieu 1984; Irala-Estévez *et al.* 2000) according to both consumption, as the quantity of food intake is more important in lower social strata than in upper, while representations of food, as reflexivity is in operation prevail in upper social strata. In this study, some traditional foods, such as processed meat, encounter a positive perception mainly from lower classes, as has been demonstrated for fatty foods in general (Corbeau 1995; Czernichow *et al.* 2005). Nevertheless, and according to national and international guidelines, although they are likely to be eaten by hypercholesterolaemic individuals, their consumption has to be reduced because their nutritional composition is not suitable for the medical profile of these persons.

On the other hand, magical thinking and the principle of incorporation can take part in the regulation of dietary deviations. Both qualitative and quantitative results have revealed that the way in which people deal with dietary lapses consists mainly in eating more lightly at subsequent meals. Thus, analysing what kinds of food are eaten during these 'special diet' days is interesting, notably when one considers green vegetables. According to the focus group discussions, French beans are considered as 'fat eliminators' and green salad as 'body cleaners', and thus, they are appropriate to counterbalance the previous intakes of 'forbidden' foods. Mineral water and plain yoghurt are also integrated into this special diet thanks to their perceived properties of expelling 'bad fats' from the body. Efficient or not, the ways in which people cope with hypercholesterolaemia and try to regulate it are often based on magical thinking. The action of this concept has also been demonstrated in the field of food-related risks (Fournier 2008).

Always keep a little space for cheese! A traditional food difficult to forget

Cheese is considered as a traditional food in France (Vial 1993) as well as in many European countries (Vanhonacker *et al.* 2008). Both qualitative and quantitative surveys have demonstrated that cheese constitutes one of the foods whose consumption is the most difficult to regulate. Since a majority of hypercholesterolaemic individuals keep on, daily, consuming cheese in spite of medical advice, its 'traditionality' has been investigated. According to in-depth interviews, cheese appears as an important cultural marker which is sometimes claimed and sometimes implicit, as the two following excerpts show:

> Ex. 1 (Male, 50, in couple; office clerk): "I eat some cheese because I am from a region of cheese". The symbolic dimension of the 'incorporation principle' is obvious in this sentence. Keeping on eating cheese although he has been advised to reduce it makes sense for this man as cheese allows him to express his roots and affirm his identity.
>
> Ex. 2 (Male, 48, in couple; worker): During a 24 hours recall interview, a man gave details about his meals in which cheese was not mentioned. In order to improve the survey, I asked him: "No cheese?", and he replied "Oh, of course some cheese, I've forgotten to name it!"

In the quantitative survey, we have seen that cheese constitutes the food which is most likely to be eaten during dietary deviations (named by 50% of the interviewed people) although only 26% of them qualified it as a food that should be avoided in regard to hypercholesterolaemia (Table 10.3). Thus, some people continuing to eat a certain amount of cheese may not consider its consumption as 'dangerous' as regards cardio-vascular risks, or may consider its traditionality (identity, region etc.) as more important than nutrition. Moreover, the gap between food eaten during dietary deviations and food to avoid with regard to the disease may also testify to an important 'nutritional cacophony' (Fischler 1993). Actually, some opposing recommendations have been imparted to hypercholesterolaemic French individuals. On the one hand, general practitioners suggest a reduction of the consumption of unskimmed dairy products because of LDL-cholesterol. But on the other hand, the National Nutrition and Health Programme[7] aims at enhancing the calcium intake by recommending the consumption of three or four dairy products a day (Hercberg *et al.* 2008).[8]

Eaters have an ambivalent relation with their food. Three forms of food ambivalence have been identified (Beardsworth 1995). The first one refers to the psychosensorial dimension of food, as eating can provoke a large range of feelings from intense pleasure to deep disgust. The second questions the relationships between life and death since eating not only constitutes the need to maintain life but also induces the slaughter of animals. The third deals with the relationship between food and health and is worth considering. British sociologist Alan Beardsworth (1995: 120) refers to the fact that: "food can be conceived of as the primary source of energy, vitality, and good health, but at the same time clearly carries the potential to introduce disease-inducing substances or organisms into the body". The consequences of these 'possibilities' are all the more ambivalent for eaters as they give rise: "on the one hand, to anxieties about acute effects [...] and, on the other, to anxieties about chronic effects" (*ibid*: 120). Concerning ambivalence towards fat products, Poulain (2008) has demonstrated that French people primarily quote "fats" when they are asked to list the foods which are prohibited or limited in order to prevent metabolic diseases, while dairy products, which generally contain a rather high fat level, except when skimmed, constitute one of the three essential foods for them. The nutritional composition of dairy products is debated. Such a calculation has been identified in the qualitative survey:

> Ex. 3 (Female, 52, in couple; researcher): "It is very difficult to give up cheese because calcium is lacking then, especially for us, women".[9]

Coping with ambivalent eating situations, hypercholesterolaemic people try to articulate in the most profitable way the symbolic, cultural and nutritional dimensions of foods. Cheese, as a traditional food in France, allows for identification of this complex process.

The French eating pattern: the culture of taste and conviviality

In this final section, I will explore taste which constitutes an important determinant of food choices in France and the role of the commensality/conviviality which is one of the main dimensions of the French eating pattern. These two factors are important as they could stand in the way of dietary advice.

The supremacy of taste

The emergence of French gastronomy in the seventeenth century can be seen as the outcome of a social context resulting, among other things, from the quest for 'authentic' taste as a vector for development of the French culinary art (Neirinck and Poulain 1988).[10] Taste was not only taken into consideration as a cultural distinction phenomenon, due to the fact that it constituted one of the conditions for recognition of the French gastronomy as a reference at the international level, but was also considered as a social distinction process which favoured the differentiation between aristocrats and bourgeois as well as between bourgeois and peasants. In this way, taste holds a central function in the French eating pattern and can be included as a traditional trait in French food (Rozin *et al.* 1999; Poulain 2002b). What is the impact of taste on the compliance with dietary guidelines of hypercholesterolaemic people?

In the quantitative survey, factors affecting food consumption were addressed, and taste was mentioned by more than 36% of individuals (Figure 10.1); health was referred to less (20%). These results are interesting because they reflect the fact that taste remains the main factor of food choice while the interviewees should be more aware of health and nutrition as they receive dietary advice for reducing their higher level of LDL-cholesterol, and they are elderly. Indeed, numerous studies have demonstrated that the relation between an individual and his/her food changes according to the stages of life (Kemmer *et al.* 1998; Devine 2005). Nutritional concerns tend to be emphasised at particular stages such as at the time of marriage (or cohabiting) or of retirement (average age of 60–65).

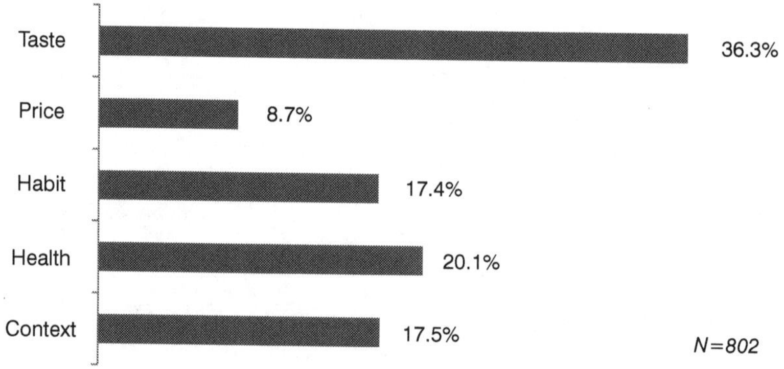

Figure 10.1 Reason behind food choices for hypercholesterolaemic French people (cohort survey)

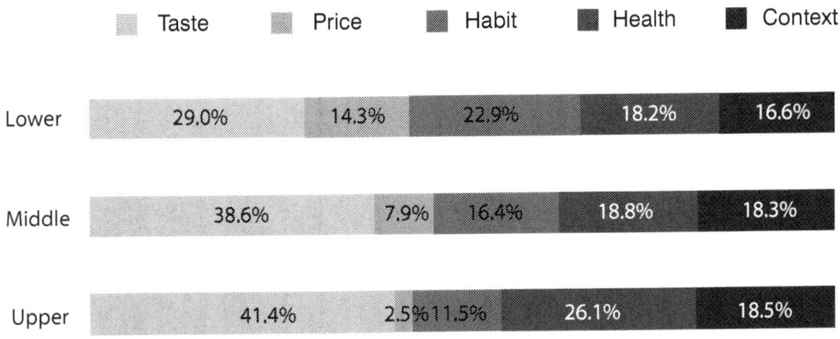

Figure 10.2 Reason behind food choices according to social classes (cohort survey)

Beyond this common attractiveness of taste, a social differentiation has to be noticed (Figure 10.2). A significant association has been identified from the crossing of the two variables: 'reason behind food choices' and 'the social position'[11] (Chi-squared = 32.116; P = 0.000). Taste in food choice is more often mentioned by people from the upper classes than those of lower status, and thus, as a social distinction in line with the French gastronomy, it continues to be relevant even today. Naming taste as the main lever of food choices within the era of food abundance and globalisation (Poulain 2002a; Ritzer 2004) would be to refer to an identity claim initiated mostly by upper class people.

To summarise, taste remains the driving force behind food choices in the sample, notably in the upper class whereas one could expect that hypercholesterolaemic people would be more sensitive to the nutritional properties of food. In a certain way, the importance given to taste may constitute a cultural resistance to food changes. It also shows the relevance of taking into account the sociological framework and cultural dimensions of food and of eating habits (Fischler 1979; Goody 1982). In addition, the supremacy of taste in respect of food choices may constitute an identity or ethic claim in the era of globalisation.

Commensality/conviviality issue in dietary compliance

In France and in a large number of food cultures, a 'proper' meal is a shared meal (Douglas 1972; Murcott 1983). According to Jeffery Sobal (2000), sociability has three dimensions: 'commensality' which means eating with other persons according to societal rules; 'interaction' which deals with social relationships during meals; and 'facilitation' which refers to the influences of social environment on personal food behaviour. Commensality has to be distinguished from conviviality. Claude Grignon (2001) explained that commensality aims at preserving the social structure of a group, i.e. establishing a frontier between 'us' and 'others'. In this way, conviviality would thus be only a possible and happy configuration of commensality. As commensality/conviviality constitutes a fundamental feature of the eating act in France (Rozin *et al.* 1999; Poulain 2002b), its influence on the compliance with diet has been investigated in this study on hypercholesterolaemic people.

The relationship between commensality/conviviality and health is ambivalent. Jeffery Sobal and Mary Nelson (2003: 187) have identified three characteristics: 1)'social facilitation' that leads to "more extensive eating and drinking in the presence of others, preventing under-consumption but risking over-consumption"; 2)'social support' from others that may "encourage eating and healthy food choices, but also may risk tempting others with unhealthy foods"; and 3)'social control' over eating "that may be exercised to sanction food choices that are unhealthy, or may guide people into eating behaviours that lead to health risks". The authors explain that these three characteristics of the relationship between commensality and health have both health promoting and health threatening potentials. As an example, social facilitation may refer either to a negative influence of a close circle of people on the nutritional status, notably with regard to over-consumption of alcoholic beverages and fat foods, or to a positive impact, as relatives may prevent under-consumption, especially in the elderly. The same process works for social support and social control. The interviews in this study have allowed for highlighting the ambivalent influence of commensality/conviviality on health.

Data from both qualitative and quantitative surveys have revealed that compliance with the prescribed diet is difficult, especially because of the presence of others during meals.

In the qualitative survey, festive meals represent a real obstacle for hypercholesterolaemic people because they are uneasy when refusing foods prepared/proposed by their hosts.

> Ex. 4 (Male, 50, in couple; architect): "I still eat some cheese when I have dinner or lunch at friends' houses. Before the meal, I never wonder about what I will eat, but during the meal, I often think about the recommendations when someone offers me more meat or cheese for example. Actually, I think that dieting is really difficult when sharing a meal with friends; it is more difficult at friends' houses because you do not know how foods are prepared and don't want to refuse dishes prepared by your friends".

This social pressure on food choices is also visible in meals in a professional context as individuals, notably men (Gough 2007), seem embarrassed when explaining to others that they follow a diet.

> Ex. 5 (Male, 64, single; contractor): "During business meals, what you eat and how much you drink expresses who you are. When I invite a client to a restaurant, I can't ask him to order what he wants and explain that I'm on a diet".

Lastly, a 'negative social facilitation' may exist at home too. For people living in couples or in a family, the organisation of meals (shopping and cooking) may sometimes cause conflicts. The presence of a hypercholesterolemic member in a family means changing the eating habits of the whole family and preparing different menus.

> Ex. 6 (Female, 40, in a family; housewife – husband office clerk): "Since I have a husband and two children, I don't want to eat my soup alone. Sharing a meal also means sharing what you eat".

During interviews, some peope pointed out that compliance with diet would be easier if they lived alone.

In the quantitative survey, hypercholesterolaemic people were asked about their 'eating style'. The responsders were classified as: 1) 'convivial', 2) 'hedonistic', 3) 'prudent', 4) 'political' and 5) 'functional'; the fourth of these was removed because it was irrevelant. People who said that the representation of eating is mainly 'being with family and friends' have been defined as 'convivial' individuals (21%). The way in which 'convivial' has been used in the following crosstab analysis refers, in general, either to 'bad' 'social facilitation' or 'good' 'social support.'

A significant association has been identified from the crossing of the 'eating style' variable with 'compliance with diet' (Chi-squared = 14.173; P = 0.003). Table 10.4 shows that individuals defined as 'prudent' are more likely to be compliant with the diet prescribed by practitioners (+4.2) than 'convivial' people (-4.6). The first association means that individuals for whom eating represents, first and foremost, 'a way of maintaining health and of protecting themselves against illness' tend to implement the nutritional recommendations. Conversely, people who think that eating pre-eminently means 'sharing with family or friends' tend to be non-compliant. Commensality/conviviality may thus be considered as a risk factor with regard to chronic food problems such as hypercholesterolaemia.[12]

Conclusions

The different interviews with hypercholesterolaemic people show that keeping on eating foods which should be avoided is not irrational because some traditional foods, such as cheese or processed meat, have symbolic properties that are part of people's social and cultural identities. That is why they try to articulate, in the most fruitful way, the symbolic, cultural and nutritional dimensions of foods. As for the French eating pattern, taste and commensality/conviviality have been taken into account. Indeed, taste may be treated as cultural resistance to food changes since it remains the driving force behind food choices for interviewees, whereas one might expect them to be much more sensitive to the nutritional aspect of food, because of age and the problem of cholesterol. The 'negative' aspect of the commensality/conviviality-health relationship is identifiable since interviewees for whom eating primarily means 'sharing with family and friends' are not very compliant with the prescribed diet. Moreover, this negative effect of 'eating together' on nutritional status works for festive meals, as well as for meals in professional contexts and for meals at home. In this way, commensality/

Table 10.4 Association between 'compliance with diet' and 'eating style'

		Convivial	*Hedonistic*	*Prudent*	*Functional*	
Compliance with diet	Number of Individuals % compliance with diet Std. Res.	53 (35.6%) 16.5% -1.8	57 (40.7%) 17.7% -0.8	69 (56.6%) 21.4% 1.8	143 (48.3%) 44.4% 0.7	
Non-compliance with diet	Number of individuals % compliance with diet Std. Res.	96 (64.4%) 24.9% 1.6	83 (59.3%) 21.6% 0.8	53 (43.4%) 13.8% -1.6	153 (51.7%) 39.7% -0.6	*P=0.003*
Total (n = 707)		149 (21.1%)	140 (19.8%	122 (17.2%)	296 (41.9%)	

Std. Res. = Standardized residuals

conviviality may be seen as a risk factor with regard to chronic food-related diseases. Because of this, tradition, when applied to foods and eating patterns, does not systematically refer to something that is 'good for health'.

In addition, the responses from interviewees are totally coherent with the 'nutritionalisation' issue of eating patterns. In France, as well as in many developed or developing countries, the nutritional aspect of food tends to overcome other dimensions of the act of eating (such as pleasure, conviviality, tradition etc.). Medicalisation process, advances in medicine and nutrition, growth of individual responsibility and eating reflexivity are equally features that favour its predominance. Some traditional foods and eating practices are healthy, and some others are not. Should only healthy ones be promoted and those recognised as health risks be banished, while both have a determining role in social relationships and cultural identities? In conclusion, I would like to stress that talking about traditional foods in order to promote food heritages seems to be useful, but talking about them in order to improve health may be more tendentious. The risk would be to emphasis only the beneficial aspects of tradition, thus reviving the famous myth of the Hunza[13] (Rodale 1948).

Notes

1 The study on which this chapter is based was commissioned by the New French Society for Atherosclerosis (la Nouvelle Société Française d'Athérosclérose). I thank the individuals who participated in the survey.

2 CNIEL: Centre National Interprofessionnel de l'Economie Laitière – Interprofessional NationalCentreofDairyEconomy.http://www.maison-du-lait.com/fr/les-organisations/cniel

3 In primary prevention, the patient is asked by his general practitioner to improve his diet for quite a long time (between three and sixth months). At the end of this time, a medicine is prescribed if the level of total cholesterol is still higher than the level recommended by the national and international guidelines. If not, the patient is invited to continue with their dietary regime. In secondary prevention (or for people with a high cardio-vascular risk), medicine and dietary measures are prescribed together.

4 This law, passed in France on 25th July 1994, aims at safeguarding the protection of volunteers involved in medical research.

5 In France, snacking mainly refers to a nibbling practice with the consumption of 'junk food' (industrially manufactured cakes, chocolate, etc.). These products tend to be marketed for young people, especially children and teenagers.

6 One of the most famous experiments Paul Rozin has carried out to demonstrate both the existence and the power of 'sympathetic magic' in the food sphere is the case of contamination of a glass of milk by a cockroach. When students were asked to drink the milk, almost all refused, justifying their refusal by saying that cockroaches are dirty insects. However, they continued to refuse to drink replaced milk in which a sterilised cockroach had been soaked. One needs to make it clear that this reasoning does not testify to the irrationality of the eaters, but rather, presents a parallel with the different forms of rationality in the food sphere already described.

7 This programme, called PNNS, was created in 2001 in France and includes nine high-priority nutritional objectives for the general population. One of these concerns the increase of the calcium intake, and consequently implies an enhancement of the consumption of dairy products.

8 Skimmed dairy products could represent a good alternative, but people who keep on eating some cheese explained during the interviews that such products are not

suitable for them because they are nothing to do with tradition. Moreover, skimmed cheeses being often industrially produced are negatively perceived by a great part of the French population.

9 In-depth interviews revealed that the attention given to calcium intake is significant for women over 45 years old due to the awareness of osteoporosis related to menopause.

10 In France, taste is an important notion which has contributed to dividing the sociology of food into two distinct theoretical approaches: one by researchers who believe in the *autonomy of the social*, in reference to the pioneer work of Emile Durkheim, in which taste is analysed as a distinction process alone, and food mainly through consumption practices (Bourdieu 1984; Grignon and Grignon 1980); and another by researchers who consider that the study of taste and food is more complex and needs an interdisciplinary dialogue (Fischler 1979; Garine 1979; Poulain 2002a).

11 Socio-professional categories were based on the French National Institute of Statistics and Economic Studies (INSEE):
Lower: independent farmer, self-employed craftsperson or artisan, independent shopkeeper or tradesperson, salaried service staff, factory or agricultural worker.
Middle: intermediate salaried professional and paramedical professional, primary school teacher or similar, salaried employee.
Upper: business owner (self-employed and with more than 10 employees), self-employed professional (except paramedical professionals), teacher (high-school and university), salaried scientist, upper level manager.
Inactive: student, disabled person, person unemployed outside.

12 Here, I deliberately emphasise the 'bad' influence of commensality/conviviality on health and nutrition. Of course, the surveys also included identifying examples in which commensality could be considered as a lever for prevention. For instance, some people described being encouraged to reduce their consumption of 'forbidden' foodstuffs or to increase that of fruits and vegetables by their relatives. This process, close to the ambivalent relationship between commensality and health defined by Jeffrey Sobal and Nancy Nelson (2000), is described elsewhere (Fournier 2012).

13 The Hunza constitute an ethnic group living in the North of Pakistan. The first researchers having met them at the beginning of the 20th century described people physically strong, happy with life and unconcerned with illness. Because of this, the Hunza have illustrated for years the virtues of a 'natural food' and a 'simple life'. However, ethnographic works led in the 1930s revealed another reality: an important level of malnutrition, numerous illnesses such as malaria and dysentery, and a regular starvation.

References

AFSSAPS (2005). *Prise en charge thérapeutique du patient dyslipidémique*, Saint Denis: AFSSAPS.

Apfelbaum, M. (ed.) (1998). *Risques et peurs alimentaires*, Paris: Odile Jacob.

Beardsworth, A. (1995). "The management of food ambivalence: erosion or reconstruction?", in D. Maurer and J. Sobal (eds), *Eating agendas. Food and nutrition as social problems*, pp. 117–143. New York: Aldine de Gruyter.

Bourdieu, P. (1984). *Distinction. A Social Critique Of The Judgement Of Taste*, London: Routledge.

CNIEL (2013). *L'économie laitière en chiffre. Edition 2013*, Paris: CNIEL. http://fr.calameo.com/read/002230051d0c12dffec73 (retrieved on 13 December 2014).

Condominas, G. (1980). *L'espace social. A propos de l'Asie du Sud-est*, Paris: Flammarion.

Corbeau, J.-P. (1995). "L'imaginaire du gras associé à divers types de consommation de gras et les perceptions de leurs qualités", in F. Nicolaïs and E. Valceschini (eds), *Agro-alimentaire : une économie de la qualité*, pp. 93–103. Paris: INRA-Economica.

Counihan, C. and Kaplan, S. (eds) (1998). *Food and Gender: Identity and Power*, Amsterdam: Harwood Academic Publishers.

Crawford, R. (1977). "You are dangerous to your health: the ideology and politics of victim blaming", *International Journal of Health Services*, Vol. 7: 663–680.

Czernichow, S., Bruckert, E., Oppert, J.-M. *et al.* (2005). "Intake of added oils and fats among middle-aged French adults: Relationships with educational level and region of residence", *Journal of the American Dietetic Association*, Vol. 105: 1889–1894.

Devine, C. (2005). "The life course perspective: understanding food choices in time, social location, and history", *Journal of Nutrition Education and Behaviour*, Vol. 37:121–128.

Douglas, M. (1972). "Deciphering a meal", *Daedalus*, Vol. 101: 61–81.

Ferrières, J., Bongard, V., Dallongeville, J. *et al.* (2009). "Trends in plasma lipids, lipoproteins and dyslipidaemias in French adults, 1996–2007", *Archives of Cardiovascular Diseases*, Vol. 102(4): 293–301.

Fischler, C. (1979). "Gastro-nomie et gastro-anomie", *Communications*, Vol. 31: 189–210.

Fischler, C. (1988). "Food, self and identity", *Social Science Information*, Vol. 27(2): 275–292.

Fischler, C. (1993). "A nutritional cacophony or the crisis of food selection in affluent societies", in P. Leathwood, M. Horisberger and W.P. James (eds.), *For a Better Nutrition in the 21st Century*, pp. 57–65. New York: Vevey/Raven Press.

Fischler, C. (ed.) (1994). *Manger magique, aliments sorciers, croyances comestibles*, Paris: Autrement, Vol. 149.

Fournier, T. (2008). "Coping with new food-related risks", *Anthropology of Food*, S0, Varia. Online 16 December 2008, http://aof.revues.org/document5303.html.

Fournier, T. (2012). "Suivre ou s'écarter de la prescription diététique. Les effets du manger ensemble et du vivre ensemble chez des personnes hypercholestérolémiques en France", *Sciences Sociales et Santé*, Vol. 30(2): 35–60.

Fournier, T., Bruckert, E., Czernichow, S., Paulmyer, A. and Poulain, J.-P. (2011). "The THEMA Study: a sociodemographic survey of hypercholesterolaemic individuals", *Journal of Human Nutrition and Dietetics*, Vol. 24(6): 572–581.

Fournier, T. and Poulain, J.-P. (2008). "Les déterminants sociaux du non-suivi du régime alimentaire : le cas des patients hypercholestérolémiques", *Cahiers de Nutrition et de Diététique*, Vol. 43(2): 97–104.

Frazer, J.G. (1995). *The Golden Bough*, New York: Touchstone, 1st publication 1890.

Garine, I. de (1979). "Culture et nutrition", *Communications*, Vol. 31: 70–91.

Goody, J. (1982). *Cooking, Cuisine and Class. A Study in Comparative Sociology*, Cambridge: Cambridge University Press.

Gough, B. (2007). "Real men don't diet: an analysis of contemporary newspaper representations of men, food and health", *Social Science and Medicine*, Vol. 64(2): 326–337.

Grignon, C. (2001). "Commensality and social morphology: an essay of typology", in P. Scholliers (ed.), *Food, Drink and Identity. Cooking, Eating and Drinking in Europe since the Middle Ages*, pp. 23–35. Oxford: Berg Publishers.

Grignon, C. and Grignon, C. (1980). "Styles d'alimentation et goûts populaires", *Revue Française de Sociologie*, Vol. 21(4) : 531–569.

Grundy, S.M., Cleeman, J.I., Bairey Merz, C.N. *et al.* (2004). "Implications of recent clinical trials for the National Cholesterol Education Program Adult Treatment Panel III Guidelines", *Circulation*, Vol. 110(2): 227–239.

Henson, S., Blandon, J., Cranfield, J. and Herath, D. (2010). "Understanding the propensity of consumers to comply with dietary guidelines directed at heart health", *Appetite*, Vol. 54(1): 52–61.

Hercberg, S., Chat-Yung, S. and Chauliac, M. (2008). "The French National Nutrition and Health Program: 2001–2006–2010", *International Journal of Public Health*, Vol. 53: 68–77.

Irala-Estévez, J.D., Groth, M., Johansson, L., Ottesdorf, U., Prättälä, R. and Martinez-Gonzalez, M.A. (2000). "A systematic review of socio-economic differences in food habits in Europe: consumption of fruit and vegetables", *European Journal of Clinical Nutrition*, Vol. 54: 706–714.

Kemmer, D., Anderson, A. and Marshall, D. (1998). "Living together and eating together: changes in food choices and eating habits during the transition from single to married/cohabiting", *The Sociological Review*, Vol. 46: 48–72.

Kotseva, K., Wood, D., De Backer, G., De Bacquer, D., Pyörälä, K. and Keil, U. (2009). "EUROASPIRE Study Group. Cardiovascular prevention guidelines in daily practice: a comparison of EUROASPIRE I, II, III surveys in eight European countries", *Lancet*, Vol. 373: 929–940.

Lupton, D. (1995). *Medicine as Culture*, London: Sage.

Mäkelä, J. (2000). "Cultural definitions of the meal", in H. Meiselman (ed.), *Dimensions of the Meal: The Science, Culture, Business, and Art of Eating*, pp. 7–18. Gaithersburg: Aspen Publishers.

Méchin, C. (1997). "La symbolique de la viande", in M. Paillat (ed.), *Le mangeur et l'animal. Mutations de l'élevage et de la consommation*, pp. 121–134. Paris: Autrement, Vol. 172.

Murcott, A. (ed.) (1983). *The Sociology of Food and Eating*, Aldershot: Gower.

Neirinck, E. and Poulain, J.-P (1988). *Histoire de la cuisine et des cuisiniers. Techniques culinaires et pratiques de table, en France, du Moyen-âge à nos jours*, Paris: Lanore.

Peretti-Watel, P. (2000). *Sociologie du risque*, Paris: Armand Colin.

Poulain, J.-P. (2002a). *Sociologies de l'alimentation. Les mangeurs et l'espace social alimentaire*, Paris: PUF.

Poulain, J.-P. (2002b). "The contemporary diet in France: de-structuration or from commensalism to vagabond feeding", *Appetite*, Vol. 39(1): 46–55.

Poulain, J.-P. (2008). "Du bon beurre à la mauvaise graisse", in C. Fischler and E. Masson, *Manger. Français, Européens et Américains face à l'alimentation*, pp. 316–328. Paris: Odile Jacob.

Ritzer, G. (2004). *The McDonaldization of Society*, Thousand Oaks: Pine Forge Press.

Rodale, J.I. (1948). *The Healthy Hounzas*, Emmaus: Rodale Press.

Rozin, P. (1976). "The selection of food by rats, human and other animals", in J. Rosenblat, R. Hinde, C. Beer and E. Shaw (eds), *Advances in Study of Behaviour*, pp. 21–76. New York: Academic Press.

Rozin P., Fischler, C., Imada, S, Sarubin, A. and Wrzesniewski, A. (1999). "Attitudes to food and the role of food in life in the USA, Japan, Flemish Belgium and France: possible implications for the diet-health debate", *Appetite*, Vol. 33: 163–180.

Sobal, J. (2000). "Sociability and meals: facilitation, commensality, and interaction", in H. Meiselman (ed.) *Dimensions of the Meal: The Science, Culture, Business, and Art of Eating*, pp. 119–133. Gaithersburg: Aspen Publishers.

Sobal, J. and Nelson, M. (2003). "Commensal eating patterns: a community study", *Appetite*, Vol. 41(2): 181–190.

Tylor, E. B. (1958). *Primitive Culture*, New York: Harper & Row, 1st publication 1871.

Vanhonacker, F., Verbeke, W., Lengard, V., Guerrero, L. and Hersleth, M. (2008). "Consumer-based definition and general image of traditional foods in Europe", in A. Banterle and X. Gellynck, *Perspectives of Traditional Food Supply Chains on the European Market*, pp. 13–30. Roma: Aracne.

Vial, A. (1993). "Le fromage: emblème d'une nation?", in F. Piault (ed.), *Le mangeur. Menus, Mots et Maux*, pp. 104–110. Paris: Autrement, Vol. 138.

Weichselbaum, E., Benelam, B. and Costa, H.S. (2009). *Synthesis Report No. 6: Traditional Foods in Europe*, European Food Information Resource Consortium.

WHO (2002). *The World Health Report 2002. Reducing Risks, Promoting Healthy Life*, Geneva: WHO.

11 Eating Ayurvedic foods

Elaboration of a repertoire of 'traditional foods' in France[1]

Nicolas Commune

Introduction

The widespread circulation and contemporary uses of so-called 'traditional medicines' have been the topic of numerous debates, both in their country of origin where they may be subjected to revitalisation policies, and in Western countries due to their growing success among the Western public. While these medicines are not recognised in the West as therapeutic systems, some food ingredients, derived from their *materia medica,* or recommended for their medical properties, are sold as foods or food supplements, labelled as 'traditional foods', and available in European organic shops, parapharmacies and on the internet. According to their promoters, these 'traditional' foods owe some of their success to their therapeutic and preventive qualities; they are used in 'healthy diets' and prescribed as 'nutritional therapies' by some Western alternative therapists for their supposed health beneficial proprieties. This emphasis on food questions the contemporary social uses and appropriation processes of these pharmacopeias by Western therapists from the world of alternative medicine.

The present chapter will focus on ayurveda, the Indian traditional medicine, recognised by the World Health Organization and regarded as one of the world's oldest medical systems by its promoters. Ayurveda is integrated into the department of AYUSH of the Indian Ministry of Health and Family Welfare;[2] it is practised in private and governmental ayurvedic and general hospitals, primary health centres and taught in universities. The ayurvedic pharmacopeia is at the heart of numerous issues: the Central Council of Research in Ayurveda and Siddha (CCRAS) of this department catalogues plants used in ayurveda and siddha medicine, and increasingly develops research to document scientifically some specific plants used in ayurveda and siddha medicines, in terms of efficacy and safety, in order to validate their use and commercialisation.[3] Pharmacopeia is also confronted with issues related to the collection and the decline of rare medicinal plants caused by high demand and deforestation (Banerjee 2004);[4] there is as well the question of its translation into biomedical terminology. The ayurvedic pharmacopeia has received a great deal of attention from Western and Indian pharmacologists and botanists, for whom safeguarding 'ethnobotanic' knowledge is essential for the protecting of biodiversity and indigenous intellectual property (Reddy 2006).

Since the 1970s, ayurveda has enjoyed a rapid growth in the United States and in Europe, highlighting the widespread circulation of a 'global' ayurveda (Wujastik and Smith 2008). In western countries, commoditised ayurvedic products are widely available on the market and ayurveda is practised by urban therapists as a mind-body medicine. Nevertheless, legislation is quite often restrictive with regard to traditional medicine so that its practice needs to be reformulated in order to fit the restrictions (Sébastia 2015b). The fact that, in the ayurvedic tradition, food is considered to play a fundamental role in therapy and prevention, is an important feature in developing ayurveda in western countries, such as France. This present chapter is therefore based on the position of ayurveda in that country.

Despite the rigid medical legislation in France which does not recognise traditional medicines, some French therapists practise ayurveda, privately and/or professionally, but they are restricted to working in preventive care in which diet and lifestyle advice play a crucial role.[5] These practitioners recommend specific diets and promote the integration of medicinal plants into daily meals. But the difficulties of prescribing ayurvedic remedies and of access to the complete ayurvedic *materia medica* lead them to reconsider their relationship with ayurvedic practice. They are constrained to formulate innovative strategies such as creating their own repertoire of plants and foods available in France that have the same ayurvedic proprieties as those in India. They juggle with various plant repertories to replace ayurvedic plants and foods unknown in France, generating the diversification of 'traditional ayurvedic foods'.

This chapter will give particular attention to the different modalities of acquisition and transmission of this therapeutic knowledge among French therapists, in order to understand how French ayurvedic therapists operate to accommodate ayurveda in the French context. It is based on fieldwork conducted for a doctorate in anthropology focusing on the appropriation of ayurvedic knowledge by French therapists. In an emic perspective, the research examines the cultural borrowing process from the point of view of French therapists. Within this framework, 15 ayurvedic therapists have been interviewed through semi-structured interviews. Ethnographic observations have been carried out on therapists, including visits to consulting rooms, kitchens gardens, encounters with patients/clients[6] and attendance at consultations. This study has also benefited from observations made at French ayurvedic workshops and ayurvedic training courses, and in interviews with ayurvedic masseurs, dieticians and alternative medical practitioners.

Ayurveda in France: its therapists and patients

In France, the use of ayurveda has increased significantly over recent decades, becoming mainstream thanks to the growing number of ayurvedic centres and training schools. Ayurvedic health centres of various size offer massage, dietary advice and/or consultations by French therapists.[7] Some of them organise ayurvedic courses, varying from a few weeks to years, to inform patients or train other ayurvedic therapists. However, as the French government does not recognise ayurveda as medicine, French ayurvedic therapists are not allowed to use the title of doctor or to treat serious diseases. Furthermore, French and European legislation on medicine restricts the importation of ayurvedic remedies, prohibiting the sales of those not scientifically tested for efficacy and safety (Rastogi 2011; Sébastia 2015b).[8] Ayurvedic therapists in France are mostly French nationals, 30 to 50 years old, who have been trained in ayurveda in France or elsewhere in Europe and/or in India. Most of them discovered ayurveda through yoga courses, or after being treated with ayurveda. Their practice is very variable: they consult full- or half-time, at home or in large or small ayurvedic centres; many of them give courses in yoga and meditation, and/or practise other alternative therapies such as Chinese medicine, naturopathy, shiatsu, aroma-reflexology or lithotherapy, etc. The scope of their medical practice includes diagnostic methods, yoga and meditation exercises, and especially daily routine and diet recommendations. Some examine more than 10 patients per week while others only a few per month. They attract essentially a French clientele (Hoyez 2012) which is mostly made up of well-educated females of upper socio-economic status (Cant and Sharma 1999; Ernst 2008). Many of their patients use ayurvedic medicine sporadically, and in parallel with other medical systems according to the typology of disease and its seriousness, but some who have established a long relationship with the practitioner consult him or her frequently for any health issue. The reasons for which patients turn to ayurveda are various, but the quality of relationship with the therapist, considered as more personalised than with a biomedical practitioner, as well as remedies using 'natural' material are the main criteria. Patients also highlight the preventive rather than curative properties of ayurveda, especially for protecting from digestive disorders, for depressive and nervous illness, and for treating chronic ailments such as migraine, allergies and skin diseases (Frank and Stollberg 2002). Other reasons, as shown in India by Brigitte Sébastia (2015a), are the desire to switch from biomedicine to alternative medicine, and attraction to Oriental philosophies. Ayurveda is perceived by patients and therapists as much more integrated than biomedicine, bringing together global and harmonious care of body, mind and spirit.

Foods and remedies in the ayurvedic pharmacopeia

Ayurveda is presented by western ayurvedic therapists as the result of the observation of the natural environment and empirical knowledge accumulated over time,[9] and passed down from one generation to the next. Its *materia medica* comprises thousands of plant, mineral and organic ingredients. Many of these ingredients are not used only to prepare medicines, they are also food (spices, vegetables, flowers, etc.), thus reinforcing the Indian medical concept that food is medicine and medicine is food (Mazars 2003; Sébastia 2015a). According to ayurveda, the emergence of diseases is largely attributed to eating habits, and thus foods are used to treat as well as to prevent diseases. This food/medicine concept does not fit Western categorisations, the European legislation on foods and medicines defining clearly foods, food supplements and herbal remedies. However, this gives therapists the possibility of using medicinal plants as food or as food supplements even though their medicinal usage is prohibited.

The importance attributed to food is clearly expressed in ayurvedic texts, notably in the Caraka saṃhita, Aṣṭānga Hṛdayam and Suśruta saṃhita, that the French ayurvedic therapists consult in their English versions. These texts classify edible ingredients according to their different qualities and therapeutic proprieties. The ayurvedic food taxonomy is based on various concepts: six tastes (sweet, salty, bitter, sour, pungent and astringent), transformation of flavours or after taste (*vipaka*), properties (hot/cold, dry/wet) and potency (*virya*). These proprieties affect the physiological principles: the five elements or *pañcabhūta* (earth, air, water, fire and ether) which compose everything; the seven bodily constituents or *dhātu* (*rasa, rakta, mamsa, meda, asthi, majja, śukra*); the three *doṣa* (*vata, pitta, kapha*) generally translated by humours,[10] and the three qualities (*guna*) related to the individual's temperament (*satva, raja, tamas*). Ayurvedic texts also present diagnostic methods, nosology and aetiology, which correspond more widely to a framework of interpretation linked to a specific worldview. In these texts, foodstuffs are codified by complex and individualised dietary rules, very different from nutritionists' prescriptions. These rules consist in *patyam* and *apathyam* 'to do' and 'not to do', 'to eat' and 'not to eat' prescriptions: some foods are recommended while others are discouraged depending on the patient's constitution (*prakriti*) and humoral disturbance (*vikriti*); some combinations are prohibited because of their indigestibility. Particular attention is also paid to the 'vital force' of foods, called *prāṇa*, by which they are considered as very healthy and revitalising if they are fresh and unprocessed. With regard to this taxonomy, ayurvedic therapists define a set of dietary rules for each patient taking into account his/her temperament, *doṣa* imbalance, life stage, gender and occupation, as well as climate, season and time of the day. This diet, in accordance with the patient's type and environment, and based on the principles of opposition (warm/cold, light/heavy, humid/dry etc...) and on six tastes, enables the maintenance and restoration of the humoral balance, the disturbance of which is considered as responsible for the disease.

French therapist and 'ayurvedic' food knowledge

French ayurvedic therapists primarily favour the prescription of traditional food from India for their patients, emphasising their importance in ayurvedic texts as well as in the Indian diet that they observed during their travels in India. First, they put forward the use of foods regarded as 'authentically Indian' and not exclusively ayurvedic, such as some varieties of rice, notably the red rice of Kerala, known as *navara* also recommended for its medicinal properties (see Marie-Vivien in this volume), dhal and chickpea, and they encourage their patients to cook French vegetables using Indian recipes. They also prescribe the use of traditional Indian spices[11] in daily meals and the replacement of cooking fat by homemade medicated clarified butter (*ghī*) belonging to the ayurvedic pharmacopeia. Then, they advise the use of ayurvedic medicinal plants as food supplements. These food supplements, made from raw material including herbs and Indian vegetables, are available in organic shops and parapharmacies or via the internet,[12] or brought from India by friends. Lastly, therapists recommend specific vegetables according to each patient's type and imbalance: while most use many common French foods selected for their ayurvedic proprieties, such as carrots or pumpkins, some recommend French vegetables or wild plants used in the past, that they consider much more 'ayurvedic' than the common ones. Most therapists do not personally collect wild plants or foods in the fields, but several have an organic vegetable garden or 'medicinal garden' dedicated to plant cultivation. Due to their particular proprieties, the prescription of these foods is highly codified: therapists provide factsheets and oral advice to patients mentioning the quantity to be eaten, and time and duration of consumption. This consumption may be on a daily basis or may consist of eating a single food over a few days, or for 'purifying' the body during seasonal changes.

For French therapists, the recommendation of Indian foods is the mirror par excellence of their identity: it represents the Indian rooting of their practice. Promotion of traditionality and exoticism (Ghasarian 2002) attributes specific qualities to the food products recommended by the ayurveda: guarantee of authenticity[13] and effectiveness and healthy values. Furthermore, social distinction is associated to foods from elsewhere, based on their strangeness, rarity and supposed powers (Bourdieu 1984). These foods are also linked to particular representations of exoticism or orientalism[14] and, according to 'magical thinking', are consumed together.[15] The Western perception of India is enmeshed in specific representations of Asia and the East, as a mysterious world of spirituality and esotericism, closer to 'tradition' and the natural world (Obadia 2009; Weinberger-Thomas 1988). This representation of 'traditional Indian plants' can be seen as a Western perception of the East, an Orientalist construction (Said 1978) of the supposed high value of ayurvedic foods and plants. Moreover, medicinal plants and traditional foods are considered by therapists and their clients as a symbol of purity and health, highlighting a particular relationship with nature and the environment (Benoist 1990; see also introduction to this volume). And their knowledge of ayurvedic plants and traditional foods gives French therapists their legitimacy and authority: it is presented as being the ayurvedic pillar of which they are the guardians, and they materialise it by establishing a herbarium and a kitchen garden, and collecting botanical books and elaborating dietary recipes. The various degrees of knowledge allow therapists to compare themselves with their peers, and to stratify the therapists' group. They also establish a distinction between specialists and laymen, so that some practitioners such as those who practice massages are not seen by therapists as knowledge-holders, but as outsiders.

However, the knowledge of 'ayurvedic foods' claimed by French therapists is heterogeneous since it draws from various fields. Therapists have to juggle with different kinds of knowledge, sometimes in opposition, sometimes complementary, in order to develop their food prescriptions for each patient, and to justify the therapeutic benefits of them. They may refer to biomedical knowledge that involves the reexamination of the ayurvedic pharmacognosy through the scientific paradigm in order to identify the active principle of plants. Occasionally, they mention studies to legitimise the use of a food scientifically validated for its proprieties, such as *guggul* (*Commiphora mukul*) for its cholesterol-lowering effects. They also may obtain knowledge from ayurvedic courses, including phythotherapy and botany courses in France and elsewhere in Europe, or from the use of a wide range of books including an index of Indian plants written by American, European or Indian ayurvedic therapists.[16] Lastly, some may rely on their practical or empirical experience (Bromberger 1986) acquired through experience and/or transmitted by Indian therapists. This individual knowledge and experience allows therapists to select particular plant foods supposedly having preventive or curative values to prevent or cure specific ailments, to realise original food combinations and, concomitantly, to gain more recognition from their clients and peers. Therapists accord different importance to this knowledge, depending on their training and background: some give primacy to practical knowledge and others to ayurvedic literature. As ayurvedic knowledge plays a key role in the process of 'adaptation' of plants and foods in France, investigating its modalities of acquisition is a means to analyse how the traditional value endowed to a repertoire of foods may be an instrument of competition between therapists in the west.

The sources of the knowledge

The acquisition of ayurvedic knowledge is the object of twofold questioning. Firstly, French therapists are outsiders as regards Indian culture and ayurvedic concepts, and secondly, the practice of ayurveda in France and Western countries generally is restricted. Because of this, to obtain ayurvedic knowledge and/or to improve their skills, some therapists use different kinds of training available in France and other parts of Europe, as well as in India.

In France, various schools of ayurveda have recently opened, offering the first opportunity for French people to acquire some ayurvedic knowledge. They offer a heterogeneous range of part-time courses spread over several years (usually three to four years): 'training modules', correspondence courses, shorts seminars or weekly sessions tackling subjects such as ayurvedic massage, dietary recommendation, herbal medicine, concepts and spiritual aspects of ayurveda. Some have also developed partnerships with ayurvedic clinics in India. These schools provide ayurvedic certificates,[17] but as Sébastia (2010) has mentioned in the Indian context, they are symbolic insignias and have no legal recognition. The first contact of future practitioners with ayurveda may be followed by a journey to India to search for an ayurvedic 'guru', a reputed practitioner of ayurveda (*vaidya*). In this quest, some French therapists use their networks to identify a *vaidya* practising in an urban ayurvedic clinic that they may have already met in France, while others travel to villages all over India to look for a 'genuine' *vaidya*, who has inherited his knowledge from his forefathers. Because of the high value attributed to traditional training, these therapists seek the 'authenticity' of ayurveda among rural practitioners whom they consider as closer to nature and more involved in spirituality than institutionally trained practitioners. Their travels in India correspond to a willingness to experience the 'full ayurvedic efficacy' that they describe as deeply emotional. This first experience with Indian ayurveda is narrated to patients and shared with other therapists as it reinforces the therapist's respectability and legitimacy. For this first contact, some French therapists may decide to study for a few months in an ayurvedic clinic or to become the disciple of the *vaidya* (*guru*) that they have chosen, according to the *gurukula* educational system.[18] Christian,[19] a French therapist of 42, trained mostly in India and established for several years in France, told of his encounter with his *guru*:

> I met my ayurvedic master in Kerala. He is a pure *vaidya*, very traditional. I began to watch him working, and I asked him to heal me so that I could test him. I realised that he was very good and I came back to him again. We have become close friends. It was fantastic to learn from him. Then, I used to visit him each year, I stayed at his place for a bit, I was living with him… and we exchanged as I could never have expected. He had great experience of things that I could never reproduce here, but to see all of his systems… it was incredible. Even though I did not speak Malayalam, and his English was poor, we managed to communicate.

The training with a master increases empirical knowledge and its content, but the modality for acquiring it is very different from the *gurukula* system. The level of deference of the student to the master is lower as the student does not live with his or her master and is free to interrupt the apprenticeship without the master's consent. The duration of training is short, varying from several weeks to a few months, but, as expressed by Christian, it may be spread over several years. During this training, a French therapist plays the role of the student, observing and noting down rigorously what the master says or does. Nonetheless, they face difficulties, notably, the language issue as they know little, or no Indian vernacular languages or the Sanskrit necessary to study texts and, moreover, the *vaidya* rarely knows English. The modality of knowledge acquisition is quite different from the model the student is familiar with, as the master reveals his knowledge according to the readiness of the student. This particularity of *gurukula* which favours secrecy sometimes leads French therapists to promote the esoteric features of ayurveda so as to distinguish themselves from other therapists.

Knowledge acquired in India is not put into practice integrally in France. French therapists are selective with their master's knowledge and they point out that they have to 'filter' it in order to retain what is important for their practice. Some of them are also critical of their master's considerations regarding Indian religion and culture that they deem aberrations, such as references to caste and gender distinctions which are not relevant in France. Nevertheless, when therapists return to France, they maintain the relationship with their master, expressing it by exhibiting the master's picture in their consulting room, and quoting the master's speeches as reference models.

The paths of transmission

The return to France compels French therapists to re-examine the therapeutic knowledge that they acquired in India. They stress the difficulty of applying it in France, as herbs and plant foods used by Indian masters are unavailable. French flora is significantly different from the Indian, and the cultivation of Indian plants in France is hardly possible due to environmental conditions. Therefore, French therapists face a dilemma: while their knowledge of Indian medicinal plants and food should underpin their competence to practise ayurveda, they cannot have full access to them in France. This obliges them to reformulate their knowledge taking into account the French context. In this endeavour, they may benefit from numerous books written recently by Indian and Western therapists. French therapists basing their work on various 'universal ayurvedic principles', put forward two key ideas: 'traditional knowledge', referring to timeless knowledge applicable anywhere, and 'naturalistic knowledge', related to the natural wisdom and therapeutic power of nature. These ideas are expressed by Françoise, a therapist trained in France, and in India by a rural *vaidya*:

> At the end of my training, I said to my guru: "I understand ayurveda very well, but in France we don't have the same foods, so what should I do?" And he told me: "Very good question". And when I went back to visit him the following year, I brought my herbarium, and he was satisfied. In fact, it is really a basic ayurvedic principle, to cure with plants that grow in the nearest environment.

This encounter between ayurvedic knowledge and universal ambition thus puts these French therapists in a particular position: they have the task of adapting and updating the knowledge so as to give access to ayurveda in France. This role places them in a cultural importer's position in which they are fully aware of the importance of the work they have to accomplish. They consider ayurveda as a treasure-trove and see themselves as the true holders of the ayurvedic wisdom or tradition, which they paradoxically consider as being lost in India. They emphasise that the value of such knowledge is today recognised, and that ayurveda is developing and expanding in the world. This claim for the universal features of ayurveda gives a particular meaning to the French therapist's work: it is not only a matter of adapting this knowledge to the French context, they have, too, to bring ayurveda out of its Indian specificities in order to bestow greater recognition on this knowledge and on its use in no matter what context. Thus, they conduct research to deepen and update their knowledge, trying to bring it into line with universal ambitions. There are those who distance themselves from the use of 'Indian ayurvedic' plants and foods, invoking a particular kind of wisdom rather than the difficulties of access to Indian plants in the French context. Some of them consider that eating Indian foods or being treated with Indian plants outside India goes against ayurvedic tenets so that, on the basis of traditional ayurvedic principles, they prescribe various French foods to replace

Indian ones. They ascribe particular powers to Indian plants which are often described as too strong for Westerners, due to Indian climatic conditions: they prescribe these only for 'serious' cases. Above all, they insist on the eating of local and seasonal products, as a 'basic ayurvedic principle'. This attention to the food's origin leads most therapists to encourage their patients to consume fresh and organic foods and to buy foods from local retailers rather than in supermarkets. As Philippe, a practitioner, told me:

> I would say that it is not necessary to use Indian plants [in France]. A local plant is quite often sufficient for the person's condition. It is always better to use European plants to treat Europeans. There are also more accessible, we like the taste, and know how to use them. Indian plants may be too strong and inappropriate (…) Europeans definitely do not get used to them. It is why I don't systemically prescribe ayurvedic food supplements, and also because of how they are produce, there. When you go to India, cultivated plants are… You have tractors which are running by pouring waste oil just nearby!

Acquisition of ayurvedic knowledge of food does not end with travels in India but continues in the French context. Attendance at ayurvedic courses, training sessions or Indian ayurvedic practitioners' conferences, facilitates the sharing of experiences. Therapists sometimes exchange knowledge and know-how from the medical/paramedical world with their patients and students, and with their masters in India. However, they also seek new knowledge suitable to be integrated into, or to complete; their approach to foods is improved mainly by interaction with other practitioners of alternative medicine; and with botanists and organic farmers. French therapists are reluctant to exchange with their French peers and prefer to 'collect' knowledge on an occasional basis from people outside the ayurvedic world in France.[20] The quest for trust based on relationship and the sharing of certain features, such as secret formulations, limit exchanges as there is too much competition involved. The work conducted by some therapists consists in adding these new components to their practices and in fitting them into a unified and coherent framework, as shown by Francoise when she justifies her research on ayurvedic foods and dietary recipes:

> I have studied botany and ethno-botany, I did a few internships here and there. I have been very interested in anthroposophy. Ayurveda and anthroposophy are interconnected disciplines, because they are rooted in the same basics. All that is very close, it works together. On the other hand, I think that it is very useful to get inspiration from what has been done in the past, and when I do botanical research on particular ayurvedic aspects of an herb or plant, such as taste. I find old Celtic recipes for example. (…) Here [in Europe] there had been the glacial era, and the Celts had developed a specific relationship with trees. There are little deciduous trees in India. There is no oak trees and oak tree' parts are interesting for their bitter taste, as well astringent taste.

This prospection involves a wide range of actors; this may be explained by the French ayurvedic context, which can be regarded as deregulated. In France, there is no authority for estimating therapists or practices, and this absence gives a certain amount of autonomy and freedom to French therapists.[21] New ways of acquiring knowledge also reinforce the specialisations of French therapists, for whom the quest for knowledge is orientated by their field of interest: *pañcakarma* (a set of five treatments for purifying the body), *jyotisa* (astrology), herbal therapy, naturopathy, yoga, anthroposophy, and so on. This use of multiple medical techniques corresponds to what Frederic Bourdier (1996) has called the *'masala'* medicine, a medicine made of a mixture of different medical systems.[22]

Re-composition of knowledge and innovations

Endowed with knowledge drawn from various sources, therapists such as Francoise undertake their own research, by elaborating their repertoire of 'ayurvedic' plants foods for their practice. The starting point of this re-composition of knowledge is to list plants foods mentioned in ayurvedic textbooks or contemporary ayurvedic handbooks in order to identify plants available in the French flora such as *kakamachi* or black nightshade (*Solanum nigrum*) or *shangeri* or wood sorrell (*Oxalis corniculata*), two herbs considered as weeds in Europe. French therapists are proud to point out that they have rediscovered these edible plants which are no longer consumed in India and France. They also highlight the fact that many vegetables mentioned in texts do not grow in France. Consequently, they have to find alternatives in order to pursue their adaptation work, by using their composite knowledge of other medical systems. Not all therapists agree, however, on the right way to work, and their training and background play a significant role in defining the methodology. Here, the dichotomy between therapists institutionally trained in ayurveda (European schools and Indian universities or clinics) and traditionally trained ones 'non-institutional' ayurveda (traditional practitioners) is a structural element. French therapists who have followed an ayurvedic institutional training are more inclined to adopt a theoretical approach to food properties than those traditionally trained. For example, Isabelle, a French therapist of 37 trained in French ayurvedic centres and Indian ayurvedic clinics explains:

> To use a plant in ayurveda, you have to know its properties. It is a really deep work which takes years, and can't be done quickly. There are researches to conduct. The properties of plants are quoted in texts; there is no need to taste the plant. It is the forefathers who wrote this, more than 3000 years ago, they gave us this; it is a part of the knowledge that we have to acquire. In olden days, sense organs were much more developed than ours; ours are blunted. So, it is no longer possible to identify the properties of plants, if we have not developed a particular refined sensitivity. It is done through texts. I base my practice on classical ayurveda. From that, it can be said that such and such a plant looks like another, but it is only superficial.

Therapists like Isabelle base their work on the descriptions of food properties found in ayurvedic texts, emphasising that they were defined by yogis with extra-sensitivity that we have lost because of our modern lifestyle. Because it is no longer possible today to decode food properties accurately, texts are the only guidelines to direct us. Using ayurveda textbooks, and also books written by Western ayurvedic therapists[23] in which are mentioned numerous correspondences between Indian and European/French plant foods, therapists look for substitutes for Indian plants in the world of European flora.

On the other hand, therapists trained by traditional *vaidya* are more inclined to conduct their research through a sensitive approach. These practitioners point out that they test the effects of French foods on their own bodies in order to investigate their properties correctly. This approach is illustrated by Christian during the visit to his medical garden:

> I am studying botany a little bit. About plants' proprieties, I taste and I try plants on me. I begin by eating very small quantities. My lab is my own body. When there is increase or decrease of *doṣa*, I can feel it very quickly. I experiment also plant flavours, tastes… Look at this nettle, it is very piquant, when you eat it you feel that there is fire. And if you look at its signature and its aspect, it looks a bit like flames.

This experimentation with plant properties varies according to the therapist: they eat different parts of the plant, cooked or raw, for several days, on an empty or full stomach. Because one plant may have various tastes, primary and secondary, substituting Indian ingredients by French ones is a very complex process. The ayurvedic semantic network, made up of homologies and metaphors, allows therapists to draw comparisons between ayurvedic proprieties and other sources of botanical knowledge, such as the signature or aspect of plant, for example, which refers to magical thinking. All agree that a good therapist must know the effects of the foods that he prescribes on his own body. Feelings may vary from one therapist to another, but this approach is not inappropriate because, from the perspective of ayurvedic therapists, each person is unique. This observation of the effects and use of foods is related to implicit and explicit categorisations made by therapists, on which they rely on establishing their food substitutions. Intuition, body listening and practice are the cornerstones of this re-composition of knowledge. Through their work which consists in defining the tastes and flavours of French foods, through the evaluation of their effects on the body and observation of their signature, these therapists are able to substitute Indian recipes for French ones that they judge analogue, as Hélène, a therapist of 47, describes:

> I gather a lot of rosehips, it is the fruit of the dog rose. Rosehips contain a thousand times more vitamin C than oranges. I like to make jam with it, sometimes mixed with other plants. It is really close to *chyavanaprasam*, an Indian ayurvedic jam made up of 18 herbs which are panaceas. For me… dog rose is a plant that should be a part of them.

Therapists attempt to verify their conclusions by accumulating evidences of the validity of their innovations. They draw comparisons between conflicting paradigms (scientific and sensory approaches, for example). Nevertheless, the implications of their work and research are limited because they are not always transferable from one therapist to another due to the fact that some therapists do not practise gardening or do not collect plants in their environment. The work these therapists carry out in their quest of food equivalences is a veritable challenge, made of multiple trials and errors. By highlighting the difficulties of their work and their innovative approach, they affirm that they protect themselves from possible errors made during the adaptation process. They emphasise that it takes an entire lifetime to be able to know ayurveda properly, and thus they are modest about their own knowledge that they describe as that of a 'simple practitioner'. Their dynamic of protection (Bouju 1995) puts them in a special relationship to the truth.

Therapists, from both institutional and traditional backgrounds, conduct as well detailed research on ancient knowledge of French foods, often highlighting correspondences between 'French recipes from grandma' and ayurvedic principles, associating and assembling different sources of knowledge. For example, some of them use lamb's quarters (*Chenopodium album*) because this vegetable was used in the European Middle Ages for its digestive qualities. This sometimes gives rise to paradoxes, as for example, in the case of the use of clarified butter (*ghī*) that therapists describe as purely ayurvedic while in fact it was used in Europe a few centuries ago as a method of preserving butter. Moreover, similar associations of knowledge match contemporary dietary prescriptions, especially those promoting the consumption of fresh and organic foods and a diet rich in antioxidants to fight degenerative diseases, such as cancer, Alzheimer's disease, or omega 3 to prevent dyslipidemia and cardio-vascular disorders.[24] Through these associations between ayurveda and other sources of knowledge, French therapists claim to practise a traditional medicine adapted to contemporary time. Thus, the various ways of accommodating ayurveda highlight the singularity of practice of each therapist, for whom a genuine approach to 'traditional ayurveda' is a means to distinguish and differentiate themselves from other therapists in order to compete with each other.

Conclusion

The acquisition of ayurvedic therapeutic knowledge presented in this chapter focusing on foods shows the importance of the context in which it takes place. Western representations and imaginary associated with Indian traditions is at the heart of the reinterpretations of ayurvedic knowledge and practice (Zimmermann 2002). Through references to basic ayurvedic tenets, French therapists bring a "paternity suit" (Pouillon 1991) on behalf of their knowledge, claiming for it a prestigious and exclusive origin. They conduct their work by selecting some part of this knowledge and leaving aside other parts that they consider anachronistic or obsolescent, in order to discover traditional foodstuffs with ayurvedic values and enlarge their own repertoire of foods qualified as ayurvedic and traditional. Their endless reference to the 'tradition' has to be understood not as a movement from the past to present, associated with the traditional ayurvedic *materia medica* and literature as a memory of the past, but as a movement from present to past, or rather to an idea that people have about the past based on contemporary standards (Lenclud 1987). This shows that 'tradition' is regarded both as an instrument of power and as a symbolic support for practising. Nevertheless, the prime objective of French therapists is to acquire usable ayurvedic knowledge, in order to provide the best ayurvedic care to their clients and to ensure their position in this profession. Their appropriation of ayurveda highlights the fluidity of medical traditions, and their utilitarian and pragmatic approaches.

The circulation of ayurvedic knowledge in the milieu of French therapists stresses the process of the transnationalisation of traditional medicines, which uses various networks and leads to their diversification (Dejouhanet 2009; Høg & Hsu 2002; Pordié 2011). Interactions between ayurveda and other medical systems are not a new phenomenon (Alter 2005; Bode 2008; Leslie and Young 1992), and anthropologists have described the construction of the "great ayurvedic tradition" in the colonial and the post-colonial context (Langford 2002: 16) as well as the process of professionalisation, institutionalisation and standardisation of 'modern' ayurveda (Banerjee 2002). However, its contemporary development in the West as 'global' ayurveda as Dominik Wudjastik and Frederik Smith (2008) call it, leads to significant and unprecedented intensifications of these interactions. In this context, Western therapists are playing an important role in appropriating ayurvedic knowledge through a 'neo-traditionalism' approach (Pordié 2008), searching for innovative strategies and producing hybridity in adapting their practices to new socio-cultural and legal landscapes (Marsland 2007; McMillen 2004). The everyday adjustments for developing a repertoire of food prescriptions are not described by them as innovations; they are seen as the logical continuity and natural extension of the ayurvedic tradition. This puts the accent on various contemporary informal uses of the ayurvedic and traditional food heritage in France, which are plural, elastic, mostly personal and seldom formalised.

Notes

1 The research is been conducted under the supervision of Patrice Cohen at the laboratory DySoLa (Dynamiques Sociales et Langagières), University of Rouen, France. I would therefore like to thank the French therapists for their warm welcome and their participation in this research project.

2 The Department of Ayurveda, Yoga and Naturopathy, Unani, Siddha and Homeopathy, was renamed in 2003 from the Department of Indian Systems of Medicine and Homoeopathy (ISM&H) created in 1995. Its goal is to promote the Indian system of medicines through the setting up of educational standards, quality control, standardisation of drugs and research on medicinal plants material (http://indianmedicine.nic.in/).

3 This research seeks to identify and analyse the active principles of plants. A number of professional critics have addressed the validation of traditional medicines through

evidence-based medicine, taking into account the inability to define the active principles of preparations composed of numerous ingredients (Barry 2006).

4 The Knowledge Database Traditional Library (TKDL) has been established by the Council of Scientific and Industrial Research (CSIR) in association with the department AYUSH to safeguard the traditional knowledge (see Reddy 2006). http://www.tkdl.res.in/tkdl/langdefault/common/home.asp (retrieved on 25 July 2011).

5 In France, people who use ayurveda in their practice are masseurs, dieticians, practitioners of alternative medicine, yoga teachers, etc. In this chapter, the 'ayurvedic therapist' refers to a practitioner who gives ayurvedic support to his or her patients, through deep consultation including diagnostic methods (observation of the body, pulse-reading) and questions about daily routines, habits, food, sleep and digestive process. According to this definition, the number of such practitioners in 2012 is estimated at between 40 and 60.

6 The use of foods and medicinal plants by patients, although they may play an important role in the circulation and reception of ayurvedic knowledge about food, will not be analysed here.

7 In France, the cost of ayurvedic consultations varies from 40 to 80 euros; this does not take into account the price of prescribed remedies. Therapists are legally prohibited to sell remedies, so they recommend their patients to buy them through various networks; medicaments are not a source of income for them.

8 In Europe and in France, the use of medicinal plants is framed by two distinct systems: the first concerns pharmaceutical products through the European Medicines Agency and the European directive on traditional herbal medicinal products, and the second, the use of medicinal plants as food supplements. See http://eur-lex.europa.eu/en/index.htm, directive 2004/24/CE (retrieved on 20 July 2011).

9 Ayurvedic texts are often considered by western ethno-pharmacologists as the accumulation of empirical knowledge accumulated over time. However, the importance of symbolism, of magical thinking and the law of similarities, and the role of culture on the perception of medicinal products have been underestimated (Mazars 2003).

10 Many translations of this concept of 'humour' have been made to draw comparisons between ayurvedic typology and others medical system such as Hippocratic and Arabic medicine (Banerjee 2002; Bode 2008; Leslie and Young 1992; Zimmermann 1995).

11 Especially turmeric, cardamom, fenugreek, cinnamon, cloves, cumin, nutmeg and coriander.

12 For a list of food supplements available in France, see a French distributor's website: www.ayur-vana.fr (retrieved on 15 October 2011).

13 The construction of authenticity, understood as a particular relationship to the time and place, is not specific to 'traditional medicine'. Similar process can be seen regarding origin-based products in France (Bérard and Marchenay 1995).

14 Virtues attributed to the exotic may be understood both in the counterculture movement of the 1970s, and in the West's fascination with Indian spirituality (Zimmerman 2002).

15 For references on the concept of 'magical thinking', see Fraser (1990 [1890]).

16 See, among other authors, Robert Svoboda, David Frawley, Vasant Lad, Atreya Smith and Deepak Chopra.

17 Various certificates are given in European and American ayurvedic schools, and also by Indian schools, but they are not officially recognised in Europe, even that of Bachelor of Ayurveda Medicine and Surgery, awarded by the ayurvedic universities after a five and a half year course and recognised by the Indian government. To gain

legitimacy and respect, some French therapists are accumulating western and Indian certificates in ayurveda and alternative therapies.

18 *Gurukula* (guru-family/clan) is the Indian traditional system of education in which the guru transmits his knowledge to his disciples. The disciples leave their father's authority to stay with the guru, living in his house in order to incorporate his knowledge, his ethic and his lifestyle, for 12 years in principle, until the student possesses the essential qualities for practising (high level of morality, pure feelings, humility and total devotion to patients). Students have to prove their patience and their motivation to the guru, a condition sine qua none for sharing the knowledge (Sébastia 2012). This mode of transmission is the subject of many changes in India, but therapists consider it as more authentic than institutional training.

19 Names and details are changed to protect the identity of therapists; translation is mine.

20 The same process can be seen among *marabouts* (Muslim holy men and healers from Northern Africa) in Paris, see Liliane Kuczynski (2000).

21 During the last few years in France, an ayurvedic association has been trying to unify the therapists and to regulate their practice (www.ayurveda-france.org).

22 *Masala* is a mix of Indian spices, condiment and herbs, which is used in everyday cooking in South India. Although it is increasingly available in ready-made form sold by various brands, some Indian families are still attached to their family formulation. They buy the spices and make them powdered in local mills.

23 See for example: Vasant Lad and David Frawley, 1986: *The Yoga of Herbs: An Ayurvedic Guide to Herbal Medicine*; Amadea Morningstar 2000: *Ayurvedic Cooking for Westerners: Familiar Western Food Prepared with Ayurvedic Principles*; Usha Lad and Vasant Lad, 1994: *Ayurvedic Cooking for Self Healing*; Atreya Smith, 2000, *Dravyaguna for Westerners*.

24 Although their food prescriptions focus on plant-related foods, French ayurvedic practitioners rarely recommend a vegetarian diet by fear of losing their clients, except when they feel the client is ready to accept it. In contrast, most of them are vegetarian, as they consider that vegetarianism contributes to the construction of the charismatic and ascetic figure of practitioner. The relation between vegetarianism and ayurveda is complicated: while animal flesh is a part of the ayurvedic *materia medica* highly valorised in the classical medical texts (Zimmermann 1992), ayurveda has been mostly practised by Brahmins and upper castes, i.e. communities who progressively adopted and promoted vegetarianism in India (Sébastia in this volume).

References

Alter, J.S. (2005). *Asian Medicine and Globalization*, Philadelphia, PA: University of Pennsylvania Press.

Banerjee, M. (2004). "Local knowledge for world market: globalising ayurveda", *Economic and Political Weekly*, Vol. 39(1): 89–93.

Banerjee, M. (2002). "Public policy and ayurveda. Modernizing a great tradition", *Economic and Political Weekly*, Vol. 37(12): 1136–1146.

Barry, C.A. (2006). "The role of evidence in alternative medicine: contrasting biomedical and anthropological approaches", *Social Science and Medicine,* Vol. 62: 2646–2657.

Benoist, J. (1990). "La *plante*-médicament, entre ses *usages* et ses *témoins*", *Ecologie Humaine*, Vol. 8(2): 53–61.

Bérard, L. and Marchenay, P. (1995). "Lieux, temps et preuves: la construction sociale des produits de terroir", *Terrain,* Vol. 24: 153–156.

Bode, M. (2008). *Taking Traditional Knowledge to the Market. The Modern Image of Ayurvedic and Unani Industry 1980–2000*, Hyderabad: Orient Longmann.

Bouju, J. (1995). "Tradition et identité", *Enquête, usages de la tradition*, Vol. 2: 95–117.

Bourdier, F. (1996). "Rencontres thérapeutiques dans l'Inde méridionale ou l'art d'élaborer une médecine masala dans les stratégies de soins", in J. Benoist (ed.), *Soigner au pluriel. Essais sur le pluralisme médical*, pp. 425–460. Paris: Les Éditions Karthala.

Bourdieu, P. (1984). *Distinction: A Social Critique of the Judgement of Taste*, London: Routledge Kegan & Paul.

Bromberger, C. (1986). "Les savoirs des autres", *Terrain*, Vol. 6: 3-5.

Cant, S. and Sharma, U. (1999). *A New Medical Pluralism?* London: Routledge.

Dejouhanet, L. (2009). "L'Ayurveda", *EchoGéo*, 11/2009, Vol. 10. www.echogeo.revues.org/11349 (retrieved on 14 July 2011).

Ernst, E. (2008). *The Oxford Handbook of Complementary Medicine*, Oxford: Oxford University Press.

Frank, R. and Stollberg, G. (2002). "Ayurvedic patients in Germany", *Anthropology and Medicine*, Vol. 9(3): 223–244.

Fraser, R. (1990). *The Making of The Golden Bough: The Origins and Growth of an Argument*, New-York: Macmillan.

Ghasarian, C. (2002). "Santé alternative et new âge à San Francisco", in R. Massé et J. Benoist (eds), *Convocations thérapeutiques du sacré*, pp. 143–163. Paris, Karthala.

Høg, E. and Hsu, E. (2002), "Introduction", *Anthropology and Medicine*, Vol. 9(3): 205–221, Special Issue, E. Hsu and E. Høg (eds), *Countervailing Creativity: Patient Agency in the Globalisation of Asian Medicines*.

Hoyez, A.-C. (2012). "L'ayurveda, c'est pour les Français? Interroger recours aux soins, systèmes de santé et expérience migratoire", *Revue Européenne des Migrations Internationales*, Vol. 28(2): 149-170.

Kuczynski, L. (2000). "Fidélité et liberté, transmission du savoir chez les marabouts de Paris", *Ethnologie française*, Vol. 30(3): 369–377.

Langford, J.M. (2002). *Fluent Bodies. Ayurvedic Remedies for Postcolonial Imbalance*, Durham, NC: Duke University Press.

Lenclud, G. (1987). "La tradition n'est plus ce qu'elle était...", *Terrain*, Vol. 9: 110–123.

Leslie, C. and Young, A. (eds) (1992). *Paths to Asian Medical Knowledge*, Berkeley, CA: University of California Press.

Marsland, R. (2007). "The modern traditional healer: locating 'hybridity' in modern traditional medicine, Southern Tanzania", *Journal of Southern African Studies*, Vol. 33(4): 751–765.

Mazars, G. (2003). "Les phytomédicaments ayurvédiques", *5ème symposium international d'aromathérapie et de plantes médicinales*, Grasse, 21–23 Mars.

McMillen, H. (2004). "The adapting healer: pioneering through shifting epidemiological and sociocultural landscapes", *Social Science and Medicine*, Vol. 59: 889–902.

Obadia, L. (2009). "The internationalisation and hybridization of medicines in perspective? Some reflections and comparisons between East and West", *Revue transtext(e)s transcultures*, 跨文本跨文化, Vol. 5 http://transtexts.revues.org/276

Pordié, L. (2011). "Savoirs thérapeutiques asiatiques et globalisation", *Revue d'Anthropologie des Connaissances*, Vol. 5(1): 3–12.

Pordié, L. (2008). "Tibetan medicine today. Neo-traditionalism as an analytical lens and a political tool", in L. Pordié (ed.), *Tibetan Medicine in the Contemporary World. Global Politics of Medical Knowledge and Practice*, pp. 3–32. London: Routledge.

Pouillon, J. (1991). "*Tradition*", in P. Bonte and M. Izard (eds), *Dictionnaire de l'ethnologie et de l'anthropologie*, Paris: PUF.

Rastogi, S. (2011). "Why and how? Addressing to the two most pertinent questions about pharmacovigilance in Ayurveda", *International Journal of Ayurveda Research*, Vol. 2: 48–52.

Reddy, S. (2006). "Making heritage legible: Who owns traditional medical knowledge?", *International Journal of Cultural Property*, Vol. 13: 161–188.

Said, E. (1978). *Orientalism*, New York: Penguin Books.

Sébastia, B. (2010). "Governmental institution versus associations. Multifaceted expression of siddha in Tamil Nadu". http://rcsi.hypotheses.org

Sébastia, B. (2015a). "Coping with diseases of modernity: the use of siddha medical knowledge and practices for diabetics' care" in K.A. Jacobsen, *Routledge Handbook of Contemporary India*, pp. 474–489. Abingdon: Routledge.

Sébastia, B. (2015b) "Preserving identity or promoting safety? The issue of mercury in siddha medicine: a brake on the crossing of frontiers", *Asiatische Studien*, Vol. 69 (4): 933–969.

Sébastia, B. (2012). "Competing for medical space. Traditional practitioners in the transmission and promotion of Siddha Medicine", in V. Sujatha and L. Abraham (eds), *Medicine, State and Society. Indigenous Medicine and Medical Pluralism in Contemporary India*, pp. 165–185. Delhi: Orient Black Swan.

Weinberger-Thomas, C. (1988). *L'inde et l'imaginaire*, Paris: éditions EHESS.

Wujastik, D. and Smith, F. (eds) (2008). *Modern and Global Ayurveda. Pluralism and Paradigms*, New York: State University of New York Press.

Zimmermann, F. (2002). "Ce qu'un hindou dit a son corps", in V. Bouillier and G. Tarabout (eds), *Images du corps dans le monde hindou*, pp. 49–69. Paris: CNRS Editions

Zimmermann, F. (1995). *Généalogie des médecines douces, de l'Inde à l'occident*, Paris: PUF.

Zimmermann, F. (1992). *The Jungle and the Aroma of Meats. A Ecological Theme in Hindu Medicine*, New Delhi: Bishen Singh Mahendra Pal Singh, 1st publication 1982.

Index